Natural Healthcare For Your Child

Trustworthy information on the prevention, causes and treatment of the diseases and ailments which are common from birth through the teenage years.

Phylis Austin
Agatha Thrash, M.D.
Calvin Thrash, M.D., M.P.H.

Family Health Publications LLC
8777 E. Musgrove Hwy.
Sunfield, MI 48890

ISBN 1-878726-01-3

Library of Congress Catalog Card Number 90-81275

First Printing 1990

Printed in the United States of America

Family Health Publications LLC
8777 E. Musgrove Hwy.
Sunfield, MI 48890

From the Publisher

This book does not intend to diagnose disease nor to provide specific medical advice. Its intention is solely to inform and to educate. The author and publisher intend that readers will use the information presented in this book in cooperation with a medical or health professional.

TABLE OF CONTENTS

NOTE TO OUR READERS

Throughout this text we have used "she" referring to the parent and "he" referring to the child. We know that children may be male or female, and believe that both parents should be involved in child care, but have taken this approach in an attempt to prevent confusion.

THE PHYSICAL EXAMINATION

Parents begin their physical examination of the child the moment they see him. They admire his two cute ears, and count his tiny fingers and toes.

The parent who wishes to take the time and make the effort to master the skills can carry out many parts of the same physical examination the doctor has been trained to perform. A few simple instruments and a few trials are all that are required to provide the parent with much information which will be helpful in the evaluation of the child's health.

Immediately After Birth

The first-time parent may be frightened the first time she sees her baby if he has not yet been cleaned up. A whitish, greasy material, often streaked with blood, covers his body, and the umbilical cord protrudes from his abdomen. His head is too big for his body, and he looks like the lightest touch might break something. The parent can take comfort in the fact that children are, for the most part, amazingly sturdy little creatures, who can, and will during their lifetime, survive a lot of parental mistakes and ignorance.

The first test performed on a newborn in the hospital is called the Apgar Test. This is used as a measure of the infant's overall well-being. It is typically performed one minute after birth, and at five minutes after birth. The child is given a score of 0, 1, or 2 on five tests, with 2 being the highest score.

(1) Heart rate: An infant with no heartbeat is scored 0; a heart rate of less than 100 beats per minute is scored 1; and a heart beat of more than 100 beats per minute is scored 2.

(2) Breathing: If the child is not breathing he is given 0, if his respirations are slow or irregular, he is given a score of 1, and if the baby is breathing well (or crying) he receives 2.

(3) Muscles: If baby is limp, and not moving, he is scored 0; if he is moving some, but not vigorously, he receives 1, and if he is actively kicking and waving his arms he is scored 2.

(4) Color: If the child is pale or blue over his entire body he receives a score of 0. If he has good body color over the trunk, but his arms or legs are pale or bluish he receives 1. If he is pink over his entire body he receives a score of 2.

(5) The last phase of the test is carried out by inserting a suction tube into the child's nose. If the child does not respond at all, he is given 0; if he merely grimaces he receives 1, and if he coughs or sneezes in response to the tube he receives 2.

The values of each of these tests are added up; 10 would be a perfect score. The five-minute test is probably of more value than the one minute evaluation. An infant in good condition will probably have a score of 7 to 10.

Birth Recovery

The newborn infant has been through quite an experience passing through the birth canal. There are many demands placed on his body, and organs which up until now have been inactive are suddenly called into service. During the first few hours after birth the child goes through a process of rapid adaptation to his new environment.

For approximately the first hour after birth the infant is wide-eyed and alert. He is likely to cry, kick and wave his arms, and make facial movements. About an hour after birth he begins to settle down a bit. His heart rate slows, and his respirations become slower. He becomes less active, and often will sleep for several hours. At about the fourth or fifth hour after birth nap time is over and he again begins exploring his new environment. He becomes physically active again, moving his head, arms and legs about. He may have his first bowel movement during this phase, and may even inform you, at the top of his lungs, that he is hungry!

The Head

The newborn's head is much too big for the remainder of his body. It now makes up almost one-fourth of his total height. As the child becomes an adult the head to body ratio will change.

Caput succedaneum is a soft, boggy swelling over the skull, which occurs as the baby's head is compressed while passing through the birth canal. There may be associated bruises. The mushy swelling consists of blood and tissue fluid which collects outside the skull bones and under the skin. It is common in newborn infants, and most often disappears within a few days. Associated bruising may take longer to resolve. This condition does not require treatment, and there are no known sequelae associated with caput succedaneum.

Caput succedaneum should be distinguished from a cephalhematoma, a collection of blood beneath the periosteum. This can usually be done by careful palpation by one experienced in these matters.

If the child has been delivered by the use of forceps there may be forceps marks. These usually disappear in a few days.

The fontanels ("soft spots") are areas on the top of the head where the bones have not yet fused. They are now covered by a tough membrane, which very effectively protects the brain from injury. The parent does not need to be concerned about causing brain damage by washing or rubbing these areas.

The parent should become acquainted with the location of the fontanels and their normal feeling. The anterior fontanel is on the top of the head, toward the front, and in the midline. The posterior fontanel is also in the midline, but further back on the head. The side fontanels are less often noticed. These areas may bulge outward when the child cries or lies down. If the anterior fontanel bulges in a sick infant it may suggest a serious illness. Greatly sunken fontanels usually mean dehydration.

Pediatricians use head measurements as

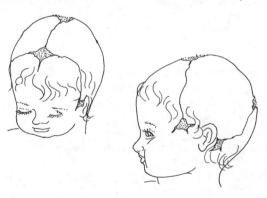

Fontanels

a guide to an infant's growth, particularly during the first six months of life. The parent can easily keep a record of this. Simply place a tape measure across the forehead above the eyebrows, and above the ears. Normal measurements are from 13 to 14 1/2 inches (33 to 37 centimeters). Some children have a lot of hair at the time of birth, others have very little. Neither condition is a sign of things to come in the hair growth department.

The newborn's eyelids are often swollen, particularly if silver nitrate or antibiotic drops have been placed in his eyes.

You may examine the child's pupillary reflexes by shining a flashlight in his eyes during one of his awake and alert phases. The pupil--the small dark area in the center of the eye--becomes smaller in reaction to the light. Some children are rather uncooperative with this exam, and close their eyes. This indicates that the child sees the light. Next, bring a brightly colored object (or your flashlight) close to the child's eyes and move it from side to side to see if the baby's eyes follow the object as you move it. Remember that the child's motor skills are not well developed, and some children do poorly at this. Even a short period of following the object demonstrates that the child can see it.

Epstein's pearls are tiny cysts in the mouth which are present in about 85 percent of infants. They frequently go unnoticed. They are firm, white or grayish-white or yellowish-white nodules, and may be mistaken for teeth. When these cysts are on the palate they are called Epstein's pearls; the same type of cyst found on the gums are often called Bohn's pearls. They are made up of the same type of material that makes up milia, which is frequently found around the nose and chin. They are more frequent in females than in males. The cause is unknown. They typically disappear spontaneously by the time the child is three months old, and require no treatment.

Epstein's pearls may be mistaken for thrush, but thrush may be removed by scratching the surface, while Epstein's pearls are immobile.

The Nose

Many young infants do not know how to breathe through their mouth. It is important to keep the nasal passages open in these children when they have colds. (See the cold section for procedure.) To determine if your child has learned to breathe through his mouth simply grasp his nose for a few seconds. If he opens his mouth to continue breathing you can be assured he has developed this skill.

Many otoscopes come with a nasal speculum. It is shorter and wider than the other "funnels." Insert the otoscope slowly and gently, watching for foreign bodies as the otoscope enters. Look carefully at the lining of the nose, which is pink in color, and covered with fine hairs. This is normally covered with clear mucus, but is present in large amounts and may be yellow in color during a cold. The nose lining may also swell and become red. If the child is suffering an allergic disease the lining of the nose may be pale in color, and the nasal discharge watery. Look at the septum, the wall which divides the nose into two sides. This wall should be smooth, straight, and no holes should be present. Check for holes by shining the light in one side and looking to see if the light shines through to the other side.

A spoon and flashlight are adequate to examine the child's throat. This can be rather tricky in a child who does not wish to cooperate. It may be difficult to get more than intermittent quick glimpses in an uncooperative child. Use the spoon (or tongue blade if you have one) to press down on the side (not the middle) of the child's tongue. Examination of the very young child requires an assistant. Place the child on a flat surface. Raise his arms over his head, holding them snugly against the sides of his head. This will prevent him from moving his head. Many young children do not enjoy this exam, so the parent must be quick.

Begin the exam by looking at the mucous membrane which lines the mouth. This should be pinkish-red in color, and moist. A dry mouth suggests dehydration. The tongue should be pink and wet. It normally has a rough textured appearance. The sides of the mouth should be pink in color, and moist. The frenulum is the small piece of tissue which attaches the tongue to the bottom of the mouth. This tissue should permit the tongue to move freely. See "tongue tie" for further discussion of this subject.

The little flap hanging down in the middle of the back of the throat is called the uvula. This functions to close off the nose when the child swallows. Look at the tonsils on each side of the throat. These become red and swollen when the child has tonsillitis. The back wall of the throat is called the pharynx. It is normally pink in color. During a cold there may be yellow mucus-like material running from the nose down into the throat.

Reflexes

Doctors evaluate two mouth reflexes in the newborn. The first is called the sucking reflex. Simply place your clean little finger into the infant's mouth. Normal infants immediately begin sucking. The second reflex, the rooting reflex, is evaluated by stroking the side of the child's cheek. The normal response is for the infant to turn his head toward the side stroked and to open his mouth on that side. Both sides are checked.

The traction reflex is checked by placing the infant on his back and gently but firmly grasping the child's wrists. Slowly pull the child into a sitting position, observing the child's head as you do so. The head normally tilts back as the body is raised, but then the child attempts to raise his head. His control will be wobbly and uncertain, but the important point is that the child does attempt to raise his head.

The grasp reflex is elicited by simply touching or stroking the palm of the child's hand. The infant will typically respond by closing his fingers around your finger.

The righting reflex is elicited by placing your hands under the child's arms and standing him up. Infants normally pull their legs upward in response to this move. Lower the child's body to place the bottom of his feet on a firm surface. The normal response is for the child to straighten his legs as if he is attempting to stand.

The stepping reflex is evaluated after the righting reflex. This is done by putting one foot flat on the table. The infant will straighten that leg, as if to step; the other foot is then put on the table, and the child will normally straighten that leg. The entire routine is a walking-like response.

The Moro reflex is also called the startle reflex. This is a common reflex until the child reaches about two months of age. The child is placed on his back on a flat surface, away from any objects that he might touch with arm or leg movements. You may slap the surface briskly several inches from the child's head, or merely clap your hands together. In response to the sudden noise the child flexes his knees, throws his arms outward, and straightens his fingers. The arms are quickly brought back close to the body. The infant often cries. During this procedure the parent should observe that the movements are symmetrical and equal on both sides of the body.

The Eyes

Newborns are typically farsighted, but develop normal vision as they mature. Most newborn infants tend toward blue-eyes, although they may develop brown, hazel, or green eyes as they grow up. Because the eye muscles have not yet learned to work together your child may have occasional jerky eye movements or have difficulty keeping the eyes from wandering.

The eye examination is begun by merely looking at the eyes. The size, shape and placement should be about equal on both sides. The white of the eye (sclera) should be clear, and white. It may become yellow (jaundiced) later on if the child develops neonatal jaundice (see section). Shine a flashlight into your child's eyes, and watch for blinking, frowning, or eye closing. Older children may attempt to follow the light if you move it from side to side, but very young children are unable to. The pupil becomes smaller in response to light. The reaction should be equal in the two eyes. It should rapidly enlarge after the light is moved away from the eye. Both pupils may become smaller even though the light is in only one eye. Hold the flashlight down and to the side of the child. The cornea, the layer over the top of the eye, should be clear, without evidence of cloudiness or spots.

Several tests may be done to evaluate eye coordination, the way the eyes work together. By the time the child is four or five months old he may be expected to have developed a reasonable degree of visual coordination.

The light reflection test is the easiest of the three tests to carry out. A small flashlight with a tiny beam is held in the midline and directed into the child's eyes. The reflection of the light should be in the same location in each eye. If the reflection is not in the same location the child's eyes may not be aligned.

The cover test is done by attracting the child's attention to an object which is held overhead. One eye is quickly covered with a card or the palm of your hand, and the uncovered eye watched for any movement. There should be no shift in position as the other eye is covered. Repeat the procedure for the other eye. If the eye shifts in position the child was viewing the object out of only one eye. The test should be done twice, once with the object about a foot away from the child, and the second time with the object about two feet away from the child. Sometimes the shift is not so apparent at close range.

This same test may be performed "backwards." Cover one eye, then attract the infant's attention to the object and observe the reaction as the cover is removed to determine if both eyes are being used.

The Ears

Parents should be alert for hearing problems in their child. Prompt treatment of any problem increases the likelihood of successful treatment, and minimizes any psychological impact on the child.

Because the hearing and balance are so closely related, some tests which measure balance are often helpful in the evaluation of hearing. The simplest of these is done by holding the child in your arms in front of your body with his head lifted up slightly so you can look into his eyes easily. Swing your body in a circle and watch your child's eyes as you move. They should swing back and forth as you move.

Simply done hearing tests may be carried out in the home but generally require two people. The tests should be done when the child is well rested, well-fed, and reasonably happy. Hold the child in your lap in a quiet room. His face should be turned toward you, providing you with a clear view of his face. The second parent should be outside the infant's range of vision. The parent holding the child should attract his attention by talking to him or showing him a toy. The second parent should make a sound such as squeezing a squeaky toy, shaking a bell, or rattling a rattle. The sound used should not be excessively loud as children with mild hearing problems will often be able to hear loud sounds when they would entirely miss softer noises. The test should be performed first on one side of the child's head, then on the other side, to check hearing on both sides. The child with normal hearing will respond to the sound. Young infants may blink their eyes or increase their respiratory rate. By the time the child is three months of age he will often attempt to turn his head in the direction of the noise, or he may become quiet, in an attempt to hear the sound better. Children six months of age often turn their head toward the sound but are typically unable to tell whether the sound is up high or down low. By eight months of age the child will turn his head in the direction of the sound and may be able to determine whether the sound came from a high or low level. The home remedies chest should contain an otoscope, and the parent should become accustomed to using it. This is a small instrument used to look inside the ears. These are often available from mail order companies or medical supply stores. Begin learning to use the otoscope by examining adults or large children in your family. Learn what the normal ear looks like. After you become comfortable with large ears you may begin practicing on smaller ones.

To examine the ears of young children use a small funnel, but use the largest funnel which will comfortably fit into the ear. Larger funnels make it easier to see the ear. Young children may be held on the lap or laid on one side on the bed. A second person should hold the baby gently, but firmly, to keep him from moving, which may cause injury to the ear. Turn on the otoscope light, grasp the ear lobe about midway, and pull it gently backward and slightly upward to straighten the ear canal. As the otoscope is inserted into the ear brace your small finger against the child's head. If the child moves this will move the otoscope away from the child's head. Insert the otoscope slowly, making sure there are no foreign bodies in the ear canal. Young children often stick strange things in their ears, and these can be pushed further into the ear by the over-eager insertion of the otoscope.

The eardrum is normally slightly cone shaped, with a small bulge in the center. The normal color is faintly tan, with a tint of pink coloring. It is easily mistaken for the ear canal, but is often shiny, and reflects the light from the otoscope back toward you. Become acquainted with the normal appearance of your child's ear, so you can evaluate the changes if he develops an earache.

Children with earache often have red, bulging eardrums. The bulging is caused by the collection of fluid behind the drum. See the section on otitis media for further discussion of this.

At the time of examination you may notice a lot of earwax in the child's ear. This wax may interfere with the exam, but probably should not be removed unless there is a lot of it present. Wax in the ear is a normal occurrence and is probably a protective mechanism. If ear wax must be removed it should not be done with a cotton swab as it can push the wax inward. It is better to irrigate to remove wax. First, plain water or a peroxide solution, available from the drugstore, may be dropped into the ear to soften earwax. Dip a clean cotton ball into the water, and squeeze it slowly into the ear, or use an ear dropper. Have the child lie quietly for about three minutes after the instillation of the drops with the ear up to permit the solution to drain down into the ear. Turn the child over on the other side and repeat the treatment for the other ear. The procedure may be carried out as many as three times a day for three days. After the wax is softened it can be easily removed with the use of an ear-syringe, available from the drug store. Simply fill the syringe with warm water, and slowly, gently squirt it into the ear canal. Do not block the opening into the ear as the water should be permitted to flush back out of the ear. As the water returns it should carry with it hunks of the softened wax. Turn the child's ear down to allow complete draining of as much water as possible from the ear. Dry as well as possible with a tissue covering the finger. For more thorough drying, pour rubbing alcohol into the ear to completely fill the canal. Then immediately turn the ear down to drain and dry with a tissue covering the finger.

The Newborn Skin

The newborn's skin is covered with a greasy coating called vernix caseosa. This material is generally washed off immediately after birth, but we usually rinse the baby thoroughly in warm water (no soap) and leave the vernix on the skin to protect it. Some infants' skin may crack and peel in a few days. This is normal. A daily rinse in warm water followed by moderately vigorous rubbing with a coarse dry towel will protect and cleanse the skin. Use no soap.

Your infant, particularly if he is premature, may have very fine hair over his body. This is lanugo hair. It normally disappears within a few days after birth, and does not mean that your child is going to be hairy.

The newborn's thermostat is often not mature at the time of birth. If a newborn develops a bluish color to the hands and feet, suggesting that the infant is cold, steps should be taken to warm him. If the child has a persistent bluish color he should be evaluated by his health care provider. Some children develop a yellowish tint to their skin a few days after birth. See the section on neonatal jaundice for a description of this.

Newborns often have skin changes, which sometimes cause parents great concern. Milia, mongolian spots, strawberry marks, port-wine stains, and capillary hemangiomas are fairly common.

Milia - Obstructed oil glands cause tiny white bumps about the size of a pinhead. Milia may be present at the time of birth, or they may appear and disappear spontaneously over the first few months of life. They are found on about half of newborns and are particularly common on the cheeks, chin, forehead, nose, and sometimes the chest and back. The skin surrounding them appears entirely normal. There may be a few, or many. Milia are sometimes felt with the fingers more readily than they are seen. They do not require treatment and typically subside spontaneously within a few weeks. Do not squeeze them.

Mongolian Spot - Mongolian spots, typically present at birth, are blue-green or slate gray pigmentations, having poorly defined margins which commonly appear on the back but may be found on the thighs, legs, abdomen, chest, palms, soles, and shoulders. They rarely occur on the head. They are more common on the arms than on the legs and occur on the left side of the body more frequently than the right. There may be one spot or many, and the patches are sometimes very large. They are found in approximately 96 percent of black children, 75 percent of Orientals, about half of Hispanic children, and about 10 percent of Caucasians. These spots may increase in size for one to two years, then gradually fade, completely disappearing by the time the child is six to eight years of age, although they persist into adulthood in some people.

Some parents, hearing the term "mongolian spot" may fear that their child is retarded, but this name is misleading. They should more appropriately be called "congenital blue spot." It is an entirely harmless condition which runs in families. The greatest danger from a mongolian spot is that someone may interpret it as a sign of bruising from child abuse. For this reason mongolian spots should be looked for at the time of birth and record made of their presence.

The cause is not understood, although it is known that the mongolian spot appears at about the fourth month of intrauterine growth.

Strawberry Marks - These bright red, raised patches are often present at birth but may appear during the first few weeks of life. They may rapidly increase in size, but usually disappear spontaneously over a course of two or three years. It is estimated that half of strawberry marks have disappeared by the time the child is five years of age, 75% of them have disappeared by the time the child is seven years of age, and 90% have disappeared by the time the child reaches his teens.

Port-wine Stain - These are purple-red or red areas on the skin, most common on the side of the face or on an arm or leg. They are flat, and may enlarge for several months. There are no apparent skin changes other than the color change. These areas do not resolve. If the port-wine stain presents a significant cosmetic problem the parents (or child) may wish removal of the defect. Many attempts at correction have resulted in less than satisfactory results, although advances, such as the use of lasers, are being made in the correction of this abnormality. The use of cosmetics to cover usually represents the most satisfactory solution.

Capillary Hemangiomas - These are often called "stork bites," and are small, red patches which appear over the back of the head, over the forehead, eyelids, nose, or lips. There are made up of tiny blood vessels located just under the skin surface. They may become darker in color when the infant cries. They gradually fade away and are generally gone by the time the child reaches one year of age.

Nearly 50 percent of children develop a rash which is red and blotchy on the second or third day after birth. A pinhead size bump in the center is surrounded by a red blotch about one-half inch wide. Doctors call this condition erythema toxicum. The cause of this rash is unknown, but it may be expected to clear up in about a week.

The Neck

Examination of the neck is begun by palpating your child's neck. Place your fingers on one side of the throat, just under the jaw, with the thumb on the other side of the throat, allowing you to feel both sides simultaneously. Gently move the fingers down the length of the throat, feeling for lumps. The lymph glands are of particular interest in the evaluation of children. Learn the location of the nodes, and their normal texture while your child is well. Use the tips of your fingers to massage in a circular motion the lymph glands,

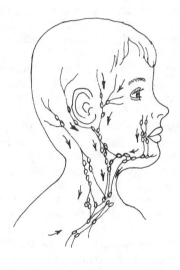
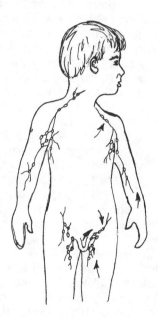

Location of Lymph Nodes

watching for hard or tender lymph nodes. These are sometimes described as feeling like B-B shot but may normally become the size of a large bean. Enlarged lymph glands indicate that your child's body is fighting a disease, usually something like a cold or inflamed gums.

The Abdomen

The child's abdomen often appears to protrude, and on top of this protrusion sits the umbilical cord stump. This stump gradually dries up and drops off over a period of seven to ten days. Leave it uncovered, out in the air. A pink area remains for a few days after the stump falls off.

This area should be watched for infection during the drying process. If increased redness, odor, or swelling appears, the area should be cleansed thoroughly during the daily bath with the fingers, extra water used to give a final thorough rinsing, and a cotton ball wet with rubbing alcohol used to wipe around the cord to remove any traces of moisture or crusting. Keep it dry between baths. A 15 minute sun bath, keeping the eyes carefully covered, will do wonders for an odor from the drying umbilical cord. If the symptoms worsen the child should be evaluated by his health care provider.

In some newborns a small lump appears in the umbilical area. This is likely an umbilical hernia, a common occurrence in newborns. See the section on umbilical hernia for a further discussion of this condition.

Examination of the abdomen should begin by merely inspecting the abdomen. Pot bellies are normal in children up until about three years of age and are generally not cause for concern. Look for skin changes, such as bruises, rashes, or other evidence of injury or illness. The bellybutton (umbilicus) normally protrudes about a quarter of an inch for several years after birth. A bulge in the umbilicus may indicate an umbilical hernia (see section). Bulges in the area where the thigh and abdomen join may be another type of hernia.

The stethoscope is also used in the evaluation of the child's abdomen. You will be able to hear the bowel sounds which are gurgling noises, made as the food is pushed through the bowel. These sounds are normally heard about every 10 to 15 seconds, but if it has been a long time since the child has eaten the sounds may be more difficult to hear. Stroking the skin over the abdomen may induce bowel sounds. Bowel sounds are sometimes difficult to hear, so listen for several minutes before you conclude there are none.

Merely feeling the child's abdomen with your fingers may provide useful information. Begin in the top right corner and move over the entire abdomen, carefully feeling all four sections. The child should be relaxed during this procedure; if he is tense you will feel tightened muscles. In extremely constipated children you may feel the feces in the colon. Children with several different types of abdominal illness will have pain when you press on the abdomen. The abdomen normally feels soft, and may be palpated without causing the child pain. Older children sometimes anticipate that they will have pain when you palpate, and instructing them to breathe slowly and deeply while you examine the abdomen will often distract them, preventing involuntary muscle tension, which will make the examination difficult.

Evaluation of Spitting Up, Vomiting and Regurgitation

There are various types of "food return mechanisms" in young children. Some of them are harmless conditions, which will resolve as the child matures. Others indicate abnormal conditions or illness and may require professional evaluation.

A young infant, when begun on solid food, has not yet learned to use his tongue to direct the food down the throat. His food is as likely to come out his lips as to go down his throat. This is termed "spitting up," and is generally outgrown.

With regurgitation food is returned from the stomach. This may occur when the child is burped. Feeding the child in an upright position and burping him often will decrease this problem. So long as the child continues to gain weight and height at a normal rate and appears happy and alert, this is not likely to be a problem.

Vomiting is more common in older children than in young infants. In some children it may be so forceful that the vomitus is propelled out of the mouth with great force. A child lying on his side may spew food for two to four feet from his bed. If he is lying on his back at the time of vomiting he may inhale some of the vomitus into his lungs, leading to respiratory problems. Any child who is likely to vomit should be kept lying on his stomach or side. Occasional vomiting is not a cause for alarm, but persistent, long-term vomiting may lead to growth retardation. Children with acute illnesses, such as the flu, may vomit repeatedly for several days and must be carefully observed for dehydration. See the section on diarrhea for a discussion of evaluation for dehydration.

Food allergy may cause vomiting in young children. If your child has persistent vomiting over a long period of time it may be worthwhile to take him off milk for a trial period to see if this is causing the problem.

If the child has blood or green bile in his vomitus he should be evaluated promptly by his health care provider. Associated diarrhea or high fever increases the risk of dehydration, and should be promptly treated. If the child has acute abdominal pain, confusion, stupor, or you are unable to touch his chin to his chest he needs professional evaluation.

The Back

The spine should be straight when the child is held upright. Some children develop scoliosis, which is curvature of the spine. This should be evaluated if you suspect it.

The Chest

The chest contains several vital organs, including the heart and lungs. The stethoscope is helpful in the evaluation of these organs. You may purchase one at the local drug store, from various mail order companies, or from a medical supply store. The stethoscope may have a bell-shaped piece at the end, or a flat disc. The flat disc makes it easier to hear sounds clearly.

To hear the child's heart, place the stethoscope on the left side of the baby's chest, immediately below the nipple and slightly to-

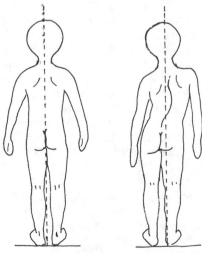

Scoliosis
A. Normal Spine   **B. Scoliosis**

ward the center of the body. This is called the "point of maximum impulse," and is where the volume is loudest. As you listen to your child's heart you will hear two sounds, the second closely following the first. These sounds are sometimes described as "lub-dup." You should listen to your child's heart when he is well to become acquainted with the normal sound. Listen to the hearts of other family members as well. The heart rate of a young child often increases as he inhales and may slow as he exhales. Doctors call this sinus arrhythmia. Most children have it; it is perfectly normal.

You may hear a heart sound that resembles "lub-shss-dup," more than "lub-dup." This is called a murmur. See the section on murmurs for further information on this.

You should also become acquainted with your child's breathing pattern when he is resting quietly. Be certain that both sides of the chest and abdomen move together in equal motions. He should not appear to struggle to catch his breath, and breathing sounds should be quiet. During periods of respiratory distress, such as croup, you may notice that the soft tissues between the ribs collapse inward as the child attempts to breathe in. Physicians call this retraction, and if it occurs the child should be evaluated promptly by your health care provider.

The stethoscope is also used to listen to the baby's lungs. If you place it on the right side of the infant's chest, immediately below the nipple, you should hear soft breathing sounds. Become acquainted with these sounds by listening to various family members' chest. Know what is normal for your child. Move the stethoscope around to listen to various parts of the lungs. Notice how the sounds change slightly as the position varies. Listen over the back of the chest, as well as the front. Breathing sounds are often louder when listened to from the back side, while the heart sounds are louder in the front. As you listen compare the sounds made on each side of the chest. They should be similar when the stethoscope is placed at about the same position on both sides of the chest. The child should breathe in about the same length of time he breathes out. A long breathing out time may indicate bronchiolitis or asthma when associated with rales. Rales are abnormal breath sounds, which may be crackling, whistling, squeaky, wheezing, or tinkling.

Know what breath sounds are normal for your child. Some infants habitually make a lot of noise while breathing; you may think they are snoring. Be aware of any unusual noisy breathing, as it may indicate illness. If your child's lips or skin become bluish or pale they may indicate a serious respiratory problem. Have your child evaluated immediately by your health care provider. Likewise, a child who is breathing in short, rapid breaths should be evaluated promptly.

The Genitals

The external genitalia are normally enlarged in newborns. There may be a bloody or white mucous discharge from the vagina. This is due to the mother's hormones and is normal. Some infants, both male and female, have enlargement of the breasts, with an associated discharge, termed "witches milk." Do not try to squeeze this discharge from the breasts. It is normal and will disappear in a few days.

The male's scrotum is most easily examined while he is in a warm tub of water. The testicles are more likely to be down in the scrotum under the influence of heat. See the section on cryptorchidism for a further discussion of this.

The Extremities

Doctors often screen newborns for congenital hip dislocation. This examination should be done carefully and gently. See the section on congenital hip dislocation for a description of the testing process.

Sucking blisters are common in newborns. They are found over the forearms, wrists, hands, index finger, thumb, or on the lip. They are felt to result from overly vigorous sucking before birth. They typically resolve spontaneously without complications.

Bowlegs are common from infancy until about two years of age. Knock knees are normal from about two years of age until about three and a half years. Tibial torsion is a term applied to the twisting of the child's lower leg.

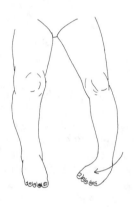

It may occur in only one leg, or both. Check for this by looking at the child's legs while he is lying on his back. Place the legs together and observe whether the feet point upward or inward. A child with tibial torsion will often point both feet in the same direction when placed on his stomach. They normally point in opposite directions.

Femoral torsion is sometimes found after the child reaches two or three years of age. Both legs are typically involved. Check for this while the child is lying quietly on his back. Gently grasp the child's feet and turn them inward. In severe femoral torsion the big toe side of the foot may be brought right down to the surface the child is lying on.

Metatarsus varus is an inward curvature of

Tibial Torsion

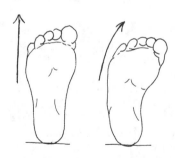

Femoral Torsion

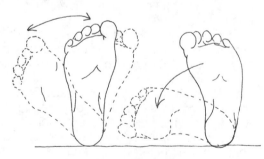

Metatarsus Varus
A. Normal   B. Metatarsus Varus

the top of the child's foot. The foot is normally straight. Pronated or turned down ankles sometimes appear after the child begins walking. Check for this by having the child stand barefooted on a flat surface. Good foot posture must be shown and insisted upon. Clubfoot is a less common problem, and is usually obvious at birth.

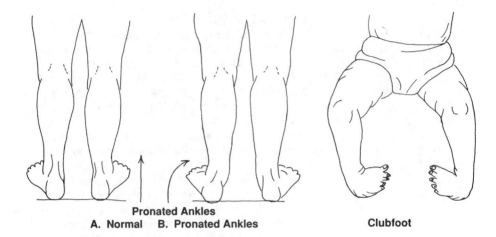

Pronated Ankles
A. Normal   B. Pronated Ankles   **Clubfoot**

The Nervous System

The parent may carry out several simple tests indicating the status of the child's nervous system. Balance and coordination may be tested by the finger-to-nose test by the time the child is four or five years of age. The child should be instructed to hold a finger up with his arm outstretched in front of him. He should then bring the finger up to touch his nose. The test should be carried out with his eyes open and repeated with them closed. A child less than six or seven years of age may miss his nose a couple of inches. The Romberg test is done by having the child stand with his heels together. He should be able to stand upright without falling with his eyes open and closed.

The child's sense of smell may be tested by asking him to identify several common odors. Test one side of the nose at a time by pinching the other side closed. He should be able to identify familiar odors with both sides of the nose.

To determine whether the nerves which move the eyes are functioning properly ask the child not to move his head but to follow the path of an object as you move it back and forth and up and down in front of his face. The eyes should move together and freely in all directions.

Several reflexes may be evaluated by the parent. The reflexes should be equal on both sides of the body. Any inequality should be called to the attention of your health care provider.

Everyone is familiar with the knee jerk reflex test. Have the child sit on a chair which is high enough that his feet do not touch the floor. Find the kneecap, then feel for a bone sticking up just a little bit underneath the knee cap. If you feel in the area between these two bones you may feel a cord-like structure. You may wish to mark this with a pen to remind you where to tap. Have the child relax, and gently tap the cord you have previously located. The lower leg will jerk upward if the test is properly done. A gentle tap is adequate. The test should be done on both legs.

The ankle-jerk reflex is done in a similar manner. The child should be in the same position, with his legs hanging freely. If you examine the back of the child's ankle you will feel the Achilles' tendon, a cord which may be felt from just above the heel bone, part way up the leg. Gently lift the front of the child's foot, and tap the Achilles tendon. The normal reflex is for the foot to jerk slightly downward.

VITAL SIGNS

Four examinations provide information on what physicians often call vital signs. These cover the pulse, the respiratory rate, the temperature, and the blood pressure.

Checking the Pulse

The pulse rate is the rate at which the heart is beating. In young children this can be checked with the stethoscope. Place it just under the left nipple, slightly toward the midline of the chest. Count each beat for 30 seconds, and multiply by two to obtain the pulse. There are wide variations in children's pulses, but you should know what is approximately normal for your child. At the time of birth the heart often beats at about 130 beats a minute. By the time the child reaches one year of age it has often slowed to 110 beats per minute; by age two it may drop to 105, and by the age of four it may have dropped to about 70, which is about the normal adult rate. Infants who are crying or moving about will have a faster pulse, so take the pulse while the child is quiet if at all possible.

The pulse may be taken at the inside of the wrist in a child over two years of age. Use your index and middle finger to take the pulse; if you use your thumb you may actually be taking your own pulse!

Checking Blood Pressure

High blood pressure is becoming an increasingly common problem in children. You should have a blood pressure cuff, called a sphygmomanometer, in the home. The ones sold in the drug store are generally designed for adults; you will need a pediatric cuff to obtain proper measurements on your child. These are available from medical supply stores. The cuff should cover approximately two-thirds of the child's upper arm. Some sphygmomanometers allow you to detach the air bulb and pressure gauge so the same equipment may be used for both the pediatric and adult cuff. See the section on home tests for the procedure for taking the blood pressure.

The Respiratory Rate

The respiratory rate is easily determined while the infant is lying quietly. Count the number of times the child's chest rises and falls with respirations for thirty seconds, then multiply by two to obtain the respiratory rate. For the first year of life the normal rate may be 30 breaths per minute; during the second year it may drop to about 25, and by the time the child is eight years of age it may be expected to slow to about 20 per minute. The normal adult rate is 16 to 18 breaths per minute.

Taking the Temperature

The child's temperature is the only one of the four vital signs that does not change markedly during the child's development. However, normal temperature varies from person to person, and you should become acquainted with what is normal for your child. Some children run a temperature below the commonly accepted normal level of 98.6 degrees F. (37 degrees C.), but others have normal temperatures above this level. You should also be aware that the temperature may vary during the course of a day, being low in the morning, and rising in the late afternoon and evening.

Temperature may be measured in the infant's armpit, mouth, or rectum. Armpit measurements are least accurate, but are often the easiest method, and least likely to transfer disease germs. Temperature measurements taken in the armpit are normally one degree lower than temperatures taken by mouth and two degrees lower than rectal temperatures.

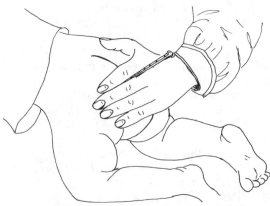

Oral temperatures can be taken only in children old enough to cooperate. The thermometer should be shaken down, and placed in the child's mouth, with instructions to hold it under the tongue for 30 seconds. Rectal temperatures should be taken with a specially designed rectal thermometer with a rounded tip, which decreases the possibility of injury to the rectal tissue during the insertion and removal of the thermome-

Taking Rectal Temperature in an Infant

ter. The thermometer should be lubricated and gently inserted into the child's rectum, and held in place throughout the entire time to prevent injury to the child.

COMMON DISEASES
ABDOMINAL PAIN

Recurrent abdominal pain is defined as more than three episodes of abdominal pain within a period of three months. Peak incidence is said to occur in 10 to 12 year old children. It is said to be more common in females. It is estimated that only 10 to 15 percent of children with recurrent abdominal pain have organic disease. That means that 85 to 90 percent of cases are benign (1). However, parents must remember that the pain is real despite the fact that it is not associated with serious disease. Pain often appears around the umbilicus but may be present anywhere in the abdomen. There may be associated nausea, vomiting, paleness, perspiration, limb pains, dizziness, constipation, and headache. Pain which awakens the child from sleep suggests organic disease, as does high fever, jaundice, bloody stools, pain with urination or urinary frequency, and weight loss. The abdomen may be tender to palpation. The severity of the pain is not helpful in the determination of the cause.

Inflammatory bowel disease, peptic ulcer, appendicitis, dysmenorrhea, milk intolerance, pregnancy, irritable bowel syndrome, pelvic inflammatory disease, urinary tract infection, ovarian cyst, intestinal parasites, kidney disease, and many other diseases may cause recurrent abdominal pain. It has been estimated that over 100 different conditions may produce abdominal pain.

Recurrences of pain may occur for several years. Some of a group followed for 20 years continued to have recurrent episodes, and some developed associated headaches or dizziness.

Treatment

Milk allergy may well be the most common cause of benign abdominal pain. Expensive, although inaccurate, diagnostic tests may be carried out, but the simplest, and probably the most accurate method of diagnosing milk allergy is to carefully eliminate all milk from the diet for a period of two to six weeks (2). A diary of symptoms should be kept during a two-week period while milk is still being used, then for a two week period while the child is on a strict milk free diet. Even a small amount of lactose, such as a bite of bread containing milk, will be sufficient to invalidate the test results in some children. A decrease in symptoms suggests that milk allergy is the cause of the abdominal pain. Onset of abdominal pain due to milk intolerance is usually about nine years of age, but may appear as early as five years of age. The pain may be present for 15 minutes or several hours, and may be severe enough to cause the child to restrict his activity. The child may have associated diarrhea, gas, and bloating. Pain episodes occur frequently, but not always about two hours after the intake of milk.

Other foods known to induce abdominal pain in sensitive children include eggs and chocolate. Food allergy induced recurrent abdominal pain should particularly be suspected if the child also has allergic manifestations such as eczema, hay fever, asthma, or has repeated "colds."

Some children have abdominal pain from the excessive intake of juices. Some juices contain large amounts of sorbitol, which is poorly absorbed by some children. This causes fermentation in the colon, with gas formation.

Fatty foods may lead to abdominal pain, as may highly spiced foods.

Stress-induced irritable bowel syndrome is responsible for some epi-sodes of recurrent abdominal pain (3). Parents should help their children learn to handle stress. Vigorous out-of-door exercise, avoiding competitive activities, is known to be helpful in stress reduction. A high fiber diet is also helpful in the treatment of irritable bowel syndrome. The abdominal pain associated with irritable bowel syndrome is often relieved by a bowel movement. Other symptoms include loose, frequent stools with the onset of pain, mucus in the stool, and a sensation of being unable to completely empty the colon with a bowel movement.

Constipation is a common cause of abdominal pain. Abdominal pain due to constipation is said to be more frequent in males. See the discussion of constipation elsewhere in this book. The child should be instructed to sit on the toilet for at least ten minutes immediately after breakfast every day to train the bowel to empty on a regular basis. Meals should be on a regular basis, and eating between meals forbidden. The application of heat to the abdomen is often helpful. A heating pad or washcloth wrung from hot water may produce considerable relief. Some prefer to soak in a warm bath.

The diet should be restricted to clear fluids during episodes of abdominal pain.

Pain associated with menstrual periods is common in teenage girls. See the section on dysmenorrhea for a discussion of this problem.

Medications, including aspirin, may cause abdominal pain.

Gas may cause abdominal pain. Chewing gum, eating too rapidly, using carbonated beverages, and food intolerance may all produce gas pains. A child who suffers from chronic nasal stuffiness which forces him to breathe through his mouth may swallow excessive amounts of air.

Children with severe, prolonged (more than two or three hours) pain, other symptoms such as fever or vomiting, or previous abdominal injury may require evaluation by your health care provider. The child with appendicitis wants to lie quietly, and often curls up in the bed. If he walks he often stoops over, and may limp. He may begin vomiting, usually has total loss of appetite, high fever, and his abdomen often feels hard on palpation. If there is any question of appendicitis or other serious illness the parent should have the child evaluated by a professional.

ABSCESS

A collection of pus anywhere beneath the skin is an abscess. Abscesses are the body's attempt to confine an infection to a small area. Children who have recurrent abscesses should be checked for diabetes mellitus.

Treatment

Hot compresses of table salt or epsom salt may be applied for an hour, left off for an hour, and repeated throughout the day. Use four tablespoons of salt to one quart of water. The compress should be as hot as the child can tolerate without burning. Heat draws blood into the area, and with it, infection fighting substances. Compresses should be changed as soon as they begin cooling off.

An alternate treatment routine is hot compresses for about 10 minutes, followed by two minutes of cold application. The changes should be repeated three or four times, with two treatment sessions each day. If the pus appears under the skin a needle may be used to open and drain the Eabscess. Do not squeeze the abscess in an attempt to drain it, but you may gently pull the sides apart with a stroking motion which will encourage drainage. Use clean towels for each treatment and sterilize the towels before laundering. Heat is most successfully used early in abscess formation. If it causes an increase in pain it should be stopped. If the abscess does not spontaneously open and drain you may need to use a sharp instrument like a needle to open it up. Hot compresses may be used afterwards. If pain becomes severe, the child experiences chills, convulsions, nausea and vomiting, diarrhea, or has a temperature over 102 degrees F. he should be seen by a physician.

Charcoal, aloe vera or garlic poultices may be used. Since garlic has antibacterial properties, using one of the commercial garlic preparations by mouth may be helpful.

ACNE

Acne is most common in adolescents, but may occur in young children or persist into adulthood. Neonatal acne appears initially at four to six weeks and persists until the infant is four to six months of age. The lesions are found on the face, upper chest and back. Neonatal acne is more common in males, and occurs in about 30% of babies. No treatment is necessary and such treatments as ointments or baby oil may worsen it.

Adolescent acne has its onset between the ages of eight and ten, with the first lesions usually found on the face. Eighty-five to ninety-five percent of children eventually develop some degree of acne, and of these about one-quarter suffer permanent scarring. Even adults are not immune--about 20 percent of adults still suffer acne. Some feel that the Western diet triggers sexual maturity earlier than the skin is prepared to cope with the demands made on it.

The sebaceous glands manufacture sebum, a substance which lubricates the skin. Obstruction of the sebaceous follicles, found primarily on the face, upper back and chest, produces the acne lesion. If sebum is permitted to flow without obstruction acne does not occur.

Drugs may cause acne and should be considered in the determination of the cause. Steroids, some birth control pills, Danazol, Danocrine, lithium, marijuana, Dilantin, adrenal stimulating hormone (ACTH), and others are known to cause acne. Tight clothing (bras, headbands, football helmets) may induce acne. Hair sprays, face creams, sunscreens, and oil-based cosmetics should be avoided, as they may induce acne. Acne cannot be cured, but can be controlled. Even if untreated it typically clears up. It may produce severe psychological problems in adolescents. It should be remembered that no one has ever died from acne, but many have died from acne treatment.

Those who are treating acne should remember that it takes about 90 days for a pimple to form, so treatment may not produce an immediate improvement.

Some studies a few years back denied a relationship between diet and acne, but most experienced dermatologists and acne sufferers will attest to the value of avoidance of such foods as fats, nuts, sweets and chocolate. In a formerly acne-free population such as the Eskimos, who had eaten little or no sugar prior to 1950, and then had a veritable explosion of sugar intake in eight years (from 26 pounds per person per year to 104 pounds per person per year), acne is now occurring in epidemic proportions.

Food sensitivities are known to cause acne. Milk, cheese, seafood, pork, bacon, cold cuts, carbonated and alcoholic beverages, chocolate, nuts, peanut and egg are common offenders. Salt restriction may help the sebum flow more freely from the sebaceous glands. Avoid high sodium foods such as potato chips, catsup, French fries, and dairy products for a trial period. A diet containing no free fats (margarine, mayonnaise, fried foods, cooking fats, salad oils and nut butters) has been found helpful. Animal fats are felt by some to be particularly harmful. A vegetarian diet will almost always help acne. Gustave Hoehn, M.D., a California dermatologist and author of the book *Acne Can Be Cured,* observed that the severe acne sufferers in his practice used a lot of milk, cheese, butter and hamburger.

Foods high in iodine may induce acne (4). These include asparagus, beef, liver, some breads, broccoli, some milk, some eggs, clams, corn, crab, haddock, hamburger, herring, kelp, white onions, seaweed, blackstrap molasses, potato chips, iodized salt, sea foods, stew meat, many fast foods and highly-processed foods, squid, tortilla chips, turkey, and wheat germ.

Wheat germ oil, peanut and corn oil all contain hormones which may stimulate acne-inducing hormone production.

Some disinfectants used in swimming pools contain iodine, as do some vaginal douches, and some surgical scrub solutions, such as Betadine. Bromine and bromides have recently been associated with acne. These substances are closely related to iodine in chemical composition. They are found in cough medicines, some soft drinks, and various vegetable oils.

Stress may play a role in worsening acne. Neutralize stress with daily out-of-doors exercise. Exercise is one of the most effective stress releasing methods known, and certainly among the safest. Today's American lifestyle discourages physical exercise, and acne may be only one of the many unwanted results. Deep breathing exercises have been used to reduce stress. Stress induces higher levels of some hormones and adrenalin, which cause an increase in sebum production, leading to clogged pores. Stress also weakens the body's ability to fight infection. Studies show a high percentage of workaholics and superachievers among acne sufferers.

Stress-inducing competitive sports should also be eliminated.

Cigarettes, caffeine, sugar, salt, fats, excessive caloric intake, and alcoholic beverages all produce elevated hormone levels. Even obesity stimulates the production of more of the hormones that contribute to acne.

Regularity in rest and exercise are essential in the treatment of acne. Some dermatologists state that young people who are up during the night and sleep during the day are stressing their bodies to the extent that their acne cannot be cured. Natural body rhythms demonstrate that man is designed to sleep during the hours of darkness and to rise with the sun. The healthiest, lowest stress sleep pattern appears to be "early to bed and early to rise."

Cleansing the skin every four to six hours will discourage bacterial growth. Washing may be done with or without a washcloth. Using lukewarm water, lather gently and thoroughly for one minute. Rinse in lukewarm water. Repeat a second time. If you use a washcloth use a fresh one daily as bacteria may grow in damp cloth.

Cosmetics

About one million dollars a day are spent on over-the-counter medications. Ironically, many of these cosmetics and lotions contain chemicals that may aggravate acne. Cosmetic-induced acne may be difficult to trace to its cause, as it may take six months to develop. Nia K. Terezakis, M.D., states that some of the most popular commercial skin care products may be the greatest culprits in skin problems. Dr. Terezakis suggests compresses of cornstarch, baking soda, or a combination of the two. Slightly moistened baking soda may be gently massaged into blemishes and thoroughly rinsed off before bedtime. A general cleansing of the entire face may be carried out in the same manner once or twice a week. Be careful not to become overly vigorous with scrubbing as this treatment can be overdone.

Some have found a tincture of capsicum to be helpful. Apply enough to cause a slight burning sensation, once or twice a day, especially at night. Put one tablespoon cayenne in two ounces of alcohol, shake occasionally for three days before pouring off the fluid. Apply fluid liberally.

A solution of 3% hydrogen peroxide may also be used to treat acne. Soak a cotton ball with the hydrogen peroxide and apply to the lesions. (Be careful where you put the hydrogen peroxide as it will bleach hair.) Because hydrogen peroxide is drying, those with dry skin probably will not benefit from its use.

If you have very oily skin milk of magnesia may be used as a facial. Avoid the flavored varieties--the fewer additives you are exposed to the less your chance of allergic reaction. Apply it liberally over the face, allow it to dry and rinse thoroughly. Do not leave it on overnight. Some are sensitive to it and cannot use it excessively.

The following table lists some cosmetic ingredients that may cause acne:

Acetylated lanolin	Lanolin alcohol
Anhydrous lanolin	Laureth-4
Butyl sterate	Mineral oil (depending
Coal tar	on source)
D & C red dyes	Myristyle myristate
Decyl oleate	Octyl palmitate
Exthoxylated lanolin	Octyle stearate
Isocetyle stearate	Oleyl alcohol
Isopropyl myristate	Propylene glycol mono
Isopropyl palmitate	stearate
Isostearyl neopentanoate	Sesame oil
Lanolin oil	Sodium lauryl sulfate

Makeup foundations are particularly likely to produce acne. Liquids are safer than creams, and less expensive products are often better than expensive ones, as the cheaper ones contain more water and less of the expensive acne-inducing oils. Some cosmetics contain oils even though they are labeled "oil-free." Semantic deceit is frequent, and government regulation of cosmetics is lax. Many other terms including "non-greasy," "natural," "organic," "hypo-allergic," and "dermatologist-tested" mean nothing in many cases.

Because the eyelids and areas immediately surrounding the eyes are not typically involved in acne, eye makeup is usually less of a problem to the acne sufferer. Oils applied to the eye area may run to other parts of the face, causing a problem if the face is not thoroughly cleansed. Some dermatologists feel that petrolatum (such as Vaseline) is the safest makeup remover.

Lip products should have a petrolatum, castor oil or mineral oil base. Avoid those with isopropyl myristate. Many blushers use dyes which may cause acne. Use a good out-of-doors exercise program for a healthy, natural blush, with unwanted side-effects.

Skin moisture is due to the amount of water in the skin. Few acne sufferers need skin moisturizers. These products often seal the skin openings and lead to obstruction of sebum flow. A diet low in proteins and fats and high in complex carbohydrates (fruits and vegetables), along with an adequate daily water intake, is the best route to adequate skin moisture. During winter months when drying occurs with heating, or in a hot dry climate, a humidifier will be helpful. For those who feel that they must apply something, petroleum or mineral oil are probably the safest products.

Cleansing soaps should be mild. Strong cleansers may actually cause acne. Antibacterial soaps are generally ineffective. The face should be thoroughly rinsed after washing.

Hair gels, pomades, cream rinses, and other hair products may contain acnegenic oils. Sunscreens, suntan lotions, shaving creams, and aftershave products may cause problems.

Some acne medications may actually cause acne! Retin-A cream contains isopropyl myristate, one of the most potent acne-inducing medications known. It is difficult to determine what substances are in cosmetics as the Food and Drug Administration does not require listing of all ingredients--only the "active" ones must be listed. Cosmetics should be used sparingly, and not worn around the house. Wash your face upon arriving home, and allow it to remain cosmetic-free as many hours a day as possible.

Dr. Terezakis also suggests the use of 100% cotton clothing and bed linen, rather than synthetic fabrics.

Do not squeeze pimples or blackheads, as this often pushes the blackhead down into the skin.

Shampoo nightly or twice a week. Keep the hair off the face, either by short haircuts or pinning it up. Hair creams and tonics get on the face when hair falls on it, as does perspiration, hair spray, and natural oils from the scalp.

Do not prop your hands against your face or even touch the face with the fingers; always use a clean tissue, even to scratch an itch.

Sunshine will help acne by increasing the peeling of the surface keratin and preventing blockage of the skin glands. Sufficient sun occasionally to induce a very slight reddening of the skin is recommended. Be sure not to overdo the sunshine as that can damage the skin. Many suntan lotions contain substances which worsen acne. The relaxation associated with sun bathing may also benefit acne.

Goldenseal tea, diluted lemon juice compresses, or aloe vera may be applied to inflamed lesions. An astringent may be made by diluting lemon juice in water.

Drink sufficient water to keep the urine pale. This assists in keeping the secretions thinner and more readily discharged.

Constipation should be carefully avoided. Food should be thoroughly chewed to assist digestion. Daily out-of-doors exercise will assist in improving blood circulation throughout the body, including the skin. Wash the face immediately after perspiration-inducing exercise.

Two capsules of garlic taken daily with meals have been helpful to some, as have red clover tea and evening primrose oil.

Ice has an anti-inflammatory effect. Rubbing an ice cube over your face for about three minutes every day may reduce inflammation. Some report that the application of ice for five to ten seconds every 30 minutes may produce rapid disappearance of an acne lesion.

Chlorinated water sometimes causes acne. A two-week trial of bottled water may indicate whether this is part of the problem. Communities who obtain their drinking water from the sea are particularly likely to have high iodine levels in their water supply.

Accutane is often given for acne. Five of seven patients taking Accutane showed symptoms and/or x-ray evidence of swelling of skeletal bones. Frank Yoder, M.D., who has been closely associated with Accutane since the first clinical study, feels that the potential toxicity of this medication has been seriously underemphasized. Other studies of Accutane revealed side effects including hair thinning, cheilitis (inflammation of the lips), conjunctivitis, cataracts, various aches and pains, rashes, skin infections, dry skin or peeling of skin, headaches, inflammatory bowel disease, skeletal abnormalities, blood abnormalities, stomach upsets, sunlight sensitivity, and disturbances in blood cholesterol. Six percent of a group of patients given Accutane developed excessive glare sensitivity and/or poor night vision. Animal studies revealed degeneration of testicles during Accutane administration. Women who become pregnant while taking Accutane may give birth to deformed children.

Antibiotics, such as tetracycline, are often given over long periods of time. Several studies have shown that tetracycline is no more effective in the treatment of acne than a placebo. Adverse effects of tetracycline include destruction of helpful bacteria, overgrowth of yeast organisms such as candida, yellowing of the teeth, decrease in absorption of some vitamins and minerals (including Vitamin A which is essential in skin health), and an increased risk for certain cancers. Recent studies indicate that people given this antibiotic, and their near relatives, may develop germs which are antibiotic resistant. If these germs get out of control it may be difficult to eradicate them because of their resistance to the antibiotic. Antibiotics applied to the skin probably do not reach the acne-associated bacteria under the skin surface. We do not yet fully understand the risks associated with long-term use of an antibiotic.

ANAL FISSURE (FISSURE-IN-ANO)

An anal fissure is a crack or tear in the lining wall of the anus, the opening through which solid wastes exit the body. The most common cause is felt to be injury with the passage of hard, constipated stools. Excessive straining or diarrhea may also cause anal fissure. Infection, overly vigorous cleaning, scratching, Crohn's disease, food sensitivity, tuberculosis, syphilis, gonorrhea and some other diseases are less common causes of anal fissure. There may be pain on bowel movement, and bright red blood on the stool or on the toilet tissue after wiping. Bleeding is generally limited and stops spontaneously. The blood is usually on the outside of the stool; if it is mixed in the stool a problem higher in the digestive tract should be suspected. Anal fissure is the most frequent cause of blood in the stool of young children. Young infants may cry, stiffen their legs and curve the spine backward during bowel movements because of pain. Older children will often resist passing their stool because of pain, thus increasing the constipation.

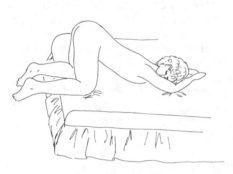

Knee-Chest Position

The parent may check for anal fissures by having the child assume the knee-chest position and gently pulling the buttocks apart. The fissure will look like a red, raw crack usually in one of the folds of the anus. A magnifying glass will help make these small cracks visible.

Treatment

Sitz baths and a high-fiber, non-constipating diet are the most effective and safest treatment (6). A study done in Denmark revealed that patients with anal fissure who were put on a program of sitz baths and bran had faster and more complete pain relief than did control groups treated with lignocaine or hydrocortisone, two medications commonly used in the treatment of anal fissure. An infant will have to be held upright with the hips submerged in a tub of warm water for twenty minutes, two to three times a day. See the treatment section for sitz bath procedure. Treatment should be continued for about two weeks after symptoms subside.

Formula-fed infants should be taken off cow's milk, as it is constipating. Breast milk is the food of choice if it is available, but soy formula may be substituted if necessary. Breast-fed infants sometimes develop an anal fissure at the time of weaning.

Older children eating solid foods should be given a diet high in fruits and vegetables. Bran (1-3 tablespoons depending on age) or bran cereals may be used. (See the section on constipation.) The child should not strain at the stool.

Children should be encouraged to drink plenty of water, particularly during hot weather or illness. Constipation may occur from dehydration. Children with fever may lose excessive amounts of water, which leads to dehydration.

Physical exercise should be encouraged, as it decreases the possibility of constipation.

A warm towel may be applied to the anus to relieve pain.

Rough toilet tissue should be avoided and the anus should be carefully cleaned after bowel movements.

Some doctors have used silver nitrate to treat anal fissure, but this causes pain and destroys tissue. Suppositories are ineffective because they pass too high in the rectum to treat the involved area.

Pain is felt to be due to spasm of the sphincter muscles. Sometimes the insertion of a gloved, well-lubricated finger into the anus will relieve this spasm. This may be carried out by the parent twice a day, or during episodes of acute pain (7). It may be done during the sitz bath if it is extremely painful to the child.

Anal fissure in children may be expected to heal within a few weeks; very few require surgical treatment.

ANAL FISTULA (FISTULA-IN-ANO)

Anal fistula occurs most often during the first year of life, and more frequently in males than in females (8). It is a complication of perianal abscess. Symptoms include tenderness, swelling, redness, and painful bowel movements. There may be pus or mucus drainage. Symptoms subside and recur over a period of time.

Treatment

Sitz baths and a non-constipating diet will resolve many of these fistulas, but surgery may be required in some.

Straining at the stool should be avoided.

ANEMIA

There are many types of anemia, but we will focus our attention only on the most common in children--iron deficiency anemia. It is estimated that at any one time 10 to 30 percent of the United States population has iron deficiency anemia (9). It is more common in the economically deprived and in black children.

Anemia is the lack of hemoglobin in the blood. Iron in the body is in the form of heme in hemoglobin and as ferritin and hemosiderin in the spleen, liver, and bone marrow. One mg. of iron is normally lost each day with body secretions. This iron must be replaced to prevent iron deficiency anemia. Approximately one of every ten to twenty mg. of iron consumed is absorbed, but when iron levels are low the body absorbs a higher percentage.

Red blood cells are manufactured in the bone marrow, liver and blood vessels before birth. After birth they are made only in the bone marrow. Red blood cells generally live about 120 days. Iron is concentrated in red blood cells and carries oxygen throughout the body.

Peak incidence of iron deficiency anemia occurs in the six-month to two-year-old group, then declines to rise again during adolescence (10). Adolescent females are more likely to become iron deficient than males because of iron loss associated with menstrual periods.

Symptoms include fatigue, pallor (paleness of skin), irritability, breath-holding episodes, short attention span, poor muscle tone, heart and/or spleen enlargement, decreased learning ability, and slow growth and spooning of nails. With severe iron deficiency there may be jaundice, cheili-tis (inflammation of the lips), itching, blurred vision, smooth or burning tongue, heartburn, glossitis (inflammation of the tongue), tachycardia, heart murmurs, angina, intermittent claudication, tachypnea, orthopnea, headache, vertigo, depression, anorexia, bone pain, nausea, vomiting, lethargy, cold sensitivity and weight loss. The oral mucosa and inner lining of the eyelids may be pale. Some develop blueness of the sclerae (whites of the eyes). Beeturia (red coloring from beets appearing in the urine after consumption of beets) is suggestive of iron deficiency anemia. If

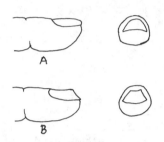

Nail Spooning
A. Normal Nail Contour
B. Spooned Nails

you are uncertain that the cause of abnormal urine color is beeturia you may test it by sprinkling baking soda in the urine. Beeturia will disappear and reappear with the addition of vinegar to the urine. This sign is felt to appear in 80 percent of iron deficiency anemia cases. Iron deficiency may be manifested as pica (see section) and adolescents often develop a craving for ice cubes.

Newborn infants rarely have iron deficiency for at least six months after birth. Even if the mother's iron supply is low the infant's iron supply is assured by a mechanism that gives the infant's requirements priority over the mother's. Low birth weight infants are at greater risk of developing anemia.

Children who have gastrointestinal problems (pyloric stenosis, regurgitation, vomiting, chronic diarrhea, ulcerative colitis, Crohn's disease, polyps, parasites) are more likely to develop iron deficiency anemia. Excessive blood loss from any cause such as frequent nose bleeds or gastrointestinal bleeding may also contribute. Aspirin may irritate the digestive system, leading to blood loss.

Many children suffer iron deficiency anemia because of the intake of cow's milk. A child who is allergic to cow's milk may develop gastrointestinal bleeding which leads to small amounts of blood loss over a long period of time. Other children drink so much milk that other iron-rich foods are excluded from the diet. More than half of iron deficient infants in the United States have "guaiac-positive stools" (stools showing blood by a chemical test). This type of anemia is so common it has been given its own name--"milk anemia." Researchers suggest that cow's milk not be given until the child is at least two years old (11). These children may actually be overweight because of overconsumption of milk (12).

Treatment

Milk should be eliminated from the diet. Infants should be breast-fed as the iron in breast milk is more readily absorbed than is iron from some other milk sources (13). Bottle-fed infants absorb only about 10 percent of the iron they ingest, while breast-fed infants may absorb 60-70 percent. Solid foods may hinder iron absorption from breast milk. Some claim that the early introduction of solid foods is essential to prevent anemia, but studies have shown that strained vegetables, egg yolk, potatoes, meat, fruits and cereals do not increase iron levels. It is felt that breast milk will provide adequate iron until the infant triples his birth weight. Iron-enriched cereals may be given if the child is on solid foods.

Vitamin C (ascorbic acid) increases iron absorption (14,15). Fresh raw fruits or vegetables should be consumed at every meal. The addition of vitamin C to a meal may increase iron absorption up to 500 percent.

Refined and sugar-rich foods should be avoided. These foods replace more healthful foods, and sugar is known to interfere with the utilization of some vitamins and minerals. Sugar has been shown to cause more tooth damage in iron-deficient individuals. Phosphorus in refined foods may hinder iron absorption, as may phosphates in soda pop.

Iron preparations, such as ferrous sulfate, are typically prescribed. These are more readily absorbed if taken between meals, but many produce stomach irritation, nausea, and vomiting. This can usually be eliminated by taking the iron after meals. Iron supplements may cause the bowel movement to become black, or may cause constipation. A diet adequate in fiber and abundant in fluids will go far in preventing this constipation. Liquid iron preparations may stain the teeth. Children should use a straw to take them, and brush their teeth immediately afterward. Keep iron preparations out of the reach of children to prevent accidental overdoses.

Ferrous sulfate cannot be taken with absolute confidence that there are no ill-effects. Iron compounds destroy vitamins A, C, and E, and several other nutrients. They may cause damage to the liver, miscarriages, or premature birth, or prolonged pregnancy, and some suggest they may cause birth defects. Excessive iron may be stored in the body. Recent studies show that extra iron stores lead to increased risk of cancer.

Good food sources of iron include wheat germ, yeast, cherries, figs, dates, grape juice, bananas, raisins, apricots, prunes, blackstrap molasses, leafy vegetables, beets, whole grain breads, legumes, pinto beans, peanut butter, walnuts, pistachio nuts, dried fruits, dark green leafy vegetables, cereals and potatoes. Dairy products (16), coffee, tea, and eggs (17) are known to hinder iron absorption. (Milk and eggs are sometimes given in iron poisoning to prevent iron absorption.)

Cold mitten friction stimulates metabolism and circulation. See treatment section for procedure.

The cooking process plays a role in determining iron levels in food. Food should be cooked with a minimum of water. Cooking in much water decreases both iron and vitamin C levels in foods.

Garlic extract has been shown effective in anemia.

Sunshine stimulates red blood cell production (18). The child should have daily sun exposure.

Cooking acidic foods such as tomatoes, spaghetti sauce, and applesauce in iron cooking utensils increases food iron.

Liver is recommended in the treatment of iron deficiency anemia, but this treatment becomes less appetizing when one remembers that the liver filters wastes out of the blood stream. These substances, along with antibiotics and pesticides found in animals, are concentrated in the liver.

ANT BITES

Treat ant bites as you would a bee sting. A cool compress, ice pack, or baking soda to which enough water has been added to make a paste, will reduce itching and swelling. Seek medical attention if the child manifests such allergic symptoms as breathing problems, hives, severe swelling, shock or dizziness.

ASTHMA

The word asthma means "breathing hard." Inhaled air passes through the trachea (windpipe) into the bronchi (large air tubes), one leading to each lung. The bronchi divide off into bronchioles (small air tubes), which divide into air sacs called alveoli. Oxygen transfer to the blood occurs in the alveoli, and carbon dioxide is picked up to be carried to the lungs. Asthma produces narrowing of the bronchi and bronchioles, hindering air movement. Three million children in the United States may suffer asthma, and approximately 100 children die of it each year. Some of these deaths are due to adverse drug reactions, rather than to the disease. Children who suffer chronic asthma may have growth retardation; this too, may be an adverse effect of drug therapy. Symptoms of asthma may include difficulty breathing, cyanosis (blue coloring of the skin due to lack of oxygen), paleness, sweating, restlessness, fatigue, abdominal pain, severe cough, low grade fever, and occasionally vomiting. The child may have dark circles around his eyes, and be a mouth breather. He may overinflate his lungs, producing "barrel chest." Symptoms are brought on by spasm of the muscles in the bronchi and bronchioles, which causes narrowing and obstruction of respi-

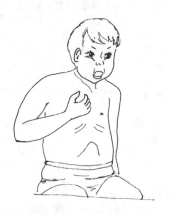

Barrel Chest

ration, with mucus production. Symptoms are often worse at night.

As many as 25 percent of children may wheeze at some time. Wheezing does not necessarily mean asthma. Asthma is present in only 5-10 percent of children who wheeze. Wheezing is often outgrown. Sixty percent of wheezers have only one or two attacks; ten percent still wheeze at 10 to 15 years of age, and 5 percent continue to wheeze as adults. Physical exercise or emotional stress may cause an asthmatic attack. The asthmatic child should be encouraged to lead as normal a life as possible. Asthma is said to be allergic or non-allergic in origin, but we believe fabrics allergies are involved in most cases. It may also be induced by aspirin or exercise in sensitive children. Onset is typically within the first five years of life, and is almost twice as frequent in males as in females in early childhood, but the proportion of males to females is almost equal in later life.

Infants should be breast-fed. Infants born to allergic mothers and fed cow's milk have a greater incidence of asthma than infants with similar histories who were breast fed. Cat dander and egg were the most common allergens in either breast or bottle-fed infants. That cow's milk may cause a flare-up of asthma has been suspected for many years. Because allergens may be transmitted through breast milk, breast feeding mothers should avoid the use of milk and eggs (19).

In allergic (extrinsic bronchial) asthma inhaled allergens such as dust, molds, feathers, mites, pollen, and animal dander set off the attack. Allergy-induced symptoms may occur almost immediately following exposure, or appear several hours later. In persons sensitive to animal dander, a morning pet exposure may produce midnight wheezing. Almost 50 percent of asthma sufferers have late-onset reactions. Dust blown from hot air central heating systems may cause symptoms. A dust-free environment is helpful to dust-sensitive asthmatics. The bed particularly should be kept clean, as the asthmatic spends about one-third of his life in it. The bedroom should be cleaned daily, preferably by someone other than the asthmatic, and the asthmatic should stay out of the room for several hours after dusting. If the asthmatic must do the cleaning he should wear a dust mask. Dusting should be done with an oiled or damp cloth on a daily basis. Furniture should be kept to a minimum and should not be so decorative it is difficult to dust. Beds should be metal or wood. Chairs should be wood--not upholstered. Pictures collect dust and if used in the bedroom must be cleaned frequently. Don't forget to dust behind them. Walls should be washed frequently. Wallpaper should be washable. Bookcases, knickknacks, and fabric-covered walls should all be eliminated, as should heavy draperies and venetian blinds. Open bookshelves and books are dust catchers. Drapes should be washable or plastic.

Dead, decomposed cockroaches were found to be the cause of asthma in approximately 40 percent of patients allergic to housedust (20).

Central air heating vents should have dust-filtering systems. Filters should be changed every two weeks. Radiators and air vents should be cleaned each fall before the heat is turned on. Do not sit in a forced air heat draft. A small electric heater may be used rather than air-forced heat. Electric fans stir up dust. Air conditioners may be helpful. Filters should be cleaned regularly. Avoid sudden temperature changes induced by keeping one room cooler than others. A ten degree temperature difference is the maximum.

Smoking should not be permitted in the bedroom. Insecticides should not be used. Flowers and plants should not be in the bedroom. The asthmatic should not be in the house during repainting, or for about two weeks afterward. They should not be involved in the painting. Avoid moth-balls, insect sprays, tar paper, and camphor. Cosmetics should not be permitted in the bedroom. Hypoallergenic products should be used.

Avoid the use of synthetic fabrics. Apparently dust collects on synthetic because of the static electricity generated by friction and motion. Static electricity develops most readily in dry material and a dry atmosphere. Cotton and wool, which are natural fibers, attract and hold moisture, while synthetic fibers do not; therefore synthetic fibers are more readily charged with static electricity (21).

The closet should contain only clothing currently being worn. Winter clothing should be placed elsewhere during the summer months. Clothing should be hung up promptly and not left lying about the room. Nothing other than clothing should be kept in the closet. Items to be stored should be kept elsewhere. The closet door should be closed, except when clothing is being put in or taken out (22).

Linoleum or hardwood floors are easier to keep clean than carpeting. Shag carpet should be removed if present. Floors should be cleaned frequently. Carpet throughout the house should be kept to a minimum. Carpet pads should be rubber and carpets should be synthetic fibers.

Use plastic coverings over box springs and mattresses, and wipe the plastic at least once a month with a clean cloth lightly dampened with half-and-half strength vinegar and bleach. Seal zippers with tape. Check plastic covers from time to time for punctures and tears. Nothing should be stored under the bed, and the area should be cleaned frequently. Bedspreads, mattress pads and blankets should be made of washable materials. They should be aired out-of-doors and/or washed frequently. Hot water is best for laundry. Wool, flannel, chenille and cotton quits are all dust producers or catchers, and should not be permitted in the bedroom. The bedspread should cover the pillow and blanket during the day to collect any dust that might accumulate. It should be removed from the bed at night.

Small children may have one non-allergic stuffed toy in bed. Stuffed toys should be kept to a minimum. Stuffed toys made with old nylon stockings are generally satisfactory if covered with synthetic materials or cotton.

The asthmatic child should store his toys in another room, bringing them into his room only to play with them. After play, they should be returned to the storage area.

At no time should pets be allowed in the home. Animal dander is difficult to remove. If exposed to animals change clothes before going into the house.

Molds in the environment may cause asthmatic symptoms in sensitive persons. Bathrooms must be carefully cleaned to prevent mold growth. Adequate ventilation will go far toward preventing mold growth. Tiles, shower curtains and areas surrounding plumbing fixtures are problem areas. Thoroughly clean the areas behind the toilet and under the sink (22). House plants may contain mold spores and should be eliminated (23).

Old mattresses or pillows, particularly foam, may contain growing mold. Perspiration may soak into these items, encouraging growth.

Air conditioners, vaporizers, and humidifiers may harbor mold. Water in vaporizers should be changed on a daily basis and the base kept clean.

A dehumidifier or bags of calcium chloride hung from the ceiling may be useful in controlling mold in the basement. Basements that become wet when it rains should be repaired, as the moisture encourages mold growth. Keeping a basement light on at all times discourages mold growth, as does a fan to keep the air circulating.

Compost piles, soil, mulch and leaves may harbor mold. Remove leaves and limbs as soon as they fall. Mold spores are released into the air when the lawn is mowed. Warm, damp weather promotes mold growth. Dried plants and flowers may contain mold. Remove debris and dead leaves from potted plants. Repotting of plants should be done out-of-doors.

Some asthmatics are sensitive to molds which grow in automobile air conditioners (33). Onset of symptoms may occur 15 to 30 minutes after turning on the air conditioner, or up to eight hours later. Fungicides may be used to kill the mold, but Dr. Prem Kumar of Louisiana State University School of Medicine in New Orleans points out that we are not certain that these fungicides are safe for human inhalation. He suggests that persons who suspect this problem avoid using their auto air conditioners.

For asthmatics sensitive to molds, a mold elimination diet may be very beneficial. The following chart shows some foods which should be eliminated:

Mushrooms	Smoked meats
Cider	Hot dogs
Dried fruits	Corned beef
Sauerkraut	Sausages
Wine, beer	Any leftover foods
Sour cream	Canned tomatoes
Buttermilk	Canned juices
Cheese	Any canned food not used immediately
Vinegar	after opening
Ketchup	Baked goods containing yeast
Relishes	Green olives
Pickles	Mayonnaise

Children who are exposed to tobacco smoke may suffer asthma. Prolonged exposure to passive smoking during childhood increases the risk of irreversible small airway obstruction as an adult. Runny nose and inflamed eyes may be present at the same time. Many of these children have positive family histories for allergies, hay fever, hives, or eczema. It has been said that as much as 34 percent of childhood asthma may be due to parental smoking (24).

Aspirin may cause asthma attacks in sensitive individuals. A single tablet of aspirin caused significant small airway obstruction in some children with chronic asthma. The attacks occurred within minutes or as long as two hours after taking the aspirin (25). About 40 percent of asthmatics are aspirin-sensitive. They may also have a runny nose and nasal polyps. In such cases, taking aspirin may be life-threatening.

Asthma is often food-allergy related, either as a cause or as a trigger. Avoid the most common food allergens (51). The top ten allergenic foods are listed in Appendix 1. Eggs, milk, fish, nuts, shellfish, wheat and berries are often incriminated. Preservatives, monosodium glutamate (MSG) often found in Chinese food, and food colorings may also induce symptoms, as may various drugs, particularly penicillin. The use of a diet free of cereals, milk, eggs, chocolate, fish and other common allergenic foods enabled a group of 50 children and 45 adults to relieve their asthma without the use of vaccines, antigens, ACTH, or corticosteroids. The diet must be strictly adhered to (26). The authors of this report state that skin test studies often fail to identify the asthma-causing foods.

Sulfites are a problem for many asthmatics (22). Eating in restaurants may be hazardous, as sulfites are often used on salad bar items, on potatoes, and in dips. There is a movement toward labeling foods treated with sulfites, but until this becomes a universal practice anyone sensitive to sulfites must eat with caution. Avoid the use of foods containing additives, tartrazine (a yellow food dye), acetylsalicylic acid, sulfur-dioxide, and sodium benzoate which are all known to provoke asthma in sensitive individuals (27). Sodium metabisulfite, found in fruit juices, alcoholic beverages, vinegar, processed meats, dehydrated vegetables, processed cheeses, syrups and toppings cause asthma in some people (28).

Fishermen often treat shrimp with sulfites on the boat to keep them from discoloring. Some fruit drinks, beer, wine, baked goods, dried fruits, and various processed foods contain sulfites. Carefully read ingredients for any packaged food you may use. Potassium metabisulfite, potassium bisulfite, sodium metabisulfite, sodium sulfite, sulfur dioxide, and sodium bisulfite are all sulfites. Sulfites are found in many medications including some heart medicines, pain medicines, antibiotics, intravenous solutions, steroids and others.

Many asthmatics, particularly those sensitive to ragweed, are allergic to melons and bananas and should avoid them (29).

A 1953 medical journal reported the successful treatment of asthma with a fat-free diet (30).

Serotonin is known to produce narrowing of the bronchial tubes in asthmatics. A Swedish study reveals that a diet low in tryptophan, the substance from which the body makes serotonin, is helpful in asthma. The patients in the study were divided into two groups. One group was given a diet low in tryptophan; the other received a diet with normal amounts of tryptophan. The patients recorded their symptoms several times daily for a month. At the end of one month the diets were switched. Both groups demonstrated improvement in symptoms while on the low tryptophan diet. Foods high in tryptophan are eggs, fish, poultry, meat, dairy products, nuts, and soybeans. Foods containing preservatives, salicylic acid, benzoic acid, and artificial colorings were eliminated in both groups during the study period (31).

Changing the diet to induce a change in bowel microflora may be effective in reducing asthma symptoms. A group of patients in Sweden were placed on a vegan diet (one containing no milk, eggs, meat or animal products of any kind) for a period of one year. The average patient in the study had suffered from asthma for nearly twelve years, and in about half of these patients allergy tests had not been helpful. Most of the patients had been admitted to the hospital during the past two years suffering from acute asthmatic attacks and their average number of medications at the beginning of the diet was 4.5 medications per person. Of the 35 patients, 20 were taking cortisone constantly and of the remaining group 7 had received cortisone at some time during the disease. The study group represented a group of patients with quite advanced disease. The diet prescribed was free of all animal products. Coffee, tea, chocolate, sugar and salt were also eliminated. Cereals were very limited, but buckwheat, millet and lentils were accepted. Citrus fruits and apples were not permitted. Patients were encouraged to drink water or herbal teas up to 1 1/2 liters every 24 hours. The patients were to spend some time every day in physical activity out-of-doors. Over 70 percent of the patients reported improvement or disappearance of symptoms after four months on the program, while after one year 92 percent were improved or well. The group as a whole reported a decrease in the number of asthmatic attacks and less severe symptoms in the attacks that did occur. Some of the patients in the study were able to completely give up their asthma medications, and others reduced medication use to up to fifty percent of the original dose (32).

Non-allergic (intrinsic bronchial) asthma may appear after respiratory tract infections, exposure to air pollution, or cold air, emotional stress, or hyperventilation. Weather changes including sudden temperature changes, wind velocity, humidity and barometric pressure changes are all known to influence asthma. Even these "non-allergic" reactions are often only triggers for a food sensitivity, and will cease to trouble the asthmatic when the offending foods are removed from the diet.

Sinus congestion or infection may cause a flare of asthma symptoms.

Episodes seem to be more frequent during the fall and winter months when upper respiratory tract infections are more prevalent. These may represent allergies to the germs that cause the infections.

Asthmatics should be encouraged to have a program of regular physical exercise. Brief exercise periods of from one to two minutes can actually open up constricted lungs according to a report from the Committee on Rehabilitation Therapy of the American Academy of Allergy (34). The asthmatic should select sports that involve only short periods of sporadic effort. Baseball and swimming in warm water 85 to 90 degrees F. are apparently excellent forms of exercise for asthmatics (35). Care should be taken to avoid exercise induced asthma.

Exercise-induced asthma comes on five to ten minutes following vigorous exercise, even though no symptoms are present at the onset of exercise. Many of these cases are felt to be food allergy related. It may be involved in over two-thirds of all asthmatic children. Exercise must be prolonged for six to eight minutes and raise the heart rate to about 170 beats per minute to be sufficient to induce symptoms. Running is the exercise most likely to induce asthma. Sufferers become short of breath, have fast heart rates, and begin to cough or wheeze. Symptoms often subside within one to two hours. Physical fitness should be encouraged, as it reduces shortness of breath on exercise, and may prevent exercise-induced asthma. Swimming is felt to be particularly beneficial. Singing lessons also help the asthmatic, as the diaphragm is strengthened and breathing control promoted. Dr. Arend Bouhuys of Emory University in Atlanta, Georgia, recommends that asthma sufferers learn to play a wind instrument or sing to improve their breathing capacity. A person at rest uses only about 10 percent of his lung capacity; hard work increases lung use to only about 50 percent. The singer or woodwind player uses his lungs almost to the fullest extent possible (36).

Exhaling forcefully through a small drinking straw into a large bottle of water forces expansion of the spastic bronchial tubes and may relieve an asthmatic attack (37).

Regular breathing exercises may be quite helpful. The following exercises are suggested and should be performed five or six times twice a day, and at the first sign of an asthma attack:

A. Stand tall with your hands on your shoulders, and elbows together in front of you. Breathe in deeply while stretching the elbows out to the side, returning them to the center as you exhale.

B. Stand straight with one arm at the side of your body, and the other curved up over your head. Breathe in while sliding the arm at the side of the body down the leg, and back up as you exhale. Reverse arm positions, and repeat the procedure.

C. Standing tall with shoulders back and breathing deeply will develop proper breathing techniques.

D. Vertical stretch and lifting of the rib cage may be achieved by kneeling so that you sit on your legs. While breathing in, stretch both hands up as you come up on your knees; breathe out while kneeling back on your legs and lowering your arms.

E. Lying on your stomach, clasp your hands together over your hips. Lift your head and shoulders while breathing in, relaxing as you exhale.

F. Turn over on your back, with your arms above your head. Breathe in as you lift both legs; lower them as you breathe out. This gives abdominal muscle control.

G. Still lying on your back, bend your knees up. Lift your hips off the floor as you breathe in, lower them as you breathe out.

H. Lie on your back with arms at your side, and your feet slightly apart. Breathe in as you lift your arms up and back over your head; breathe out as you sit up to touch your toes. Breathe in while lying back and breathe out as you relax (38).

I. For ten minutes and at the first sign of an asthmatic attack, sit up straight in a chair. Inhale through your nose, and exhale through pursed lips. Pursing the lips assists in opening the bronchial tubes (39).

J. Lie flat on a firm surface with the knees bent. Slowly raise the right knee to the chest while breathing out and tensing the abdominal muscles; lower the right leg, inhale and relax the abdominal muscles. Repeat the procedure with the left leg (40).

Postural drainage will assist in clearing the mucus from the lungs. (See treatment section) Lie on your stomach with your head and chest draped over the edge of the bed. Bring up the sputum by coughing gently for two to three minutes. During an attack some people cannot tolerate this position. These people may lie face down in bed with two or three pillows under their hips (39). Children with frequent bouts of asthma may benefit by a daily coughing and postural drainage program. See treatment section for routine.

About 40 percent of asthmatics are aspirin-sensitive. They may also have a runny nose and nasal polyps. In such cases, the taking of aspirin may be life-threatening.

Treatment

Pouring cold water on the back of the neck is helpful in controlling asthma (41). The patient bends over and cold water is poured on the back of the neck from a pitcher holding about a gallon of water held about 24 inches above the neck for 30 to 90 seconds. The treatment is repeated two to three times daily.

Fever therapy was helpful in over half of a group of patients given four treatments on a weekly basis. Body temperature was raised to 104 to 105 degrees F. and kept there for five to seven hours. The first or second treatment often brought relief (42). Another researcher successfully used a course of two to four treatments each of three hours duration, raising the temperature to between 102 and 105 degrees F. (43).

Hot fomentations to the back of the neck and thorax and front of the chest are helpful, along with a hot foot bath. Keep the head cool by sponging with cool water or use a fan. The treatment should be continued until the attack subsides, generally within 15 to 30 minutes. Finish off with a shower or alcohol rub, and have the child rest in bed until sweating subsides.

A cool air vaporizer may be used during an acute attack. Menthol or oil of eucalyptus may be used if desired.

Garlic has been used for hundreds of years in the treatment of asthma. Blend one clove of garlic in one cup of hot water. Some patients vomit after drinking the solution which assists in loosening the bronchial secretions. Give a second cup if the first is vomited, as the active ingredient is excreted through the lungs after intestinal absorption.

Adequate fluid intake will assist in secretion removal. Pure, fresh water may be the very best asthma medication available. Milk, iced drinks, caffeine, and chocolate beverages should be avoided. Cold beverages or food may cause a reflex bronchospasm.

A cup of hot water, mullein, or catnip tea may be given each hour. Camomile tea has an antiallergic action. Drink one cup morning and evening (44). Anise tea is especially helpful in bronchial asthma attacks (45).

Some find a neutral bath (94 to 97 degrees F.) helpful. Patients may remain in the tub for up to two hours.

Expectorants are of dubious value in the treatment of asthma. Garlic tea, however, can be very helpful. Use one-half to one whole clove of garlic to a small glass of boiling water. Blend until smooth. Drink while still slightly hot.

Antihistamines have little effect on source of asthma and should not be used. Apparently histamine is not a major factor in the allergic reaction (52).

Aerosol nebulizers have been shown to produce a rebound similar to that produced by nosedrops, forcing the patient to use more and more medication while obtaining less and less relief. Some authorities in the field of asthma are discontinuing the use of this type of medication. These medications may also dry the secretions in the lungs, producing thick mucus plugs. There is also the possibility that these medication will interact with other medications, producing what could be a fatal heart irregularity (46).

Oral steroids may be given to treat asthma. The accompanying table shows some possible adverse effects of these medications:

Weight gain
Moon face
Fat distribution changes
Blood sugar changes
Hair growth on face and hands
Stretch marks on skin
Glaucoma
Cataracts
Salt retention and edema
Suppression of adrenal gland
Irregular menstrual cycles

Osteoporosis
Increased bone fractures
Growth retardation
Acne
Thinning of the skin
Muscle wasting
Diminished infection
  resistance
Increased risk of stomach
  ulcers
Mental changes

The asthmatic child should live in the country, in an area with minimal air pollution. Sulfur dioxide may produce an immediate increase in airway resistance in even normal persons, and one study revealed an increased number of asthmatic attacks during times of high atmospheric pollution (47).

The child should sleep outdoors if possible. This is more beneficial than sleeping in a room with the windows and doors open (48). The child should sleep on his stomach. This aids in natural drainage, removing secretions and infection from the lungs, and makes it easier to keep the mouth closed. The parent should insist that the child breathe through his nose rather than his mouth at all times. Approximately 90 percent of asthmatics are mouth breathers (49). Organisms in the mouth and throat are more readily transmitted to the lungs in mouth breathers, increasing the incidence of respiratory tract infections. Mouth breathing also brings cold air into the trachea which may result in wheezing. Allergenic particles may penetrate further into the respiratory system with mouth breathing.

Children should be taught "sleep breathing" and should begin it at the first sign of an attack (50). Sleep breathing is slower and deeper than usual, with a three second pause at the top of the inspiration and at the end of the expiration.

Parents should be instructed to avoid overprotection and excessive parental anxiety. Teach the child to calmly begin breathing exercises and pursed lip breathing if an asthmatic attack begins. The child should also be taught to start drinking a glass of water every 10 minutes for an hour, the size of the glass determined by the size of the child.

An onion chest poultice may be helpful. See treatment section for procedure.

The child should be protected from chilling, cold air, and sudden barometric changes, which may precipitate an attack (53). Particular attention should be paid to keeping the limbs well clothed.

ATHLETE'S FOOT (TINEA PEDIS)

Athlete's foot, also called *Tinea pedis* and ringworm of the feet, is the most common superficial infection. The skin between the toes is most commonly involved, and becomes itchy, scaly, and may crack. With severe infection skin fissures may occur and a foul odor may be present. The soles and sides of the feet may become infected, as may the hands. Athlete's foot is uncommon in parts of the world where people never wear shoes (54).

Prevention

Do not go barefoot in public areas.

Apple cider vinegar (or any vinegar) or lemon juice has been found curative in most cases. Apply every time itching begins, and always after every bath to stop fungus growth. Usually this is the only treatment needed.

Cornstarch dusted on the feet will help control moisture.

Treatment for Infected Athlete's Foot

Use one of the following solutions as a 20 to 30 minute foot bath twice a day:

    A. Four ounces of thyme to a pint of alcohol
    B. Goldenseal tea. After drying, dust with goldenseal powder
    C. Sea water or saline
    D. Red clover tea
    E. One clove of garlic blended in one quart of water
    F. Comfrey tea
    G. A diluted solution of bleach (follow directions on bottle) (55)

Do not use B, E, or G if there is severe cracking, or if the areas between the toes are raw.

Wash the feet, particularly the area between the toes, with soap and water and dry carefully twice a day. Some use a hair dryer to remove moisture (56). Put on clean socks.

Wear shoes that allow moisture evaporation (57). Sandals are best. Leather shoes with cotton socks allow the feet to breathe. Avoid shoes with plastic lining. Change shoes every other day to allow them time to dry.

Small pieces of cotton may be placed between the toes at night to absorb moisture. Some claim that soaking cotton balls in honey and placing them between the toes at night is helpful. Cover the feet with socks to keep the bed clean.

Use white cotton socks (58). Cotton absorbs perspiration better than synthetic materials. Coloring dyes may produce an allergic reaction, further complicating the problem.

Expose the feet to sunshine at least 10 to 15 minutes a day.

Rub the infected area with a cut clove of garlic.

Hot and cold foot baths may be used. Fill a foot tub with enough hot water to come up above the ankles. The water should be as hot as can be tolerated, and more hot water should be added as the foot bath cools. Keep the feet in hot water for six minutes, then use a one minute ice water soak. Repeat the hot and cold three times. Dry feet thoroughly, and dust with cornstarch or goldenseal powder. The treatment may be repeated every two hours in severe cases.

Equal parts of garlic oil and olive oil may be rubbed into the feet five times a day. To make the mixture peel eight ounces of garlic and puree in a blender. Add an equal amount of olive oil, and allow it to set for three to five days, shaking it daily. Keep refrigerated (59).

A drop of olive oil may be rubbed between the toes each day after bathing. Leave only a thin coating of oil (60).

A poultice of red clover may be helpful.

Athlete's foot tends to recur. After the initial attack clears the child should be careful to keep his feet clean and dry and to avoid going barefoot in public areas.

Avoid the use of over-the-counter athlete's foot remedies. In one study 40% of the people using these products were found to be allergic to one or more of the ingredients. Boric acid is readily absorbed into the body through broken skin and may produce toxicity. It is found in many over-the-counter athlete's foot remedies (61, 62). Ointments may trap moisture, providing an environment favorable for the growth of the organisms which cause athlete's foot.

Griseofulvin is often prescribed for stubborn cases of athlete's foot, but studies have shown that this medication produces cancer in laboratory animals. It is felt very likely that it does the same in humans. We know that it is toxic to offspring and should never be given to pregnant women. More immediate side-effects of griseofulvin include headache, mental confusion, blood changes, and gastrointestinal disturbances.

At times, overly vigorous or excessively strong treatments may cause an "id reaction," an itching or painful rash involving the hands. Parents may become alarmed, fearing that the fungus is spreading throughout the body by the bloodstream. The id reaction is merely an allergic reaction to the fungus products caused by the too-vigorous treatments, and will subside with milder treatment of the feet.

BAKER'S OR POPLITEAL CYST

Baker's or popliteal cysts appear as smooth, firm lumps on the back of the knee. Size may range from ping-pong ball to grapefruit size (63). They may be painful. They usually appear on only one side. They are more common

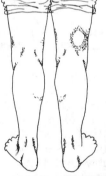

in boys. Illuminating the cyst by holding a bright light against it may reassure the parent that it contains only fluid.

Baker's cysts may occur in association with juvenile rheumatoid arthritis in some children, but most cases are felt to be associated with injury to the back of the leg, such as might occur when the legs are dangled off chairs which are so high the child's feet do not reach the floor (64). They seem to be most common in six and seven year olds, with the incidence decreasing after nine years of age. Baker's cysts in adults seem to be different from those of children. Despite the high frequency of recurrence and high rate of complications (65), many physicians recommend surgical excision. Some writers feel that

Baker's or Popliteal Cyst

children should never undergo surgical excision, as the cyst is very likely to resolve spontaneously. A study of 120 cysts revealed that 51 of 70 untreated cysts resolved without treatment over a period of 20 months (66). Recurrences occurred in nearly half of those cases operated on, and some cases required three or more operations. Some feel that popliteal cysts, even in juvenile rheumatoid arthritis, should not be surgically treated as they assist the body to protect the involved joint (67).

BALANITIS AND BALANOPOSTHITIS

Balanitis is an inflammation of the end of the penis; if the inflammation involves the foreskin it is called balanoposthitis. Symptoms may include swelling, redness, itching, yellowish or whitish discharge, foul odor,and discomfort or difficulty on urination. There may be red streaks up the penis. Poor hygiene, irritation of the penis from soiled or wet diapers, trauma, or masturbation injury may predispose to infection. Circumcised babies may suffer balanitis from irritation caused by rough clothing, laundry soaps or detergents, ointments, or urine. Drug reactions are a common cause of balanitis. A diaper rash often occurs at the same time.

Treatment

In the uncircumcised child, when the foreskin has become loose from the head of the penis, it should be pulled back gently two or three times a day and the area carefully cleaned (68). If the foreskin remains stuck tightly, there is no need to loosen it unless there is irritation under it. Just as baby cats' eyes do not become unstuck for a while after birth, neither does the foreskin for several months or even years. Use soap and hot water, or an irrigation of hot saline. Test the water with your hand to make sure it is not too hot. Return the foreskin to its original position after cleansing.

Sitz baths may be given two to three times a day.

Cool or wet compresses may be applied for discomfort.

Diaper rash, if present, should be treated.

Candida albicans infection may cause balanitis (69). Children of mothers with candidial infection may acquire the infection during birth. It may manifest itself as thrush, balanitis, or several other types of skin manifestations. Children who are given antibiotics are at increased risk of developing **Candida albicans** infections.

Circumcision has been recommended as a method of preventing balanitis, or as treatment after an acute episode. Recent studies do not show a significant difference in balanitis rates between circumcised and uncircumcised boys (70).

BEDWETTING (NOCTURNAL ENURESIS)

Bedwetting, or nocturnal enuresis, is a problem all too common to parents. At the age of two, half of all children wet the bed at night; by age four the figure drops to 10 to 15 percent. Less than 5 percent still wet at age 12. Boys wet more often than girls, blacks more than whites, and children who were underweight at birth wet more than children who were normal weight. Bedwetting tends to run in families and is more common in large families (71). Bedwetters tend to be slightly shorter than non-wetters but are more likely to be overweight. Some children wet only on schooldays and are dry over the weekend.

Bedwetting is classified as primary or secondary. In primary enuresis the bedwetting continues from infancy; the child has never stopped wetting the bed. In secondary enuresis the child has achieved nighttime bladder control, but starts wetting the bed again. Secondary enuresis may be due to stress, illness such as urinary tract infection, or excitement. Our discussion will be limited to primary enuresis.

Most bedwetters have a small bladder capacity, and this small capacity makes it difficult for them to go through the night without emptying the urine. Bedwetters pass urine frequently during the day. The bladder is generally normal anatomically; the small size is because the bladder is in spasm, and when the cause of spasm is removed the bladder enlarges and bedwetting ceases.

The parent may easily estimate the child's bladder capacity by having him retain his urine as long as possible, then urinating into a container so the urine can be measured. The normal child has a bladder capacity in ounces of his age in years plus two. In other words, a four year old child should have a bladder capacity of six ounces.

Treatment

Parents should try to be patient with the child. He does not wet the bed deliberately. His body has not yet matured to the point that he has sphincter control. He should not be scolded for wet nights. The treatment plan must be one of cooperation between parent and child, with the child taking the primary responsibility, if he is old enough.

There is much evidence that the primary cause of bedwetting is allergy. Bedwetting in children occurs in families in which there is a much higher incidence of hay fever, hives, urinary tract infection, and food and drug allergies in both parents (72).

A 1978 study of 100 bedwetting children revealed that removing milk from the diet stopped the bedwetting in over half of the children. The investigators felt that milk lowers the voiding reflex threshold by its action on the inhibitory center of the brain stem (73).

The American College of Allergists reports that about 5.5 million American children wet the bed each night because of food allergy. Cow's milk was the offending agent in about 60% of cases; chocolate, eggs, cereals, bread stuffs, and citrus fruits were also incriminated (74). Removing the food from the diet brought an almost instant cure to bedwetting. An earlier study revealed that in a group of 60 bedwetters, 24 were sensitive to milk, 20 to wheat, 17 to egg, 13 to corn, 4 to chick and orange, and smaller numbers to pork, tomato, peanut, beef, apple, fish, berries, peas, chocolate, rye, and cauliflower.

One researcher reported success with a diet which eliminated milk, chocolate, foods containing salicylates (Appendix 3), and foods and drinks containing additives (including sugar and honey) (75).

Dr. Benjamin Feingold, famous for his work with hyperactive children, reports that hyperactive children have a high incidence of bedwetting, and that his diet is often helpful (76).

Carbonated drinks and citrus fruits may cause bedwetting (77). Chocolate and cola drinks stimulate urine output, and should be avoided.

To assist in determining whether or not food allergy plays a role in the child's bedwetting the parent may measure the urinary output for one week on the child's regular diet, then place him on a diet free of the common food allergens and again record urine output for a week. If the child goes longer between voidings, and eliminates more urine with each voiding on the allergen free diet, this suggests that allergy is a contributing factor.

Some children develop bedwetting during hay fever season. Molds, sting.

animal danders, pollens, cigarette smoke, and house dust may also cause enuresis in the child sensitive to them.

Constipation may contribute to bedwetting (78). A large mass of fecal material can decrease bladder capacity by pressure against it. Treatment of constipation may cure the bedwetting. It should be remembered that constipating foods are meat, milk, eggs, cheese, sweets, white flour products and white rice. Give children fewer animal products and more fruit, vegetables and whole grains. Generally speaking, the fewer animal products a child gets the better.

Various exercises have been recommended in the treatment of enuresis. Probably the most common is merely to repeatedly stop and start the flow of urine each time the child urinates. Some bedwetters will benefit in six weeks, but others will require longer. To train the bladder to hold more urine some authorities suggest that the child put off going to the bathroom as long as possible after they feel the urge.

Diseases such as pinworms, anemia, upper respiratory tract infection, urinary tract infection, or any toxic condition may predispose to bedwetting. These should be treated (79).

Many children have a temporary cure of their bedwetting during the summer months when they are out-of-doors and more physically active than during the school year. The bedwetter should be encouraged to have vigorous exercise out-of-doors daily. People who perspire heavily excrete less urine because the fluid is lost through perspiration (80).

Some children who have stopped bedwetting have a return of the problem during the winter months. Dress the child warmly when out-of-doors (81). Chilling increases bladder tone. The child should be warm enough at night.

Bedwetters should be encouraged to take abundant fluids early in the day. Large fluid intake increases bladder capacity. Liquid intake should be tapered off in the late afternoon and evening. However, if a child is thirsty he should not be refused fluids, but should be given small amounts of fluid.

Concentrated urine may also irritate the bladder, causing bedwetting. The child should take sufficient water to keep his urine pale in color.

The child should empty his bladder before he goes to bed. Before the parent goes to bed he should awaken the child to allow him to empty his bladder. Bedwetting tends to occur within one to three hours after going to bed.

Some say that bedwetting occurs only when the child is sleeping on his back (82). Having the child sleep on his stomach or side may help. This can be accomplished by sewing a child's sponge ball on the back of sleeping clothes. The ball need not be removed for laundering.

Medications should not be given to treat bedwetting. Although inconvenient for the parent, the condition has never killed a child, but medications bring the risk of many varied and unwanted side-effects (83).

BEE STINGS

Wash the area with soap and water. Apply cold to stop itching. The stinger should be removed without squeezing. Use tweezers or fingernails. Apply a charcoal poultice as soon as possible, preferably within seconds after the

It brings quick relief. A baking soda bath may be soothing. Add one cup of baking soda to 20 to 30 gallons of water. Meat tenderizer moistened with water, a slice of raw onion, witch hazel, alcohol, vinegar, and honey have all been reported effective in decreasing pain and swelling.

Dr. Bob Evans, a University of Georgia Extension Service insect specialist, says that wet salt should be applied immediately to bee stings, and left in place for 30 minutes. He states this pulls the bee venom out by osmosis.

Seek medical attention if the child manifests such allergic symptoms as breathing problems, hives, severe swelling, shock, or dizziness.

BLEPHARITIS (INFLAMED EYELIDS)

Blepharitis, an inflammation of the eyelids, is one of the most common eye diseases (84). Symptoms include swelling, redness, burning, itching, irritation, crusting and scales at the base of the eyelashes. There is sometimes a sensation of something being in the eye. There may also be a discharge. Swelling may be severe enough to close the eye entirely. Swelling usually resolves in 24-48 hours. There is often associated conjunctivitis. In severe cases the eyelashes may fall out. It tends to be recurrent and chronic. The upper and lower eyelids of both eyes are usually involved. It may be associated with cradle cap, eczema, dandruff, or seborrheic dermatitis.

Allergy may induce blepharitis-like symptoms. Elimination of the most common food allergens (See Appendix 1) may be helpful. Cosmetics, medications, dust, air pollution, tobacco smoke and gasoline fumes may induce blepharitis in those sensitive to them.

There are two general types--seborrheic and staphylococcal. In seborrheic blepharitis the scales are oily or waxy, and easily removed. Scales of staphylococcal blepharitis are drier, and more difficult to remove. There may be associated ulcers or blister-like lesions.

Treatment:

Hygiene is the key to the treatment of all types of blepharitis. Removal of eyelid debris, and increase of blood flow in the eyelid is the goal of treatment. Scales should be removed twice daily by applying hot compresses of normal saline for 10-15 minutes to soften them. A cotton-tipped swab or soft toothbrush may be dipped into a 50:50 solution of baby shampoo and water, rolled against a dry, clean swab to remove excess shampoo, and then used to remove the crusts (85). Use a fresh swab for each eye. The motion should be downward from the eyelid margin to the tip of the eyelash. The shampoo should be thoroughly rinsed off at the conclusion, using a fresh washcloth. A solution of 2% sodium bicarbonate (baking soda) is recommended by some (86). Olive oil or castor oil may be used to soften the crusts for removal. Cool compresses are often helpful (87).

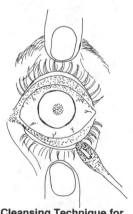

Cleansing Technique for Blepharitis

Seborrheic blepharitis is often associated with oily skin, dandruff, or acne. These conditions must be treated before the blepharitis can be cleared. The diet should be balanced, and free from sweets, alcoholic beverages, hot drinks (88), oils, pork (89), refined carbohydrates, spices, and foods to which the child is sensitive. Overeating should be avoided, as should irregularity in meal time, eating between meals, insufficient chewing of the food, and constipation.

The eyelids should not be rubbed and dirty handkerchiefs and fingers must be kept away from the eyes (90). The scalp must be kept clean, and water should not be permitted to run over the eyes while washing the hair. Keep the fingernails short, and wash the hands frequently.

Lice may cause blepharitis-like symptoms (91). Tiny white eggs (nits) are seen, and itching may be severe. The lice and nits should be removed with tweezers. Some recommend applying a thick layer of petrolatum jelly twice a day for up to eight days to smother the lice, which are then picked off easily.

BLISTERS

A blister is an elevation above the skin level which is filled with fluid. They are often caused by friction, and are most common on the toes, heels and hands. Blisters should be kept clean to prevent infection. Do not break the blister. It will gradually resorb in ten to fourteen days. If the blister breaks spontaneously, carefully trim off the excessive skin, and keep the area clean. A bandage may be applied to decrease rubbing and irritation of the raw skin.

Two pairs of socks may prevent foot blisters. If the child repeatedly develops a blister in a specific location, a piece of adhesive tape may be placed over the area to prevent blistering. Inflamed blisters may be soaked in warm water twice a day for ten to fifteen minutes.

BOILS

Boils are collected infections which occur beneath the skin. They are generally caused by "staph"--hemolytic Staphylococcus aureus bacteria. Symptoms include pain, redness, and pus. The boil comes to a head and drains through the skin. Because the draining pus contains both dead and live bacteria the pus may cause spread of boils. A large boil, with multiple heads, is called a carbuncle. A boil which appears on the edge of the eyelid is known as a stye. Sometimes many boils appear at the same time and this condition is referred to by physicians as furunculosis.

Some children have repeated bouts of boils, while others never have them.

Treatment

Warm soaks of Epsom salts solution made by adding one-half cup of Epsom salts to one quart of water (92); or saline soaks made by adding one teaspoon of salt to a quart of water, often help bring the boil to a head, causing it to drain. The soaks may be continued for one hour at a time, four times a day. The drainage should be caught in a clean bandage, which is changed frequently to keep the surrounding skin clean. The area around the boil may be wiped with 70 percent alcohol or a bleach solution made by adding one tablespoon of bleach to one quart of water to keep the skin clean (93). After the boil has drained the area may be soaked in hot water to reduce swelling, pain, and redness.

A child who suffers from boils should restrict his sugar intake, and drink plenty of water. He should have daily out of doors exercise, fresh air and sun exposure. Red clover tea taken daily is said to be helpful. Some recommend alternating hot and cold baths twice daily as a general health measure.

Boils should not be squeezed, as it may cause them to spread. When the boil comes to a head you may open the boil using a sterile needle to make a large opening. Gently pull the skin away from the boil on both sides at once if necessary to promote immediate emptying. The boil will probably continue to drain for two or three days.

Care should be taken with laundry and eating utensils to prevent the spread of the infecting organism. All bandages should either be burned or carefully discarded in plastic bags.

Boils on the face or head, particularly around the nose, may cause internal infection, and should be carefully treated. If the child develops associated fever or chills, or a red streak from the boil he should be treated promptly with hot soaks for 30 minutes every two hours until the streaks disappear.

Garlic has been shown to have antibacterial properties, and may be helpful in recurrent infections. There are a number of good garlic preparations on the market, either in the form of capsules or dehydrated powder tablets. Depending on the child's size and the ability to secure cooperation in taking the pills, use one to four of the garlic tablets or capsules three times a day.

BOWLEGS (GENU VARUM)

Bowlegs are common in normal young children due to their position before birth. As the child matures, his legs will straighten, often progressing to knock-knees before straightening into the normal adult position. Children who begin walking early, or are overweight may be more likely to have bowlegs, (94) but even in these children, most cases may be expected to resolve without any treatment whatsoever (95). The bowlegged child's parents, brothers and sisters may have also been bowlegged, as it tends to run in families.

The peak incidence of bowlegs appears to be between one and two years of age (96). It may not be apparent until the child begins to walk. Many children appear bowlegged because of thick diapers, and after the diapers are outgrown, the legs begin to straighten.

Probably thousands of children have been subjected to treatment for bowlegs that they would have outgrown given the time. This is probably why any treatment for bowlegs appears to be so effective. Children often have bowlegs until they are about two to four years of age, then develop knock-knees (97). As the child approaches his teens, the knock-knees straighten.

A few children require treatment for bowlegs. Rickets used to be a common cause of bowlegs but with the vitamin D fortified diet found in the United States today, rickets is a rare cause of bowlegs (98). Children with kidney disease or Blounts disease should be seen by their health care provider.

BREAST ENLARGEMENT (GYNECOMASTIA)

Breast enlargement occurs in about 60 to 80% of all boys during puberty, with the peak incidence in 12 to 15 year olds (99). In females the peak incidence occurs earlier--in 8 to 12 year olds (100). It may occur on only one side, or on both. The breasts may be tender, and the boy may attempt to hold his clothing away from his breasts. Boys who have been wrestling or tussling with others may feel that they have sustained injury during the physical contact. It is a developmental process and does not necessarily indicate that anything is wrong, although some diseases (testicular or adrenal tumors, thyroid disease, some liver disorders, and other diseases) and some drugs may induce breast enlargement. Estrogens fed to food animals may contribute (101).

Gynecomastia is less common in black males, and involves only one side in about 25% of cases. The right side is involved more often than the left when it occurs on only one side.

Newborns often have breast enlargement, which is attributed to maternal hormones. This resolves over the first few months of life. Parents are often tempted to try to express the milk which is often found in the breasts of newborns but this stimulation will only encourage the production of even more milk (99).

Treatment

Most breast enlargement in young males will subside spontaneously over a period of two or three years (102). It does not require treatment. If it is due to drugs they should be eliminated.

Obesity may cause breast enlargement. This gynecomastia is treated by a weight reduction program. All milk and dairy products as well as free fats (mayonnaise, margarine, fried foods, cooking fats, and salad oils) must be removed from the diet.

Cold compresses may be applied to the breasts if they are excessively tender.

BREATH-HOLDING

Breath-holding (apnea) episodes, common in infants and young children, can be frightening to parents. Most infants hold their breath briefly during crying episodes (103), but about five percent of children aged 6 to 24 months have breathholding episodes in which they cease breathing, turn blue, and may lose consciousness for a few seconds. There may be muscle jerks or blueness around the lips. Crying, often from a minor injury or frustration or an attempt to have his own way, is a precipitating event. The child begins to cry with anger, frustration, or surprise. He may cry briefly and then stop breathing. One study reported that the longer a child cried the less likely he was to hold his breath (104). There is a gasp as the child begins breathing again and he rapidly regains his color (105). Children often use these episodes in an attempt to manipulate and control the parent. The parent becomes so anxious over the non-breathing child that she gives in to his demands.

There are two different types of breath-holding attacks. The most common is called a cyanotic attack. Anger, fright or pain often induce this type of episode. The child stops crying to hold his breath, turns bluish in color, and may lose consciousness. He may have some muscle jerks. In the other type, pallid attacks, the child becomes pale and may have muscle spasms or arch his back and extend his legs during an attack.

These episodes usually begin when the child is between 6 and 18 months of age. Children in one study had peak incidence of episodes between the ages of two and three. They occur irregularly and usually cease by the time the child is four years old (106). About one-third of these children have one or more attacks a day, but some children have been reported to have ten to fifteen daily episodes. They are more common in boys, perhaps because of slower physical maturation. There is often a family history of similar behavior (107). If the child is normal neurologically and has no epilepsy the outcome is always favorable (108). Parents may be helped to distinguish epileptic seizures from breathholding episodes by the following factors:

(1) Breath-holding episodes are typically initiated by crying; epileptic seizures are not typically induced by crying.
(2) Seizures may occur during sleep, breath-holding never does.
(3) The child with epilepsy will often wet his pants, this rarely occurs during breath-holding.
(4) Seizures generally last longer than one minute, but breathholding usually lasts for less than one minute.
(5) After a seizure children are often confused, while breathholding does not produce confusion (108).
(6) A child having an epileptic seizure is hot and sweaty, and has a rapid pulse. A breathholding child is cool, clammy, and has a slow pulse.

Parents should not become overly anxious as this may worsen the problem. They should consider these episodes a form of temper tantrum. The parent should not react to the child during a breathholding episode. If she leaves the room the child is deprived of what he is trying to gain (109). Ignoring the attacks typically initially increases, then as the child learns they do not gain the desired result, the frequency decreases (110). Children cannot hold their breath until they die; if breathholding leads to loss of consciousness the child will spontaneously resume breathing and will shortly regain consciousness (111).

The child should have a daily program that eliminates stress as far as possible. He should be on a regular schedule for rising, meals, and bedtime. Excessive mental stimulation from television, video games, movies and radio should be avoided. Excessive fatigue should be guarded against. There should be daily out-of-doors exercise with sun exposure (112). Discipline should be firm and consistent.

Iron deficiency anemia is a common finding in these children (113). Daily sunshine exposure and a diet high in vitamin C (from fresh, raw fruits and vegetables) and iron (see section on anemia) will be helpful to these children. Excessive milk intake may cause anemia (114), therefore milk should be eliminated from the diet of breath-holders. Pica (see section) may also produce anemia.

A developmental study of 36 breath-holding children revealed that none still had episodes after three years. There is no association with epilepsy or low intelligence, and these attacks are not felt to cause brain damage.

Breath-holders may manifest other behaviors such as temper tantrums or head banging when they are unhappy (111).

BRONCHIECTASIS

Bronchiectasis is a sac-like enlargement of the ends of the small bronchi with a chronic inflammation. Some of the small branches become partially or entirely blocked by mucus, scarring, or inflammation. Repeated infections, pneumonia, asthma, allergies, inhalation of an foreign object, or chronic bronchitis may lead to bronchiectasis. It is often associated with cystic fibrosis.

About 20 percent of cases are said to initially occur in children under one year of age, and 75 percent of cases occur before the child reaches five years of age (115). The primary symptom is a chronic cough, which is often associated with sputum production. Coughing is often worse with change in position, and may occur when the child lies down, rolls over, or sits up. The coughing may be severe enough to produce vomiting. Very young children may have stridor or wheezing. If the disease is of long duration the child may develop an enlarged chest, clubbing of the fingers, anemia, and easy fatigability. The child may grow slowly.

Treatment

Postural drainage will assist in clearing mucus from the dilated sacs (116). See treatment section for procedure. This should be carried out twice a day for twenty minutes at a time. Secretions are sometimes easier to move in the morning. The child should be placed in the postural drainage position which stimulates the most coughing and raising of sputum. During periods of active disease the postural drainage should be increased to as much as three hours per day. The child may forcefully cough to bring up the sputum. Following the postural drainage the child should breathe slowly and deeply for about ten minutes (117).

The child should be as active as his condition permits (118). Regular out-of-doors exercise should be encouraged.

The diet should be free of sugar and low in fats. If the child is overweight he should be placed on a weight control program (118). Extremely hot or cold foods should be avoided as they may provoke coughing.

Mist inhalations are helpful in thinning mucus (119). It is felt that a humidity of 30 to 50% encourages best mucociliary function.

Irritating substances such as tobacco smoke, pollen, aerosols, and dust should be avoided.

Abundant fluid intake should be encouraged. The child should take at least eight glasses of water every day (118). This assists in thinning the secretions, making them easier to cough up.

Sudden changes in temperature should be avoided (118). Wear a mask or scarf over the mouth and nose to warm air in cold weather.

Laughing, loud talking, exertion, and crying may trigger attacks.

See the treatment section for instructions on an onion chest poultice. This may be very helpful to relieve cough.

Special attention should be given to keeping the mouth and teeth in good condition (118).

Some children benefit from raising the foot of the bed three to five inches (118). This discourages mucus collection in the lower lung lobes. Sleeping without a pillow may help.

Allergy is a common factor in bronchiectasis. Children may benefit from allergen-control. An elimination and challenge diet should be instituted to determine if secretions are reduced when certain foods are eliminated, and return when they are again eaten. Mouth-breathing should be discouraged.

Deep breathing exercises should be carried out every day.

The child should have regular, adequate rest.

Children with bronchiectasis should be kept out of large crowds where they may be exposed to various types of infections.

Cough medications and antihistamines often dry bronchial secretions, making them more difficult to remove.

BRONCHITIS AND COUGHS

Bronchitis is an inflammation of the bronchial tubes. These tubes are the branches off the trachea or windpipe.

Symptoms of bronchitis include cough, fever, shortness of breath, chest discomfort, blueness of the skin, and sometimes nausea and vomiting. The cough is typically worse at night, and is often worsened by changing the child's position, such as when he first lies down at night, or gets up in the morning. Vigorous exercise also may induce coughing spasms.

Bronchitis is most common in young children less than two years of age. Males are more frequently affected. It is most common during the winter and early spring. Onset may be with a one or two day history of mild cold symptoms followed by the development of a cough. Bronchitis may follow a cold, croup, influenza, measles, tonsillitis, or pneumonia. Young children may have a rattling sound as they breathe. Symptoms of uncomplicated bronchitis typically resolve in about two weeks, but sometimes a chronic bronchitis develops which may persist much longer. There are sometimes recurrent episodes, with several bouts during the course of a year.

Acute bronchitis may be caused by allergies, chemical substances such as dust, fumes or smoke, and viral or bacterial infections.

Treatment

Good fluid intake should be ensured. Adults may take as much as 8 ounces of water every hour. This fluid is essential to thin and loosen the bronchial secretions, making it easier to cough them up. Fluids other than milk should be given. Warm drinks may be comforting to the child, and may be given frequently.

A cool vaporizer will increase humidity, sometimes making it easier for the child to breathe. Eucalyptus oil may be added to the vaporizer. The child may be placed in a steamy bathroom (run hot water) if a vaporizer is not available. Pans of water may be placed about the child's room to add moisture to the air.

An onion chest poultice may relieve cough. See treatment section for procedure. It may assist breathing to raise the head of the bed on five inch wooden blocks (120).

Activity should be limited during episodes of bronchitis, but the child may be up and mildly active if he feels up to it. The resultant increased respiratory rate assists in freeing the mucus in the lungs (121).

Cough medicines should be avoided as it is important to cough up and remove the sputum (122). Chest heating compresses are helpful for coughs, as are hot fomentations (see treatment section). The parent may simply apply a towel wrung out of hot water (not so hot as to burn the child) over the chest for three minutes, remove the towel and quickly wipe the area with a washcloth dipped in ice water, then apply another hot towel for another three minutes. Continue the alternations for three to five changes. Gargling or sipping hot water may also help. Encourage the child to breathe through his nose rather than his mouth. A hot foot bath (see treatment section) will assist in relieving chest congestion.

Expectorants may produce gastric irritation with associated nausea and vomiting. Their value in the treatment of bronchitis has never been demonstrated. Water is the very best expectorant available.

Children whose parents smoke are more likely to suffer bronchitis (123). If both parents smoke the child is at even higher risk. Smoking should not be permitted near children. Exposure to cigarette smoke during the first year of life doubles the risk of the child developing either pneumonia or bronchitis (124).

Postural drainage may help remove secretions from the lungs. (See treatment section.) The child may hang his head over the edge of the bed while the parent percusses his back with cupped hands to loosen secretions. Even massage of the chest and back with olive oil will assist in improving circulation (125).

Fever can be treated with a hot half bath (125). Finish off the bath with a cold mitten friction (see treatment section for these techniques.)

Infants who are breast fed are at decreased risk of developing bronchitis.

A bulb syringe may be used to clear an infant's nasal passages if he is too young to blow his nose. (See section on common cold for procedure.)

The diet should be light and consist mainly of fresh fruits, vegetables and whole grains. Refined sugars and milk should be strictly avoided. Milk produces mucus and should be avoided in all its forms--cheese, butter, yogurt, ice creams and ice milks (127). Nuts, coffee and chocolate are also suspected of causing mucus formation in some people.

Steam inhalations (see treatment section) may be done several times a day (127). Nausea and even vomiting may result if the child swallows his secretions instead of spitting them out (127).

The child should be carefully protected from drafts and chills. The neck, shoulders, and chest should be kept warm (127). The child should not walk barefooted on a cold floor.

The child should not breathe fumes of any type. Children who live in homes where gas stoves are used for cooking have higher rates of bronchitis than in those living in homes which use electricity for cooking (128).

Anise tea and almond milk have been reported helpful in bronchitis. Make the almond milk by blending six tablespoons of almonds in a pint of water (129). A tea made by boiling dandelion greens in water until half the water is boiled away may be helpful in bronchitis. A tea made from steeping a teaspoon each of slippery elm and mullein can be quite soothing and expectorant. Non-productive, paroxysmal coughing may be helped markedly by sipping on fenugreek tea throughout the day or night.

BRUXISM (TOOTH GRINDING)

Bruxism, or tooth grinding, is said to occur in 7 to 88 percent of children (130). Frequency increases up to the age of seven to twelve, then decreases. Bruxism has been observed in young infants with eruption of the first teeth. Parents may hear grating or clicking sounds and notice the child tightly clenching his teeth. The average bruxer has five episodes a night, each episode lasting eight to nine seconds. Episodes may occur during dreams.

Bruxism during sleep is common in normal children, but tooth grinding during the day may be a sign of mental deficiency or extreme stress (131). Tooth grinding may occur as a side effect of some medications, including amphetamines.

Bruxism and TMJ (temporomandibular joint) symptoms show a positive correlation. Symptoms of TMJ dysfunction were 50% greater in bruxers than in non-bruxers. Older children may report headaches; and bruxism may produce dental wear, exposure of the tooth pulp, muscle tenderness, bite changes, limited ability to open the mouth, bone loss, hypermobility or hypersensitivity of teeth, and recession or inflammation of the gingiva.

Bruxism seems to run in families and children whose parents ground their teeth as children are more likely to do so (132).

Causes of Bruxism

Many factors are felt to be the cause of bruxism. A diet low in magnesium may contribute, as may vitamin deficiencies.

Allergy is probably the most common cause (132). Children with allergies have a three-fold increase in bruxism rates when compared with non-allergic children. Mouth breathing, producing a dry mouth, is felt by some to cause bruxism. A stuffy nose from allergies may lead to mouth breathing. Episodes of tooth grinding are more frequent during exacerbations of such allergic conditions as allergic rhinitis, asthma, and upper respiratory tract infections. Parents sometimes report that their child grinds his teeth more often after the intake of foods to which he is allergic (132).

Many hyperactive children grind their teeth; hyperactivity has been associated with allergies. Always try to discover foods to which the child is sensitive by a trial period of elimination.

Other oral habits such as chronic chewing of toys, finger- and thumb-sucking, mouth breathing, and tongue thrusting, all common in allergic children, are also common in bruxers (132).

Some researchers have claimed improvement in bruxism by training the tooth grinder to clench his teeth tightly until pain is felt for five seconds, then to relax for five seconds, many times a day (133).

It may be necessary for the dentist to fit a plastic bite plane.

Stress is sometimes given as a cause. Children who grind their teeth during sleeping hours may be reacting to stress in their daily life. Parents should study the causes of this stress and attempt to relieve it. Spending time with the child before bedtime allowing him to talk about his fears and anxieties may be helpful (134). Reducing television time, competitive sports, and stimulating activities is often helpful.

BURNS

Burns are a common occurrence in children as well as adults. Small burns may be readily managed at home. Extensive or severe burns, and burns which involve the eyes, fingers, or face, should be treated by your health care provider.

Treatment

Cold applications applied as quickly as possible are probably the most effective treatment for burns (136). If applied within the first ten seconds after the burn they may be sufficient to greatly reduce the amount of injury. Dip the burned area in cold water or apply cold packs for at least 30 to 45 minutes, but the cold applications may be continued until the pain does not recur when the affected area is removed from the cold water.

A bandage is not required unless the area is likely to be rubbed or bumped. A thin layer of sterile petrolatum may be applied over gauze to prevent the gauze from sticking to the burn.

Elevating the burned part will often decrease pain and discomfort.

Blisters should be broken and opened along one side quite a long distance to allow drainage and prevent the development of irritating ammonia in the fluid. Do not remove the loose skin unless it becomes infected.

A poultice of comfrey leaves, raw potato, aloe vera, or ordinary black tea may be applied. A study from India reported the use of boiled potato peel in the treatment of mild burns. Potatoes were soaked, washed, and boiled for 20 minutes in clean water. Peels were removed without any adherent pulp. The inner surface of the peel was placed against the burn, and two layers of saline-soaked gauze applied over the peel. A bandage was used to hold the peel in place. If there was no infection present the peel was changed every four to eight days, but daily in infected cases (135).

A recent study revealed that aloe vera gel decreases bacterial counts and speeds healing of burns. Aloe-treated burns healed in an average of 30 days, while burns in the control animals required 50 days to heal (137).

Do not apply greasy substances such as butter. These substances may cause infection.

Over-the-counter anesthetic sprays may induce allergic reactions, and should be avoided.

If the burn becomes increasingly painful, produces pus, or redness or swelling appears, or if high fever develops, the child should evaluated by your health care provider.

CANKER SORES (APHTHOUS ULCERS)

Canker sores are round or oval white ulcers surrounded by an area of redness. They are found most commonly on the cheek, tongue, inner lips and gums (138). There may be one or several. One may be healing as others are developing. For one to three days before onset of the ulcer there may be a sensation of tingling, burning, pain, or roughness of the skin (139).

The ulcers generally heal within seven to ten days, but while present may interfere with eating or talking. About 20 percent of the population are said to suffer from them, and they are common in school aged children. They are more common in girls than in boys.

The cause is not clearly understood, but many people report that the intake of specific foods will induce them. Stress also probably plays a role, although this may be more true in adults than in children.

Canker sores tend to run in families. Onset is generally before 20 years of age, and as the person ages episodes often become less frequent.

Treatment

Recent studies have shown a relationship between celiac disease and canker sores (140). One group of patients being treated by a gluten-free diet for their celiac disease, noted disappearance of their canker sores. Another group of celiac patients were found to be sensitive to milk and they reported decrease in canker sore incidence when milk was eliminated from their dietary (141).

English walnuts or other nuts, citrus fruit, tomatoes, peanuts, peppermint, acidic foods, salted foods, fresh pineapple, honeydew melon, cinnamon, shellfish, and chocolate have all been associated with canker sores. The person should keep a list of foods eaten for several days prior to the onset of the canker sore, and try to determine if the canker sore is due to food sensitivity. Preservatives and food colorings may also cause problems.

Injury to the lips or cheek may also contribute to canker sores. Overly vigorous toothbrushing, biting the lip or cheek, and trauma from toothpicks should be avoided. Stress can increase muscle tightness of the lips and jaws, increasing risk of injury from the teeth. To refrain from talking while chewing or turning the head to one side during chewing, or during conversation, can help avoid injury from the teeth.

While the canker sore is present it may be difficult for the child to eat. Cold or hot foods or carbonated drinks may cause pain and some prefer to take fluids via a straw (142). Young children taking a bottle may need to be switched to a cup. Generous fluid intake should be encouraged. A soft diet, which does not require much chewing, may be taken better. Some find cold foods soothing. Older children may suck on ice for a while before eating to decrease the pain (143).

A cotton applicator dipped in 2% hydrogen peroxide may be touched to the canker sore several times daily, or a mouth wash, made of one-half teaspoon to eight ounces of water used several times daily and after meals to cleanse the mouth (144). Some obtain pain relief by rinsing the mouth with milk of magnesia or antacid (145).

Goldenseal or bayleaf tea may be used as a mouthwash and gargle. Goldenseal powder may be applied to the ulcer. Make the bay leaf tea by simmering five fresh or dried bay leaves in two cups of water for twenty minutes, strain, stir back in the oil which forms on the surface of the water, and cool. Warm the tea slightly before use. The tea should be made fresh every two days.

We have found that many a canker sore can be stopped in its tracks, at its very beginning, if the child will start drinking a glassful (size of glass proportional to size of the child) of water every 10 minutes for one hour. If the water drinking begins within one hour of feeling the first sign of the sore it will usually not develop.

CAROTENEMIA

A diet high in carotene may produce yellowing of the skin which may be mistaken for jaundice. In true jaundice the whites of the eyes become yellow; they remain white in carotenemia (146). The greatest risk of carotenemia is that the child will be subjected to an unnecessary work-up for the possibility of liver disease (147). Carotene is excreted through the sweat glands, and pigmentation is particularly noticeable in areas of the body which contain many sweat glands (148). The incidence is not known, but it appears to be a rather common occurrence. Peak carotene levels apparently occur about age five, and gradually decrease afterward (147).

Treatment

The cure for carotenemia is to decrease certain foods such as alfalfa, apples, apricots, asparagus, beet greens, berries, broccoli, butter, cantaloupes, carrots, chard, collard greens, cucumbers, endive, escarole, figs, lettuce, mangoes, milk, mustard, oranges, palm oil, papayas, parsley, papaws, peaches, pineapple, prunes, pumpkin, rutabagas, sweet potatoes, yellow squash, tomatoes, yams, yellow corn, yellow turnips, parsnip, spinach, green and yellow beans, kale, watercress, and eggs all of which contain high levels of carotene. Carotenes are present in all pigmented fruits and vegetables, but the color may be masked by chlorophyll. As a general rule, the deeper the color the higher the level of carotene (149). Pureeing, cooking, or mashing foods breaks down the carotene-containing cells, allowing greater absorption (149). Children fed a diet of pureed foods have higher carotene levels than do similar children fed the same foods in a non-pureed form (148). Carotene-containing vegetables are used as bases or coloring for many commercially prepared baby foods (149). This is probably why children six to eighteen months of age are more likely to develop carotenemia.

The body converts carotene to vitamin A.

Breast-feeding mothers who consume large amounts of carotene containing foods may produce orange milk, causing carotenemia in their infants. One mother gave birth to children who were already pigmented, and remained so until they were weaned off breast milk (150).

CAT SCRATCH DISEASE

Cat scratch disease is generally a benign disease which resolves over the course of several months. It is often associated with young cats, but may come from any sharp object which penetrates the skin, and carries the infecting organism. The disease is felt to be carried by rodents or birds, natural prey for cats, and the cat is merely a carrier which does not become sick (151). He is probably capable of spreading the disease for only two or three weeks and for that reason most authorities do not insist on destroying the cat. The infectious agent may be spread by mouth secretions when the cat bites or licks the child (152). Several cases have been linked to exposure to pet birds. Sharp objects, such as thorns, fishhooks, splinters, or pins may be contaminated with the organism (153), which is carried into the human body when the skin is broken by these sharp objects. It is much more common in children, about 75 percent of all cases being in young people.

It was initially reported in 1931, with incidence increasing since then. The true incidence is unknown as many cases are so mild they are not recognized as cat scratch disease and the parents do not seek medical attention for the child, who does not appear seriously ill (154). It is now considered by some to be among the most common causes of one-sided lymphadenopathy (disease affecting the lymph glands) (155). Lymph glands anywhere in the body may be affected, but most commonly the glands in the neck and under the arms are involved (155). This may be because the injury is most typically on the arms. It does not seem to be carried from person to person but several members of the family may develop cat scratch disease, probably from the same source of infection. It has been estimated that only 10 percent of the individuals scratched or bitten by an infected cat will actually develop the disease (156). Most cases occur during fall and winter months (157).

The disease begins with a small elevated area of skin over the site of a scratch or other injury which has broken the skin. The area may be swollen and red and an ulcer may form. These ulcers are often slow healing. Fever, headache, loss of appetite, nausea, vomiting, abdominal pain, chills, generalized aching, a sensation of not feeling well, and enlargement of the lymph glands follow in 10 to 30 days (151). The low grade fever may persist for months. Lymph gland involvement, which is the only symptom in about half of all cases, often persists for about two months but may last for over a year. In the majority of cases only one lymph node is involved. In some cases the lymph glands retain sufficient fluid that they appear ready to rupture. These lymph glands may require aspiration by your health care provider. Complications, which are rare, include arthritis-like pain in joints, enlargement of the spleen, and inflammation of the brain.

Treatment

Antibiotics are ineffective (157), and should not be administered. The most effective treatment is warm, moist soaks to the involved lymph glands (155).

Bed rest or minimal physical activity should be maintained while the fever persists. Vigorous activity should be prohibited as long as the lymph gland enlargement persists, because of risk of injury to the swollen glands (158).

Parents should insist that their children wash any cuts or scratches immediately and that the cat not be allowed to lick any area of broken skin. The child should wash his hands immediately after petting the cat and should be taught to handle cats gently so as to prevent bites or scratches (158).

One episode of cat scratch disease seems to confer life-long immunity (159).

CATERPILLAR STINGS

Caterpillar hairs often become embedded in the skin. Cover the area with cellophane tape, then lift off, pulling the hairs out of the skin. Meat tenderizer or charcoal compresses may be used for pain relief.

Seek medical attention if the child manifests such allergic symptoms as breathing problems, hives, severe swelling, shock, or dizziness.

CELIAC DISEASE

Peak incidence of celiac disease is between 9 and 18 months, with the onset of symptoms after gluten is added to the diet (160). Gluten is found in wheat, rye, barley, and oats (161), and may be one of the very first solid foods given to a child.

The disease is rare in blacks and Asians, and occurs equally in both sexes (161). It tends to run in families.

Symptoms include diarrhea which often smells bad. Stools may be pale, bulky, and oily (162). Stools may look like oatmeal. The stools often float on top of the water in the toilet. There may be one or several stools per day. However, not all celiac children have diarrhea (162). These children are chronically malnourished because of malabsorption, and appear much like starving children. They have protuberant abdomens, with spindly arms and legs. They are often irritable and may not want to eat. Growth is hindered with long-term uncontrolled disease. Some children have vomiting or abdominal pain. There may be sores in the mouth, a smooth tongue, easy bruising, edema, and finger clubbing.

The intestinal mucosa is lined with tall villi (finger-like projections) which function to absorb nutrients from the food passing through the intestine. In celiac disease these villi flatten out, decreasing their ability to absorb nutrients (160).

Children with uncontrolled celiac disease often grow slowly, but they usually catch up within a year or two of starting on a strict gluten free diet.

Treatment

There is usually weight gain and improved behavior within two weeks of removal of gluten from the diet (162). The child must be on a gluten free diet all his life. It has been observed that those who eat gluten are at increased risk of developing certain types of cancers later on in life. Gluten is found in many commonly used foods and the celiac child should be taught how to avoid these foods. Grains are used as fillers in many foods (160). The commonly used "vegetable protein" contains gluten, as does monosodium glutamate.

All grains given to children should be thoroughly cooked for two to three hours. The child must be strict in his gluten-free diet. Coffee and coffee substitutes may contain malt, wheat, rye, barley, or oats. Almost all commercial breads, bread mixes, crackers, muffins, cupcakes, rolls, Ry-Krisp, and pretzels contain gluten. Commercially prepared puddings, cakes, candies, cookies, ice cream, and sherbets may contain gluten, and salad dressings are sometimes thickened or emulsified with products containing gluten. All breaded meats, luncheon meats, frankfurters, and canned chili must be avoided. Macaroni, noodles, spaghetti, bread stuffings, many commercial soups, vegetables cooked with cream sauce thickened with flour, bottled meat sauces, condiments, flavoring syrups, gravies and sauces, and cocoa mixes may contain gluten. Breads and cereals made from rice, corn, millet, soybean or potato starch may be used.   A low fat diet should be given. Fat is poorly absorbed by these children. Spicy foods should be avoided, as they may further irritate the already inflamed bowel (161).

These children often show allergic responses to other foods. Most common are milk (163), egg, and oatmeal. They often benefit from a sugar-free diet.

Ripe bananas are said to be well tolerated (164). Corn, rice, buckwheat, quinoa, and millet are acceptable (165). Many pharmaceutical products contain gluten, and may cause adverse effects in the unsuspecting medication taker.

Breast feeding seems to delay the onset of celiac disease (167). Breast-fed infants first manifested symptoms of celiac disease at 16 months of age, while bottle-fed children had symptoms at 10 months of age. Children formula-fed from birth or breast-fed for less than 30 days may be four times more likely to develop celiac disease than those who are breast-fed for longer periods (168). Breast-fed infants who do develop celiac disease develop it later.

Sun exposure may improve calcium metabolism and absorption (169).

Infections and stress may induce exacerbations of symptoms (170).

Garlic has been shown helpful in celiac disease. It may be taken raw, cooked, or in tablets or capsules.

CENTIPEDE BITES

Centipede bites may very painful and may be associated with swelling of the lymph glands. Symptoms usually subside within 48 hours. Apply a charcoal compress as in bee stings. An ice cube may be applied for pain relief.

Seek medical attention if the child manifests such allergic symptoms as difficulty breathing, hives, severe swelling, shock, or dizziness.

CHALAZION

A chalazion is an inflammation of one of the glands in the eyelid. It appears as a small, hard, slow-growing bump on the eyelid. Chalazions sometimes resolve spontaneously. They are more common in adolescent girls who do not clean off their eye makeup at night. Hormonal influences, dehydration, and food sensitivities are also felt to contribute.

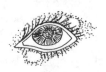

Chalazion

Treatment

Hot compresses may be applied at the first indication of a chalazion. A clean cloth may be folded in layers, dipped in warm water, and wrung out until it no longer drips water. Apply over the affected area, refreshing the compress as it drys. Continue the application for at least 20 minutes. Repeat every four hours. Apply a charcoal compress every night. It may require several months for the mass to absorb. In some cases surgical removal is required.

Girls should be instructed in the proper removal of eye make up. The eyelids should be cleansed with a mild soap and thoroughly rinsed with clean water.

RED, CRACKING LIPS (CHEILITIS)

Cheilitis, also called perleche, is an inflammation of the lip or lips, with symptoms of redness, a burning sensation, scaling, tenderness, and sometimes cracks in the lip. These cracks often occur at the corners of the mouth and may be due to excessive lip licking or drooling. Nutritional deficiencies are known to cause some types of cheilitis. Mouth breathing may cause drooling, which keeps the lips wet constantly. In adults, poorly fitting dentures may produce cheilitis. Allergic reaction is a common cause of cheilitis in children. Reactions to medications, chewing gum, cosmetics, mouthwash, and toothpaste may cause lip soreness, and cheilitis may be associated with skin conditions such as psoriasis or seborrheic dermatitis. Trauma from braces or other dental appliances may cause cheilitis. It may be found in association with a fever.

The condition usually clears in three to four weeks, even without treatment, but the child must be instructed not to lick his lips. Excessive wind or sun exposure may worsen the condition. The child should discontinue the use of toothpaste and use salt or baking soda to clean his teeth.

Cheilitis may be prevented by coating the lips with a bland ointment or petroleum jelly.

CHICKENPOX (VARICELLA)

Chickenpox is a highly contagious disease readily spread by direct contact, air-borne virus, or virus-contaminated linen or clothing. Poor appetite, a sense of not feeling well, cold-like symptoms, headache, and fever

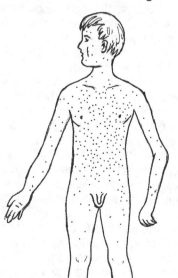

may be initial symptoms, followed by onset of lesions. The pox begin as small red bumps which may look like insect bites, become blisters, and dry to form brown crusts within a 24 hour period. New crops may occur for four to five days as old lesions resolve (172). The rash typically begins on the back, chest, and head. It spreads over succeeding days to the trunk, arms, and legs. Lesions may appear inside the mouth, rectum, vagina and urethra. Cool baths are often helpful in relieving itching in the genital area. A long hot bath at the onset of the lesions may be used to bring out the pox more rapidly and shorten the duration of the disease.

Fever is often present, with a higher fever occurring in a child with a greater number of lesions. Some children have low grade fever and only a few pox;

Distribution of Chickenpox Rash

others have many pox and a high fever. Fever is typically highest on the third or fourth day of the illness (172).

Sores may occur in the mouth and may interfere with eating (173).

In a typical case the child may have fever for a week and the rash for about five days, followed by crusting for about five days.

Treatment

Itching is the most troublesome symptom. Children should not be permitted to scratch, as infection may develop. The child may be placed in a cool tub of water to which one-half to one cup of cornstarch, baking soda or apple cider vinegar has been added. Pat dry afterward to avoid rubbing off the scabs. Spray starch (find cornstarch, not sizing agents) is soothing to itching lesions (174). Avoid brands which contain large amounts of nitrates and borates as they may induce allergic reactions. If your child develops a reaction stop the use of spray starch. Do not spray the starch near your child's face to avoid getting starch in the eyes.

A paste made of baking soda and water may be applied to the lesions to reduce itching (173). Aloe vera applications are soothing. Calamine lotion may be used for itching. Olive oil may be applied to the drying crusts to cause them to drop off sooner.

The child should be kept in bed only during the most acute phase of the illness. Keep him as quiet as possible to avoid sweating, which may increase itching (175). Clothing should be soft and lightweight. After the fever begins to drop he may play in the yard if shade is available and the weather is nice. He should indulge in only quiet activity to minimize perspiration. Sun exposure is felt to increase the incidence of lesions in chickenpox (175). Be sure adequate warm clothing is worn to prevent even a slight degree of chilling, as chickenpox pneumonia is more likely to occur after chilling.

Instruct the child to wash his hands often during the day to prevent infection (172). Picking and scratching should be discouraged. You may wish to put soft gloves or socks on the hands of young children to prevent scratching. Older children may need them during the night. Fingernails should be kept short and clean. Bed linen should be changed daily.

Fever and itching may be treated with hot baths at 106 degrees, one minute for each year of the child's age several times a day (see treatment section). Never use aspirin to reduce fever, as it has been associated with Reye's syndrome (172). An interesting study from Johns Hopkins revealed that acetaminophen (Tylenol) use caused prolongation of the illness and did not produce symptomatic relief (176). The researcher, Dr. Timothy Doran, feels that fever is helpful to the body in its effort to fight the disease. Children in his study group given Tylenol had a one day increase in illness duration. Antibiotics are neither necessary nor helpful (177). Mouth sores may be treated with saline mouth washes or gargles. Add one-half teaspoon of salt to eight ounces of water. The child should be encouraged to drink plenty of fluids, particularly while he has a fever. Cold foods are often taken more readily than hot foods. Avoid salty or spicy foods and citrus fruits.

Lesions may occur on the eyelids but do not represent a risk to vision (172). If lesions occur on the eyeball a physician should be contacted immediately.

Temporary skin discolorations may persist for up to a year after the illness. These color changes may be more pronounced in black children, and may remain for several years.

The child can spread the infection from 24 hours before the onset of the rash until a week after the rash appears. Disease onset occurs anywhere from ten to twenty-one days after exposure, but most often within two weeks. Severity of the disease seems to be related to the intensity of the exposure. Chickenpox is relatively mild in young children while children ten years of age or older are often much more uncomfortable during their illness.

Chickenpox seems to occur most often in winter and spring in the temperate regions of the world, while it occurs year around in warm climates (178). Outbreaks often begin with school exposure or in areas where housing is crowded.

CHIGGERS

Chiggers are tiny but mighty annoyances. They are found in all parts of the world and are most active during spring, summer, and fall months (179). In temperate climates they may be active year around but become less active after temperatures drop below 60 degrees F.

These tiny mites have four pairs of legs. They suck, rather than bite. They attach themselves to the host with claws, and secrete powerful digestive juices, which liquify skin cells. The fluid is then sucked up by the chigger. Their diet consists of dissolved skin cells, rather than blood.

Chigger eggs are laid in soil and after hatching, the larvae climb up onto vegetation. When they sense a nearby host (animal or human) they drop off the vegetation and onto the host. They remain on the host, feeding for about three days before they drop off. After this feeding, the larva reaches adulthood, when it is no longer parasitic. The entire life cycle is two to three weeks long (180).

Chiggers prefer bottom land areas which are overgrown with vegetation, although they may be found in well-kept lawns.

Itching is the most obvious symptom and may begin three to six hours after the mites attach themselves to the body. Symptoms may persist for three to ten days with the most intense itching often on the second day. Itching may be severe enough to interfere with sleeping. A warm bed may increase itching (180).

Treatment

Prevention is the treatment of choice. Long clothing should be worn if one goes into woods expected to contain chiggers. They often attach themselves near the tops of socks, or on underwear leg bands, waistbands, or near other clothing which causes an obstacle to their travel over the body. Clothing should fit snugly at the wrists, ankles, and about the neck (180).

After being in woods likely to have chiggers one should shower vigorously, using a brush or coarse washcloth to scrub loose any chiggers which have not yet become attached. All clothing should be laundered in hot water.

Chiggers do not burrow into the skin and drop off after feeding. Attached chiggers, which look like a red fleck on the skin, may be removed with the fingernails or tweezers. Some prefer to paint them with petroleum jelly or castor oil, which clogs their breathing apparatus and will hopefully cause them to detach from the body.

Itching from chigger bites may be controlled by several different methods. A twenty minute bath as hot as can be tolerated will usually bring several hours of relief. Starch baths are also often helpful. Some people find cold baths or compresses effective in relieving itching.

Charcoal poultices are helpful to some. (See treatment section for procedure) A paste may be made by adding a little water to finely ground oatmeal, and the mixture applied over the chigger bites. If they are widespread over the body, powdered oatmeal may be added to bathwater for a soaking bath (181). Some report good relief with the application of banana or banana skin (182). Clear fingernail polish is also reported to relieve itching (180). Rubbing a stick deodorant over chigger bites is also reported to provide almost instant relief of itching (183).

The child's fingernails should be kept short, and scratching should be discouraged as it may lead to secondary infection.

Some people use over-the-counter local anesthetic medications to control itching, but these carry a high risk of sensitivity reaction, worsening the symptoms.

Insect repellents are generally effective in preventing chiggers, but these are known to have adverse effects, even in low doses (180). Citronella oil, available at some drugstores, may be a safe and effective deterrent.

Hikers and campers may decrease their risk of chiggers by staying on open trails and away from areas with heavy growth.

COLD

The common cold, called an upper respiratory infection by physicians, is due to a viral infection of the nose and throat. It is the most common of all childhood illnesses (200). Spread of the virus may be by airborne germs or from direct contact with germ carrying objects such as telephones, toys, doorknobs, or hands (201). Many of the more than 100 different cold viruses are able to live for three days on objects. The virus is carried into the nose or eyes by the fingers, and begins to spread down the throat. Symptoms of the common cold include fever, loss of appetite, red watery eyes, sore throat, runny or stuffy nose, irritability, sneezing, cough, headache, muscle aches and hoarseness.

Most newborns do not catch cold during the first three months of life. At about three months of age the infant's own immune system begins to function, and the child loses the immunity acquired from the mother. A child may catch several colds during the first year of life. Young infants do not know how to breathe through their mouths, and a stuffy nose will make them very uncomfortable. He will be unable to breathe and breast-feed at the same time and may decrease feedings because of the difficulty.

Colds in infants and young children tend to persist about three days longer than do colds in older children and adults. Some perfectly normal children suffer one cold after another; others seem to have a perpetual cold. The incidence of colds seems to be in proportion to the number of exposures. One study suggested that children less than one year of age average seven colds per year, one to five year olds suffer seven or more per year, with the incidence decreasing after five years of age (202). Boys catch more colds than girls. Children in school and day care facilities, or from large families have more frequent colds, as they have greater potential for exposure to others who have them. Colds are more frequent during winter than summer. Children in overcrowded living conditions suffer more colds than those in healthful environments. Children whose parents smoke are more likely to catch cold. An interesting Australian study revealed that individuals who ate a vegetarian or high fruit and vegetable diet had fewer colds than those on a "typical" diet.

Treatment

The room should be kept at a comfortable temperature and free from drafts. The child should not be overdressed, but chilling should be avoided. Chilling of the legs causes contraction of the blood vessels in the nose, worsening nasal congestion.

A cold-water humidifier or a pan of water on the radiator may be used to humidify the air. Water in humidifiers should be changed daily to avoid mold growth. Robert Solomon, M.D., chief of the University of Michigan Medical Center allergy division, cautions that vaporizers should be scrubbed daily with a rough object such as a plastic pan scrubber and that the unit be rinsed carefully afterward (203). He cautions against the use of chemical agents which may remain in the vaporizer and be sprayed into the air. Even bleach may produce a respiratory allergy in sensitive individuals. Humidifiers should be placed out of the child's reach. Wet towels hung in the room will add moisture to the air.

Encourage fluid intake, particularly in a child with a fever. Small amounts given frequently are often taken more readily than large amounts of fluids occasionally. The child should not be awakened from a sleep because the parent feels it is time for more fluids, nor should fluids be forced on a child who does not want them. Hot fluids assist movement of the nasal mucus. Milk should be avoided as it thickens the respiratory secretions in some. The diet should be light and should consist largely of fruits. Spices, fats, sweets, and condiments should be avoided.

A runny nose is nature's attempt to remove the virus from the body (201). Medications to dry up secretions inhibit the body's efforts. Blowing the nose is the only treatment needed. Some feel gentle sniffing is better, as blowing may force the virus into ears or sinuses (204). Until about four years of age a child is generally unable to either blow or sniff. The parent can make the child much more comfortable by clearing his nasal passages for him.

Several times a day, particularly before feedings and at bedtime, suction the infant's nose if he is not yet old enough to blow it. This can be a very effective method of making the child more comfortable. You will need a rubber ear bulb syringe, salt water nose drops, a medicine dropper, and tissues. To make the salt water solution add one-fourth teaspoon of ordinary table salt to one cup of boiled water (204). Measure the salt carefully, as excessively strong solutions can damage nasal tissues. Allow the solution to cool before using it. It may be refrigerated and saved for a day or two, but should be brought to room temperature before being used. These nosedrops are very effective in shrinking nasal membranes and liquefying mucous, making removal easier.

Place the child on his back with his head tipped backward. Some children resist this treatment with great effort and an older infant may need to be restrained by a second person. An older child may lie on his back and hang his head over the edge of the bed. Place one-half to one dropper full of saline solution in each nostril. It may seem like a lot of fluid, but you want to cover as much of the nasal membranes as possible. Allow the drops to remain in place a couple of minutes. Sometimes the saline drops induce the baby to sneeze, clearing his nose. Compress the ear syringe to remove air, insert it into the nostril, and suction the solution out of each nostril (205). If there is only a small amount of fluid, a cotton swab may be used to clear the passages. Be certain the child does not move while the swab is in his nose. Adding drops, waiting one to two minutes, then clearing the nose may be repeated several times in succession to clear the back of the nose. To effectively suction the back of the nasal passages insert the bulb tip, close off both nostrils with your fingers, and suction. Empty the secretions into a tissue, and repeat the suction. At the close of the procedure clean the bulb with warm soapy water, rinse in clear water and allow to dry.

Rubber bulb syringes should be boiled for at least ten minutes before being used by anyone else. Bacteria may collect in the bulb and spread to other users (206).

Commercial nose drops may cause excitation, hallucinations, agitation, and even convulsions in small children, even when used in recommended doses (207).

Decongestants have never been proven effective in preventing complications from colds, and should be avoided because of the possibility of adverse effects. While they may initially shrink the swollen blood vessels, and make breathing easier, the effect soon wears off, and the blood vessels often swell worse than before treatment. The treatment is repeated and rebound swelling again occurs. The cilia, tiny hair-like structures in the nose, serve to move fluid and mucous over the surface of the mucosa. These structures may be damaged by nasal decongestants, hindering their ability to work.

Red, irritated eyes can be rinsed frequently with wet cotton balls (201).

If the nose and upper lip become red from wiping, apply a thin layer of petroleum jelly to protect the skin.

Antibiotics are useless in the typical cold and do not relieve symptoms, shorten the course of the illness, or decrease complications (208). On the contrary, they often add to the problem.

Hand-to-hand contact is probably the most common method of cold virus spread. Washing the hands frequently during cold season and keeping the hands away from the eyes, nose, and mouth, will decrease a person's chances of catching cold (209). Wash hands carefully after caring for a child with a cold, to decrease the likelihood of spread.

Pouring cold water over the back of the neck has been shown helpful in relieving nasal congestion. Cold cloths applied to the neck do not seem as effective (210).

Steam inhalations often improve nasal congestion. Place a pan or tea kettle to boil on the stove. Form a cone from newspaper to contain the steam. This may be used for ten minutes every hour. Be careful that the child does not burn himself or set the newspaper on fire. Children too young to inhale steam through the cone may be taken into a closed bathroom with all the hot water faucets turned on until the hot water runs out. This will steam up the bathroom.

Garlic has natural antibiotic properties, but children may not like to take it. A lemon and garlic tea may overcome this problem. Cut a garlic clove into small pieces and mash with the bowl of a spoon. Place one teaspoon of peppermint or mint in a teapot, add the mashed garlic and the juice of one-quarter of a lemon. Add boiling water and steep for about five minutes. Strain and serve. Drink one cup three times a day.

Those who don't mind the taste of garlic may eat a clove two or three times a day.

Sore throat pain may be helped by hot salt water gargles. Add one teaspoon of salt to one-quarter cup of hot water. Use water as hot as possible without burning oneself. Gargle three to four times a day. Use a throat heating compress at night, and in children too young to gargle.

Fomentations to the chest with a hot foot bath (see treatment section) are helpful for lung congestion. A hot half bath is also useful in treating fever.

Nasal stuffiness is often relieved by exercise. A Japanese study demonstrated that ten minutes of exercise produces a striking increase in norepinephrine and relief of nasal stuffiness (211). A hot foot bath with a little mustard powder in the water is also effective in head congestion.

Some feel that coughs are best treated with increased fluid intake and air humidification, rather than with cough medications. The cough is nature's way of clearing phlegm from the lungs and airways, and in some people this will accumulate in the lungs, producing pneumonia. An onion chest poultice (see treatment section) may be very helpful for cough.

A panel at the ear, nose and throat disease symposium of the Children's Hospital of Pittsburgh noted that antihistamines should not be given in the treatment of common cold as they are ineffective. They have not been shown to relieve cold symptoms or shorten the course of the illness. Rest, fluid intake, and time are as effective in the treatment of a cold as is any type of antihistamine. Americans spend about $775 million dollars a year for over-the-counter non-prescription antihistamines (212).

Antihistamines are one of the most frequently used medications and many are available over-the-counter, without prescription. A study of adverse effects of antihistamines listed nearly 100 side-effects, including high blood pressure, insomnia, coma, delirium, dizziness, drowsiness, confusion, delusions, hallucinations, paralysis, ringing in the ears, lack of appetite, constipation, diarrhea, irritability, headache, muscle twitching, nervousness, rapid heart rate, tremor, fatigue, lassitude, weakness, hysteria, depression, nightmares, blurred vision, double vision, heart murmurs, vomiting, nausea, cerebral edema, electrocardiographic changes, low blood pressure, palpitations, nasal stuffiness, bronchial spasm, urinary frequency, painful urination, dermatitis, dryness of the mouth and respiratory passages, bone marrow depression, hemolytic anemia, early menses, breast enlargement, hypoglycemia, birth defects, syncope, urinary retention and skin rashes (213).

Fever may be controlled with wet sheet packs, neutral baths, and sponging. The body should be rubbed during all these treatments to prevent vasoconstriction, which will hinder heat loss (214).

Bed rest is not essential in a child who feels well enough to be up. However, activities should not be excessively vigorous.

COLD SORES (SEE FEVER BLISTERS)

COLIC

Colic, defined as episodes of crying more than three hours a day for more than three days a week, is estimated to occur in 10 to 40 percent of all infants during the first four months of life. Onset of symptoms may appear before the child is one week of age. Premature infants do not develop colic until they mature somewhat physiologically (184). Symptoms include irritability, distended abdomen, crying, or fussing. There may be belching and burping, and rumbling in the abdomen. The infant may become red, clinch his hands tightly and kick his feet. The feet are often cold. A bowel movement or gas passage often seems to bring relief. Symptoms typically occur during the evening hours (from 6 to 12:00 P.M.) when the mother is often tired, making it more difficult to deal with a child who cannot be consoled. Some children cry for 12 hours a day. The cause of colic is not clearly understood, but several factors, including allergy, parental smoking, and medications, are known to be associated. The parent should be sure that the child is not crying from earache or other health problem.

Mothers often feel that they are inadequate as caregivers because they cannot stop the child from crying. Unfortunately, this is probably one of the most common causes of child abuse, as the mother is driven to total frustration with a situation entirely beyond her control. Mothers should remember that colic typically subsides by the time a child is four months of age and that it is no reflection on her ability as a mother. If others can care for the child for an hour or so during the crying episode, allowing the mother to get out of the house it will often help her endure the situation until it passes. Parents can comfort themselves with the knowledge that these children are usually healthy children, who will outgrow colic (185).

Treatment

Breast-fed infants are less likely to have colic, although those who are sensitive to cow's milk may receive the allergenic substances through the breast milk if the mother drinks cow's milk. The first step in the treatment of infantile colic should be to take both mother and infant off cow's milk and all other dairy products. The likelihood of allergic reaction to these foods is probably decreased if the child is exclusively breast-fed for at least six months, although they may receive antigens through breast milk if the mother eats them. Cow's milk is the most common offender but chocolate, colas, tea, coffee, fatty, fried or spicy foods, cabbage, broccoli, ham, bacon, sausage, pork, shellfish, beans, banana, apple, orange, eggs, citrus, nuts, strawberry, corn, tomatoes, onion, legumes and sweet potato may produce symptoms. The risk of infant colic increases as the diversity of the material diet increases. Nursing mothers should use a simple diet of whole grains and fresh fruits and vegetables.

Vibration producing mechanisms are often helpful. Some take their child for a ride in the automobile, others rock the child in an old-fashioned cradle or rocking chair, and still others place the child in an infant seat placed on top of a running clothes washer or dryer. Children who are carried are less likely to cry (186). Parents may try keeping the child in a front carrier during the day, when mother's activities permit. The front carrier is preferred to the back carrier, as the child can look into his mother's eyes, and hear her heartbeat from the front position. Sometimes skin-to-skin contact is beneficial. Three to four hours a day of carrying may reduce crying 50 percent within one week. The child less than three or four months of age cannot be spoiled by excessive carrying. Those infants whose mothers respond promptly to their cries tend to fuss less when they are older. Speaking to the child in a soothing, quiet tone, gentle movements, avoiding vigorous jiggling or bouncing, and swaddling the infant in a warm blanket may all be tried. Snug swaddling, which restricts the child's movement decreases the incidence of crying.

The child should not be permitted to sleep for long periods during the day (184). If the child sleeps longer than three hours at a time he should be awakened, and bathed, fed, or played with. Discouraging sleep during the daytime encourages nighttime sleep and assists the child's body to adjust his circadian rhythm. Particular efforts should be made to keep the child awake during the early evening hours.

The baby should be fed while in an upright position and burped frequently during feedings (187). Never feed the child while he is lying down, and do not prop up his feeding bottle. If formula is used it should be given at body temperature. The child should not be overfed, as distending the bowel increases discomfort (188). Feeding should be done in a quiet, calm environment. Swaddle the child securely after feeding (189).

Some report that infants receive comfort from a pacifier. It is felt that some infants cry because of inadequate opportunity to suck.

Position changes are often helpful in relieving colic pain. The child may be more comfortable on his stomach or right side. A well covered heating pad or hot water bottle (be careful not to burn the infant) is often soothing (190).

Children who are suffering from gas pains may be relieved by the insertion of a petroleum-coated little finger or well-lubricated thermometer into the rectum, to assist in the passage of gas. A one to two ounce warm water enema may also be helpful. "Bicycling" the infants legs on his abdomen may also help release gas (191).

Infants whose mothers receive drugs during labor and delivery are more likely to suffer colic than are those who have unmedicated deliveries (192).

One or two ounces of warm water will bring relief to some. Warm fennel, anise, peppermint, chamomile, thyme, or catnip tea may bring comfort to the distressed baby. Make a cup of any tea and give one tablespoon at a time to the sufferer. Bay leaf tea may be prepared by boiling a cup of water and one-quarter of a bay leaf for 15 minutes. Remove the leaf and allow the tea to cool before giving it to the infant. More bay leaf may be added if the quarter leaf is not effective, but more than one leaf should not be used. Give one tablespoon at a time.

Charcoal is helpful in relieving gas. Powdered charcoal may be mixed in water and given to the child in a bottle. Charcoal can be constipating and may make the stools black, so mothers should not be alarmed should either occur.

A 15 to 20 minute warm bath, making sure the warm water covers the abdomen, may be soothing (189). An ordinary bath towel, wrung out of warm water, may be placed over the child's abdomen (194). Cover it with dry towels to retain the heat as long as possible. The towel may be refreshed as it cools.

Some infants respond to abdominal massage (190). Massage in a clockwise direction. Simultaneous rectal stimulation with the other hand is recommended by some.

Some overly-eager eaters benefit by being limited to about ten minutes on the breast (190). If they insist on more sucking, a bottle of warm water or pacifier may be readily accepted. Overeating may cause colic. Some mothers attempt to feed an infant every time he becomes fussy. Sometimes the child merely needs a little attention from the parent. A fussy child who has recently been fed should be checked for wet or dirty diapers, played with, given a drink of water, repositioned, or distracted in other ways before he is given more food. Breast fed babies probably do not need to be fed more often than every two hours, and bottle fed infants should not be fed more often than every two-and-a-half-hours, as long as they are growing and gaining weight normally.

The feet should be kept warm at all times (195). Dr. John Harvey Kellogg observed that pain in the bowels may result from cold feet (196). Booties should be kept on the feet of colicky infants 24 hours a day, removed only for bathing. Three-quarters of infants who were treated for colic in this manner were cured by this simple measure.

Some children are soothed by being taken out of doors, perhaps because they are distracted by the new sights. Mobiles over the crib are also recommended (197).

Children whose parents smoke in the house are more likely to have colic. Ninety-one percent of children in homes where the father smoked 20 or more cigarettes per day suffered colic. Colic rates increase as the number of cigarettes smoked per day increase (198).

Drugs are generally ineffective in the treatment of infantile colic, and some drugs which have been given in the past have caused seizures, coma, and respiratory collapse. One study showed placebo medications to be more effective than the medication.

One physician reported that giving a breast-fed baby three ounces of cold water before a feeding will assist in the prevention of colic (199).

Placing the child on a lambskin rug may be calming. Provide as much skin to rug contact as possible.

Infants given iron-fortified formula are more likely to develop colic, according to one study. Breast-feeding mothers should not take iron supplements. Vitamin supplements and fluoride should also be eliminated for a few days to see if any change occurs (188).

Overly concentrated formula may cause carbohydrate overload, causing gas and irritation (192).

Excessive environmental stimulation as from bright lights, loud noises, and young siblings may cause the child to become overly fatigued (193).

The breast-feeding mother should not consider colic a reason to stop breast-feeding. It is not an indication that the child should be switched to formula, as this will only increase the possibility of exposure to allergens.

CONSTIPATION

Constipation is the irregular passage of very hard or sticky stools. It occurs in five to ten percent of children. The child who does not have a bowel movement every day is not necessarily constipated if his stools are large and soft.

There are many causes for constipation: painful passage of stool because of diaper rash, diarrhea, or anal fissure; poor appetite, lack of adequate fluid intake, over-heating, fever, or other illness, inadequate dietary intake, fear of strange toilets, improper toilet training, lack of exercise, medications, physiological abnormalities, and mental handicap, among others. Bottle fed infants may have hard "rabbit-pellet" stools; constipation rarely occurs in breast-fed infants, although after two or three months of age some go two to five days between bowel movements. So long as the stool is soft, and passed without pain there is probably no reason for concern.

Symptoms include small hard stools, abdominal distention, pain in the abdomen, loss of control of liquid stools, vomiting, nausea and lack of appetite. Persistent or severe constipation may lead to a condition known as encopresis (see section).

A child who grunts and strains, becomes flushed, and pulls his legs up while passing stool may not be constipated (215). The involved muscles have not learned to work in a coordinated fashion, and may require some practice before they do (216). Also remember that lying down is not the most convenient position for passing a stool. You may assist the child by holding his thighs up against his abdomen (217). If children cry during the bowel movement a physical cause, such as anal fissure, should be looked for.

Sometimes the insertion of a well-lubricated fifth finger or rectal thermometer into the rectum may induce sufficient stimulation to cause a bowel movement in a young infant. If the finger is inserted, the rectal wall may be gently massaged much like rubbing the inside of the mouth.

Young children may be given pureed fruit to stimulate bowel function. If the child has recently been started on solid foods it may be well to leave them off for a while (218). Similarly, if a new food has just been added and the child suddenly develops constipation which was not present before, eliminate that food from the diet for the time being.

Cow's milk should be eliminated from the diet. It is a common cause of constipation in people of all ages (219). Cheese, ice cream and ice milk should also be eliminated.

If the child has diaper rash or anal fissure these should be treated. The child may attempt to retain his stool to avoid the pain associated with these conditions.

Adequate fluid intake should be encouraged, and fiber and fresh fruit should be emphasized in the diet. Whole grains should be used, and the child should never be given refined foods. Raw food should be included with every meal.

Medications, including aspirin, may cause constipation. Even one five grain aspirin tablet is sufficient to induce constipation in sensitive people (220). Many other medications are also guilty of inducing constipation--any medication should be suspect. Even over-the-counter medications, such as cough syrup, antihistamines, and decongestants, should be avoided.

Improper toilet training can lead to constipation. The child should be the one to initiate toilet training. The child suddenly has some control over the parent, and some defy the parent by refusing to pass their stool. A child may not be ready to begin toilet training until two years of age. If he is not ready maintain him in diapers until he matures sufficiently to be so. Girls usually are ready earlier than boys. Attempts at forcing the child to pass stool are usually in vain. Feed the child foods high in fiber to keep the stool soft and bulky.

The child should be given water on arising in the morning, and adequate fluids should be taken throughout the day. The child should drink enough to keep the urine almost colorless.

A teaspoon or two of dark corn syrup may be added to four ounces of formula if the child must be bottle fed (221). Water may be offered in the bottle three or four times a day. Prune juice, diluted grape juice, or apple juice are often effective in producing a bowel movement.

A child who has begun solid foods may be given strained prunes, apricots, peaches, plums, pears, beans or peas. Mashed cooked carrots or squash have been recommended for chronic constipation (222). Some children become constipated with foods such as apples, chocolate, cocoa, tea, meats, hot and spicy foods, white rice, and bananas. A high fat diet may lead to constipation (223).

The child should be encouraged to have a regular toilet time. Place him on the toilet for 10 minutes after every meal, but do not make a big scene if he produces nothing. If his feet dangle off the edge of the toilet, place a box so he has firm support to press against. This motion straightens the rectum. Success should be rewarded with lavish praise.

Abdominal massage may be helpful for some children. Place your hands one on top of the other, beginning under the rib cage, and massage down over the course of the colon, applying firm pressure.

Warm castor oil massaged over the abdomen is said to be as effective in the treatment of constipation as is taking it by mouth (224).

Out-of-doors physical activity will stimulate bowel activity in children (225). See treatment section if enemas are necessary.

CRADLE CAP

Cradle cap is a common scalp disorder in infants, but may be seen up to the age of five years. Symptoms may be thin, whitish, flaky scales or thick, yellow, greasy crusted material. The inflammatory process may spread from the scalp to the eyelids, outer ear canal, and sides of the nose. In some cases scales may occur on the forehead, behind the ears, or even in the diaper area. The child occasionally temporarily loses some hair. About half of all infants suffer from it at one time or another.

Allergy may play a role in cradle cap. Removal of milk and other common food allergens may be helpful (see Appendix 1 for Common Food Allergens). Onset of cradle cap in one group of 187 studies revealed that onset was often within three to four months after introducing a new food to the infant's diet. These children had clearance of their cradle cap after the new food was removed the diet. The foods most often felt to cause symptoms were milk, wheat, egg, oranges, beans and peas. Sometimes oatmeal was involved (226, 227).

Parents are often afraid to wash over the fontanels (soft spots) of the child's head. This may allow the start of cradle cap. Parents (and grandparents) should understand that the skin over the soft spot is like skin anywhere else on the body, and it will not break with reasonable pressure, nor will the brain be injured, as several very tough layers protect it.

Frequent shampooing will help clear cradle cap. Use a mild soap, and massage the scalp firmly enough to loosen the scales, which then can be shampooed out. If the flakes or crusts are stuck to the skin one may gently rub vegetable or mineral oil into them, allow it to set for a few minutes, then shampoo it out. A fine-toothed comb may be used to remove the crust (228).

Some prefer the use of an olive oil shampoo. Dissolve the shampoo in hot water to form a thick lather. Apply the lather to the head, then rinse thoroughly (229).

Strong shampoos or medications should be avoided, as the child may absorb some of the substance through his skin.

CROHN'S DISEASE

Crohn's disease and ulcerative colitis are often grouped together and called "inflammatory bowel disease." The two diseases have many similarities, but some differences. Crohn's disease is also called regional enteritis, as only regions, or sections, of the bowel are involved in the inflammatory process.

Onset of symptoms in Crohn's disease is often slow, coming and going over a period of many months. Symptoms vary in intensity over time. Diarrhea and abdominal pain are the most prominent symptoms. Pain is generally cramping in nature, is worse after meals, and is often relieved by a bowel movement. Diarrhea may consist of only one loose stool per day, or there may be ten or more episodes per day. The diarrhea is often most intense in the morning and then gradually decreases throughout the day. Children with Crohn's disease may grow slowly and frequently lose weight during exacerbations of symptoms. There may be fever, lack of appetite, rectal bleeding which may lead to anemia, and joint pains and/or arthritis (230). Canker sores are common in Crohn's disease patients, and they are at increased risk of developing kidney stones and gallstones. X-ray examination of the colon shows thickened walls, inflammation of the lining, and sometimes the presence of scarred bands or rings. The lining of the colon may take on a "cobblestone-like" appearance.

The peak incidence of Crohn's disease is felt to be between 10 and 30 years of age, but ten percent of children with inflammatory bowel disease have symptoms before they reach ten years of age (231). The disease appears about equally in both sexes. Statistics show that the incidence of celiac disease is decreasing, but Crohn's disease appears to be occurring more frequently. Several factors point to its being a sensitivity or allergic disorder. Crohn's disease patients in one study were more likely to have been hospitalized to treat a respiratory disease (more common in allergic persons) than were normal controls, and the use of antibiotics is more common in Crohn's disease patients.

Treatment

Breast feeding for long periods has been shown to decrease the incidence of Crohn's disease (232). Breast-fed children who do develop Crohn's disease have a later onset of symptoms than do children who were fed cow's milk. Many feel that milk allergy may play a significant role in Crohn's disease. A two to three month strict milk-free diet may produce considerable relief of symptoms. Soy milk may be helpful for those who are allergic to milk. Goat's milk is recommended by many, but the parent should be aware that goat's milk also contains lactose.

Several studies have shown that patients have prolonged periods of remission of symptoms when they use a diet free of foods to which they are sensitive. Wheat and dairy product allergies were most common in these patients, but other foods, including corn, citrus fruits, tea and coffee may cause symptoms (233). Gluten is felt to be the substance which causes the adverse reaction. Gluten is found in wheat, oats, rye, and barley. A trial diet eliminating the most common food allergens (see Appendix 1) may be most beneficial.

The diet should be low in fat, as these children absorb fats poorly. High fat diets may worsen diarrhea. Low fat diets decrease fluid loss, and improve zinc, magnesium, and calcium absorption. A German study suggests that chemically processed, polyunsaturated fat (e.g., shortening, margarine, homogenized peanut butter) may play a role in the development of Crohn's disease. Researchers observed that as the use of chemically processed polyunsaturated fats increases, rates of Crohn's disease increase (234). They point out that there are no areas of the world with a high incidence of Crohn's disease and low use of chemically processed polyunsaturated fats. Laboratory animals given chemically processed polyunsaturated fats developed changes consistent with the changes observed in the intestines of humans with Crohn's disease.

Professor E. Guthy, of the City Hospital in Weiden, West Germany, reports that margarine and chocolate creams may induce or worsen Crohn's disease (235). He reports that Crohn's disease is much more frequent in countries where margarine consumption is high, and low in countries where little margarine is used. After 1920, when hydrogenation of fats began in Germany, the incidence of Crohn's disease increased. When butter replaced margarine use under Third Reich food policies, and all fats were scarce, Crohn's disease incidence decreased. Dr. Guthy cautions that margarine is frequently used in food preparation in cafeterias and that Crohn's patients should avoid eating in these establishments. Patients also need to be cautious in the use of rectal suppositories, which are often made with hydrogenated fats. Dr. Charles Bates of British Columbia, has presented research showing that many people are low in one or more enzymes that break down the polyunsaturated fatty acids to beneficial prostaglandins. Instead, harmful inflammatory prostaglandins are formed, leading to inflammatory bowel disease and other disorders.

In the past the Crohn's disease sufferer has been given a low fibre diet, but the trend today is toward a high fiber, whole grain, low refined sugar diet. Thirty patients recently diagnosed as having Crohn's disease were compared with 30 healthy individuals, matched for age, sex, marital status, and social class. A comparison of the diets of the two groups revealed that those who had developed Crohn's disease had consumed a diet containing substantially more refined sugar, considerably less raw fruits and vegetables, and slightly less fiber than the healthy control person. The authors of the study concluded that a diet low in raw foods and high in refined sugar may contribute to the development of Crohn's disease (236). One researcher who placed Crohn's disease patients on a diet with a normal amount of fiber and low in refined sugar, observed that the patients on the trial diet had fewer hospitalizations for their disease (237). The hospitalizations in the diet group were shorter than those in the control group. Most Crohn's disease patients tolerate bananas and cooked fruits and vegetables well.

Spices and seasonings are irritating to the colon, and should be avoided (238).

Cold and hot fluids stimulate bowel activity, and should not be used.

Smoking appears to increase the risk of Crohn's disease. They should not be around smokers (239).

The indiscriminate use of antibiotics for such conditions as earache and sore throat may be at least partially responsible for the increased rates of Crohn's disease now being seen in the United States, according to Dr. John F. Sessions, professor of Medicine at the University of North Carolina School of Medicine (240). Those who have had ready access to medical care are probably at increased risk for Crohn's disease. It is possible that these antibiotics alter the normal flora in the colon, predisposing to disease. Nonsteroidal anti-inflammatory drugs have been shown capable of inducing changes in the small bowel which are very similar to those of Crohn's disease.

Regular out-of-doors exercise to tolerance should be encouraged, but the child should not be allowed to become overly fatigued. Competitive sports are stressful and should be avoided. The child should be encouraged to live as normally as possible within the limitations of his disease. Discipline should be consistent; the child should not be permitted to have his own way because of his illness.

Sunbathing, early morning and late afternoon, is often helpful, but sunburn should be avoided. This will strengthen the body's immune system, increasing its ability to resist disease.

Adequate water intake should be given priority. Large amounts of water will be needed to replace that lost in diarrhea.

Gas-forming foods should be avoided. These gases may further irritate the colon. Laxative foods and all condiments such as pepper, mustard, horseradish and vinegar should be avoided, as should all types of food additives.

Surgery is often recommended, but should not be entered into lightly. The quality of life in non-operated patients is better than those who have undergone surgery (241). About half of all patients who undergo surgery have rapid progression of their symptoms following surgery (242).

Heat may assist in relief of abdominal pain. Use a heating pad, fomentations (see treatment section for procedure) or hot water bottle.

Charcoal may be helpful in control of diarrhea. Two or three tablets or one or two capsules may be taken two to three times a day between meals. Charcoal powder is less expensive and sometimes more effective, but not so convenient. Use one teaspoon two to four times daily. If the charcoal seems to irritate the colon one to three tablespoons of powdered charcoal may be stirred into a glass of water, the charcoal allowed to settle out and, when it is almost clear, the water drunk. The almost invisible particles can be somewhat helpful.

Evening primrose oil and freshly ground flaxseed will provide gamma linolenic acid and the omega-3 fatty acids necessary to produce the anti-inflammatory prostaglandins lacking in these patients.

CROUP

Croup is a term applied to a group of inflammations of the respiratory tract. It was formerly associated with diphtheria. It is a common childhood illness, and is estimated to occur in about 15 percent of one-year-old children, 5 percent of one- to three-year-old children, and only about 1 percent of children over the age of eight. It often runs in families. It is more common in temperate zones of the world, and in areas with rapid changes in air humidity. Some believe that air pollution is also a contributing factor. Others believe cow's milk drinking to be an important factor. It is often associated with measles, occurring on the third or fourth day of the illness. Episodes typically occur at night.

Laryngotracheobronchitis

Laryngotracheobronchitis, or viral croup, often begins with an upper respiratory infection (cold) of one or two days duration (243). There may or may not be an associated fever. The child is put to bed without signs of acute distress, but during the night develops a harsh, high-pitched, barking cough, hoarseness of the voice and difficulty breathing. His face may become red, or bluish colored from lack of oxygen. Symptoms may subside with treatment, and the child appear well the next day, with recurrence of the symptoms for the following two or three nights. Parents should run the humidifier for several nights after an episode of croup. The humidifier should be cleaned with soap and water every day to discourage mold growth.

Peak incidence is during the cold months, with high rates in October and November. Children between the ages of 3 months and 3 years are most commonly affected, as their respiratory organs are smaller and more easily obstructed than those in older children or adults. Laryngotracheitis is slightly more common in boys than in girls. There may be repeated episodes, but the child eventually outgrows them. Children with allergies seem to develop croup more often than non-allergic children, and excitable, hyperactive children are more likely to suffer from croup.

Epiglottitis

This form of croup is more common in children from three to six years of age, and is less likely to recur than laryngotracheobronchitis. However, it is the more serious form of croup. Onset may begin with an upper respiratory infection, with rapid development of high fever and difficulty swallowing. The child may drool because he is unable to swallow his saliva. He may refuse to talk. He may have severe respiratory distress, and sit upright in a tripod position, with his chin pushed forward.

Treatment

Most cases of croup can be treated adequately in the home (243). Treatment should begin at the first sign of croup. Humidification of the air should be accomplished as quickly as possible. The child may be taken into the bathroom with the parent, the doors and windows closed, and the hot water faucets turned on, in an attempt to steam up the room (244). Do not use additional room heaters as the cooler room temperature will produce more steam from the hot water. While one parent is in the bathroom caring for the child, the other parent should set up the humidifier in his bedroom, where he will be transferred after the hot water runs out, and the bathroom is no longer steamy.

Cool or warm mist is the first step in treatment of croup (243). Cool air humidifiers are preferred over warm air, as it is less likely the child will be burned accidentally, but parents may use whichever they have access to. Medications should not be put in the humidifier, as these may further irritate the respiratory passages. A simple croup tent may be made by draping blankets or a sheet over the rails of the crib and directing the humidifier under the blanket. If there are no bed rails an umbrella may be placed at the head of the bed and a sheet draped over this. Some children are frightened at being closed in, and the parent may need to encourage the child to pretend that he has a private play tent. Physical contact is important to the frightened child, and the parent should remain nearby at all times.

Several pots of water may be put on the stove to boil with the escaping steam captured in a newspaper cone which is directed toward the child's face (245).

If there is no humidifier in the room, towels and sheets may be dipped into water, wrung out to prevent dripping, and hung about the room to give off their moisture as they dry out.

Instant humidification may be provided by placing a warm, wet washcloth loosely over the child's mouth and nose, and having him breathe through it (256). This may frighten some children, who already are anxious about their ability to breathe.

If humidification of the air does not relieve the symptoms within ten to thirty minutes, you may try taking the child outdoors into the cool night air. Many a parent has rushed his child to the hospital emergency room in the middle of the night, only to have his symptoms subside with exposure to the cool air in transit (243). Taking the child for a ride in the car with the windows down may produce relief of symptoms (247).

Fluid intake should be encouraged to liquify secretions, and make them easier to move. Cold fluids may induce spasm, and should be avoided (247). Small amounts should be offered frequently. Milk and citrus juice should be avoided. Do not be concerned if the child does not want solid food.

The inability to breathe easily is frightening to the child and parent. Caretakers should be calm, and attempt to soothe the child. Holding the child in the arms, reading a story, or talking quietly will assist the child to relax. Crying worsens the problem, and should be avoided (248). Rocking or rhythmic movements are sometimes soothing to these distressed children.

A hot half bath (see treatment section) with a cold water pour afterward may be given (249).

Fomentations (see treatment section) may be applied to the upper back and neck for five to ten minutes, alternating with a cold neck compress for ten to twenty minutes may be useful (249). Cold mitten friction may be carried out every three hours (see treatment section) (249). Sometimes simply sprinkling cold water on the child's face and chest brings prompt relief (250). A piece of ice may be rubbed over the neck and upper chest. Keep body parts not being treated covered to prevent chilling.

A cold compress may be applied to the throat, and changed every ten minutes. Place two washcloths in a basin of ice water, wring one washcloth out and place it over the front of the neck. As it begins to warm, wring out the second washcloth, remove the first, and replace with the second. Change washcloths every few minutes, as they begin to warm up (251).

Older children may benefit from a cold shower (252).

An onion chest poultice may be helpful. See treatment section for procedure.

An alternating hot and cold bath is considered one of the more effective treatments (250). The child should be placed in a tub of water at 100 to 102 degrees F. The heat may produce relaxation of the spasm of the larynx within a few seconds. If relief does not occur, the child should be lifted from the warm water and a basin of cold water poured over his body, then the child returned to the tub of hot water. This procedure may be repeated several times.

Alternating hot and cold compresses may be used if a tub is not available (250). A cloth should be wrung from hot water and placed over the throat and upper chest, fitting it snugly to the jaws and up over the ears. After fifteen or twenty seconds remove the hot compress and apply a similar compress from a cloth dipped in cold water. Reapply the hot compress after ten to fifteen seconds, repeating the hot and cold cycle several times.

Dr. John Harvey Kellogg reported relief of symptoms by holding the child upside down and slapping him on the back (250).

Chilling should be carefully avoided during any treatment. The bedroom should be kept warm, but not overheated.

The child should be encouraged to be out-of-doors during the day if the weather is such that chilling can be prevented. Sudden temperature changes should be avoided. Dress warmly at all times, but avoid overheating. Bed clothing should be changed if it becomes wet from the high humidity levels (253).

Water makes an excellent cough syrup. Give the child a small glass of water with every coughing episode.

A heating compress may be applied to the chest at bedtime. Squeeze a thin piece of cotton fabric from cold water, place it against the chest, cover well on all sides with a piece of plastic, and hold in place with long strips of material such as bed sheeting, or a tight-fitting sweater.

Sponging the child with tepid water for about 15 minutes may help reduce fever if is present. If the child develops chills, irregular heart beat, shallow respirations or blueness of the skin, the sponging should be discontinued immediately, and the child warmed (254).

Antibiotics and steroids are of no value in the treatment of most cases of croup, and induce the risk of adverse effects (255).

Some feel that vomiting is valuable in breaking up the spasm, but others caution that vomiting should not be induced, as it may lead to aspiration of the vomitus into the lungs.

A child who suffers croup should not be near anyone who smokes (256).

Children should be observed closely; if severe shortness of breath, extreme paleness, or blueness of the skin develop, he should be evaluated by his health care provider.

CRYPTORCHISM

Cryptorchism is failure of a testis to descend into the scrotal sac. It is one of the most common congenital abnormalities in males. It is common in premature infants, and occurs more frequently in males delivered in the breech position. Infants born before eight month's gestation almost invariably have non-descended testes. It is most often unilateral in full-term infants, and most often involves the right testis. It is bilateral in only about 10 percent of cases (257). Its cause is not clearly understood. Its frequency is very difficult to ascertain, as recent studies suggest that many boys who in the past have been diagnosed to have this problem actually have retractile testes.

Cryptorchism

Retractile Testes

Retractile testes are testes which temporarily ascend, but which normally lie in correct anatomical position. The cremasteric reflex, induced by cold or fright, pulls the testis back up into the inguinal canal (258). This is a common finding in boys one to twelve years of age, and does not require treatment. This phenomenon has probably frequently been diagnosed as cryptorchism, and led to many unnecessary surgical procedures. The cremasteric reflex is inactive at birth, so examination at birth, or within six months afterward, revealing proper testis descent, should assure the parent that inability to locate the testis on later examination is most likely a temporary condition. The cremasteric reflex is fully active at about six months of age.

Examination

Proper examination is essential in the evaluation of cryptorchism. The room and examiner's hands should be warm. The child should be relaxed. If the child sits cross-legged the cremasteric reflex may relax, permitting the examiner to manipulate the testis into the scrotum. Placing the child in a tub of warm water may aid in relaxation and examination, as may the application of warm compresses over the scrotum. Children old enough to cooperate may be seated in a chair and their legs drawn up to their chest for the examination. Young infants may be examined with the child lying quietly. Examination should begin in the inguinal canal area, and the hand gently moved down to the scrotum.

Some examiners like to apply soap to their fingers, which facilitates examination. Others apply talcum powder to the child.

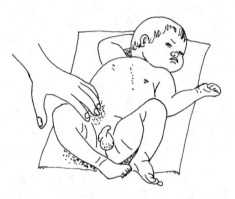

Treatment

About 75 percent of testes which have not descended at birth do descend by the time the child is one year old (259). Less than one percent of males one to three years of age have undescended testes. Surgery should be delayed to permit natural

Technique of Examination for Cryptorchism

descent. Many suggest that the child be at least eight to ten years of age before surgery is carried out.

DIAPER RASH

Diaper rash is a common problem in infants. At least 50 percent of infants are bothered with it at least once. The skin becomes red and shiny, rough bumps may appear, and the skin may appear thickened. It may be due to a variety of causes but regardless of the cause, the basic principles of treatment remain the same. Diaper rash is most common in the nine to twelve month old.

Treatment

The diaper area should be kept dry and warm. Diapers should be changed frequently, and the child should be allowed to go without a diaper to permit drying of the area when possible. Infants may be placed on several layers of diapers to absorb any urine passed while diaperless. Any ointments should be removed to allow the skin to dry. Special attention should be given to skin folds.

All urine and stool should be carefully removed at each diaper change. Plain water is generally adequate to remove urine, but a mild soap may be required for complete removal of stool. Harsh soaps should be avoided. Mineral oil may be used to remove stool.

Cornstarch or ordinary flour may be used as a powder on the skin to assist in absorbing skin moisture (262). This should be carefully removed and freshly applied with each diaper change. In the past some have said that cornstarch encouraged the growth of Candida albicans and should not be used, but recent studies suggest this is not the case (260). Cornstarch is as effective as any commercially prepared product and is much less expensive. A paste may be made from cornstarch and water. Alcohol may upset the natural skin flora and should not be used on a regular basis (261).

Children who have thrush (see section) may develop simultaneous diaper rash. Children who have been given antibiotics are more susceptible to this type of infection. Camomile tea is said to be very helpful in Candidal diaper rash (337). Make the tea, allow it to cool, and use it to gently wash the area. Pat dry. One-quarter cup of vinegar should be added to a sinkful of water for baby's bath to make the skin more acid, an unfavorable condition candida growth. Plastic or rubber pants retain moisture in the diaper area providing an environment favorable to the development of inflammation. A thin coating of plain petrolatum jelly keeps moisture away from the skin.

A hair dryer set on low may be used to hasten drying of a wet bottom (262). A lamp, placed a safe distance from the baby and from bed clothing, will have a drying effect (263). Do not place a baby boy face up under a lamp, as his urine may hit the hot light bulb and cause it to explode. The child may be exposed for about 20 minutes at a time, two or three times a day. All ointments should be removed from the skin before light treatments, as they may make the skin more sensitive to the light.

Commercially prepared diaper ointments may cause allergic reactions. A 12-month-old boy, who was allergic to milk, developed severe allergic reaction after a casein-containing ointment was applied to treat his diaper rash (264). Some diaper rash medications have been shown capable of producing nerve damage. One eight-month-old infant developed precocious puberty, with early development of breasts and pubic hair, while being treated with a veterinary salve for his diaper rash (265).

A diaper rash ointment may be made by placing one-fourth cup of vitamin E oil in a container and adding approximately one-half cup of cornstarch, mixing thoroughly (266). This may be stored for about a week in a tightly closed jar. Apply with each diaper change. Make a fresh batch after a week.

Food allergy may contribute to diaper rash. Milk allergy may be a common cause, as diaper rash is less common in breast-fed than formula-fed infants. Allergy to cow's milk, citrus fruits, and wheat have all been associated with diaper rash. Breast-fed infants may react to an allergen eaten by their mother. Diaper rash often appears with the introduction of solid foods.

Two or three diapers are recommended for nighttime use. The illustration

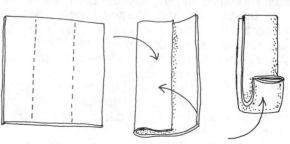

Triple Fold Technique for Diaper Rash

shows how to fold a diaper for maximum urine absorption. Place the thickest portion in the front for a boy, and in the back for a girl.

Diarrhea increases the risk of diaper rash (267). A child with diarrhea should be treated to prevent diaper rash. Petrolatum may be applied over the area with every diaper change. The diapers should be changed frequently. Air exposure should be encouraged to keep the area dry between diarrheal episodes.

Liquid lecithin has been reported useful in the treatment of diaper rash. Tepid compresses made by adding 1 level teaspoon of table salt to one pint of water are helpful. They may be applied for ten minutes at a time, four times a day (268).

Fluid intake should be encouraged in infants with diaper rash. Concentrated urine has a higher acidity level, and is more irritating to the skin (246). Some suggest that the child be given cranberry juice (269).

Diapers should be washed in very hot water, using a mild detergent. Some like to boil the diapers for 20 minutes before laundering them. Dirty diapers should be soaked in a solution using one-half to one cup of borax or Borateen to a gallon of water. This solution should be rinsed out by running the diapers through a rinse cycle, then the diapers washed in a mild soap. The diapers should be rinsed twice, using bleach or one-quarter to one cup of vinegar in the last rinse water. Diapers should be sun dried if at all possible. If they must be machine dried, fabric softeners should be avoided, as they may cause allergic reactions (270).

Newborns are said to have less diaper rash if they are kept on their stomach, rather than on their back (271).

An overheated room or bed may contribute to diaper rash.

The parent should wash his hands thoroughly before and after diaper changes (279).

DIARRHEA

Diarrhea is a symptom, rather than a disease. It is defined as an abnormally frequent discharge of fecal material and fluid. Parents should be aware that what may be normal for one child may be abnormal for another. One infant may have four to six stools per day, while another may have only one or two. Breast-fed infants have more frequent stools.

Diarrhea is a common problem in young children. Fortunately, diarrhea in children is often self-limited and brief. In many cases it is the body's method of ridding the body of viruses, toxins, or other cause of inflammation of the bowel. The parent should think twice before medications are administered to treat diarrhea, as these medications may handicap the body in performing a very important protective function.

Acute diarrhea in a child less than one year of age may quickly lead to dehydration, the excessive loss of body fluids.

Acute diarrhea in infants is most commonly caused by improper feeding. Overfeeding is felt to be a common cause (272). An irritable or fussy child should not be given food or fluid to soothe him. Overfeeding may also lead to vomiting.

Chronic diarrhea may be due to cow's milk intolerance. An artificial diet, high in polyunsaturated fats, will produce looser stools than a formula high in saturated fats. Changing formulas may induce diarrhea-like symptoms. A high sugar content in the diet may produce watery, soft stools. Some mothers add honey to milk which may induce looser stools.

Infections and medications may induce diarrhea. Antibiotics 273) and various prescription and over-the-counter medications are offenders. The sugars added to medications to make them more palatable to children may produce diarrhea. Infections such as urinary tract infection, may cause diarrhea. These infections should be treated promptly.

Childhood diarrhea may be due to gastrointestinal infections or disease such as Crohn's disease or ulcerative colitis. Diarrheas due to these diseases often contain blood in the stool.

Food poisoning is typically associated with diarrhea of sudden onset and a number of people (everyone who ate the food) may suffer onset of symptoms almost simultaneously. There may be associated abdominal pain, nausea and vomiting.

Some children have diarrhea in association with teething, although teething in itself is not felt to be the cause. The child often produces excessive amounts of saliva in association with teething, and this swallowed saliva dilutes the stool, making it more watery.

Food allergy may cause chronic diarrhea (274). Cow's milk, egg, and chicken are common factors in food allergy induced diarrhea.

Toddler's diarrhea, also called chronic nonspecific diarrhea, is diarrhea of an undetermined cause. The child suffers intermittent episodes, with clearing of symptoms, and normal growth between episodes. Symptoms typically appear between six months and 20 months of age, and disappear by the time the child is 40 months of age in about 90% of children. These children often have a large, formed stool the first stool of the day, but stools become looser and smaller as the day goes on. Vegetable fiber and mucus may be observed in the stool.

Some children develop diarrhea in reaction to unusual anxiety or excitement. This diarrhea subsides spontaneously.

Medicines or antibiotics are not necessary in many cases of diarrhea. The child should be given clear fluids for 24 to 48 hours. Milk should not be given.

Children cared for in day-care centers are at greatly increased risk of developing a viral diarrhea (275). Inadequate hand washing between diaper changes readily spreads the infection.

Treatment

Eliminating the cause and preventing dehydration are the primary goals in therapy of diarrhea. Allowing the bowel to rest by fasting or light meals is often beneficial. The child should be given only clear fluids for 12 to 24 hours. Fluids should not be cold, as cold stimulates bowel function (276). If ice chips are given they should be melted in the mouth and warmed before being swallowed. Cow's milk in any form should be carefully avoided. Many children have diarrhea as an allergic reaction to milk; those who suffer diarrhea from other causes often react unfavorably to milk even though it is not the initial cause of the diarrhea. Fluids should be administered in small amounts (a teaspoonful at a time), and given frequently. If the child vomits the fluid, he may be given another teaspoonful immediately, as there is often a refractory period following a vomiting episode, during which the fluid will be retained. If the teaspoonful of fluid is well tolerated, the amount may be gradually increased, depending on the age of the child. The older the child the more fluid he is likely to be able to tolerate. Under one year of age the child may be given one-half ounce of water every 20 minutes; over one year of age one ounce of water may be given every 30 minutes (277).

The parent may make an oral rehydration fluid which will assist in restoring electrolytes and minerals to the body. One level teaspoon of ordinary table salt, and four heaping teaspoons of sugar may be dissolved in one quart of boiled water (278). The formula should be carefully measured, as excess salt may increase dehydration, and lead to seizures and possible brain damage (283).

Others suggest a solution of four tablespoons of sugar, one-half teaspoon of baking soda, one-quarter teaspoon of potassium chloride (salt substitute) and one-half teaspoon of table salt added to a quart of warm water (280).

Home-made rice water is another effective rehydration solution (281). Cook one part rice to 30 parts water until about a third of the water evaporates. Add one level teaspoon of salt to the solution, after it has been strained.

Boiled barley water is also reported helpful, as is red raspberry leaf tea and camomile tea. Blueberries may be given to older children. Red raspberry leaf tea is made by placing one ounce of dried red raspberry leaves in a pan of water and boiling for five minutes (283). The tea is then removed from the heat and allowed to steep for five minutes. Strain and cool the tea before administering. The child may be given one-half cup of tea at a time.

Carbonated beverages often contain sugar which may worsen diarrhea (283). Cola drinks, although often recommended in the treatment of diarrhea, contain very low amounts of electrolytes, and have high osmolality, which may worsen diarrhea (284).

Frequent feedings stimulate gastrocolic reflexes which encourage diarrhea. Feedings should be several hours apart. Children who want solid foods should be given mashed ripe banana, cooked carrots, beets, blended raw apple, carob pudding, or rice cereal. Both green and over-ripe (black) bananas contain substances which may cause diarrhea. To prepare cooked carrots, chop and cook one pound of washed and peeled carrots in a pressure cooker for an hour, mash the carrots, then blend them. Carrots contain phosphorus and potassium, both of which may be lost during diarrhea (285). A child who does not want solid food should not be forced to eat, but fluids should be encouraged. Give them frequently and in small amounts.

The parent should be alert to signs of acute dehydration. Weight loss, changes in behavior, reduced urine output, fever, sunken

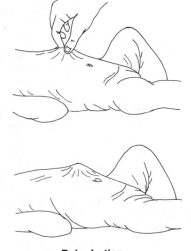

Dehydration

eyeballs, lack of tears when the child cries, dry skin, tongue and lips, poor sucking, rapid breathing, fast heart beat, gray skin color, and depressed soft spot on the top of the child's head are all indications of dehydration. If the parent pinches up the abdominal skin, and the skin remains up rather than returning to its normal position, this suggests dehydration.

The child should be kept cool, as excessive body heat encourages even more fluid loss through perspiration. However, the child should be protected from chilling.

Breast-fed infants are less likely to develop diarrhea than are children given an artificial formula. The breast-milk contains antibodies to many of the viruses which cause diarrhea. Breast-feeding should be continued if the child develops diarrhea. It is known that foods the mother consumes may cause diarrhea in breast-fed children. The mother should examine her diet for the use of cow's milk, beans, gas-forming foods, and eggs. If the mother eliminates these from her diet, the child's diarrhea may clear (286). If breast milk is available it may be used in the treatment of diarrhea in children who are not being breast-fed (274).

Charcoal is the treatment of choice in an attempt to get rid of the cause of diarrhea (287). One tablespoon of charcoal powder may be mixed in a little water and given to the child using a straw in the glass or baby bottle for infants. Older children may be given six to eight charcoal tablets or three or four capsules. The dose should be repeated every four hours or with every loose stool. Carob powder, available at the health food store, may be mixed in water to form a paste, or made into pudding, and given to the child with diarrhea.

Hot and cold fomentations may be applied over the abdomen, if the child is having associated cramping discomfort. Cold abdominal compresses, changed every 15 minutes, are said to be helpful to some (288).

Children who are receiving phototherapy for neonatal jaundice sometimes develop diarrhea. It is felt that this may be due to lactase deficiency.

Excessive fluid intake may overwhelm the bowel, and cause diarrhea. Large amounts of fruit juices are common causes of diarrhea. Apple juice has high osmolality, and large amounts of sorbitol which is poorly absorbed by the body, and may cause diarrhea if given in large amounts (289).

Sorbitol and mannitol, commonly found in sugar-free foods, may cause diarrhea. Sugar-free chewing gum may cause childhood diarrhea (290).

Cold foods of any type should be avoided, as cold food in the stomach is capable of stimulating colonic motility (291).

Up to 83 percent of blacks are allergic to milk (291). There are no laboratory tests which are accurate in the diagnosis of milk allergy. The best test is to carefully avoid the use of milk and all milk products for several days to see if the diarrhea subsides. If milk is causing the diarrhea improvement may be observed within 72 hours of starting the milk free diet. The diet must be strict in order for the test to be accurate. Other foods known to induce allergic diarrhea include eggs, chicken, fish, wheat, and soy products (339). Some children are allergic to rice and should not be given the rice rehydration solution described above.

The bottle-fed infant may develop diarrhea due to overfeeding (273). Bottle-fed children are often urged to finish their bottle and this causes overfeeding, which taxes the digestive system.

Children with diarrhea must be carefully watched to prevent irritation of the anus and diaper area. Petrolatum may be applied over the area to protect the skin from irritating fecal material or moisture. Soiled or wet diapers should be changed immediately. Care should be taken to wash the hands after each diaper change to avoid spread of the disease.

EARACHE (OTITIS MEDIA)

Otitis media is a common childhood infection. It is exceeded only by well-baby visits as the most common reason for trips to the doctor's office during childhood. One of three children seen by a physician is diagnosed as having an ear infection (292). It is estimated that thirty million physician visits are made each year for otitis media. The number of visits is said to have increased approximately 52 percent between 1981 and 1984. About 900,000 children in the United States may have an ear-related condition on any given day. One-half of all children have had at least one ear infection by the time they reach 12 months of age; one-third of all children have had three or more ear infections by three years of age. By their fourth birthday about 70 percent of children have had at least one attack. An estimated 90 percent of children in the United States have at least one ear infection by the time they are six years of age. Annual medical costs for otitis media alone are estimated to be two billion dollars in the United States alone.

The eustachian tube is a small canal which runs from the middle ear to the nasopharynx, the space immediately behind the nose. This tube opens frequently throughout the day with such activities as swallowing and yawning. The child's eustachian tube is shorter and more horizontal than the adult's and this predisposes the child to ear infections. As the child matures, and develops an "adult" eustachian tube, ear infections become much less frequent.

Short, hairlike cells, called cilia, which line the middle ear, move fluid and mucus from the ear into the eustachian tube, where it is transported into the nasopharynx to be removed from the body. These cilia require oxygen to function. Their oxygen supply comes from the periodic opening of the eustachian tube. If the eustachian tube fails to open and close normally or becomes entirely blocked, these cilia are deprived of oxygen and are unable to function. The fluid, which they are unable to remove, collects in the middle ear and may cause the ear drum to bulge (292).

A number of factors may produce blocking of the eustachian tube. Mucus or inflammation produced in association with a cold, or other respiratory infection, allergies, food sensitivities, or several common childhood diseases such as measles, chickenpox, and strep throat may block this small tube.

Middle ear infection may be caused by viruses or bacteria. Our experience with dairy products indicates that most or all dietary products increase the incidence of ear aches. When we have removed the milk products from the diet of a population of children in an institution in Alabama, we have seen a complete disappearance of ear aches among the staff and patients. We believe the viruses and bacteria follow the inflammation brought on by the sensitivity to milk products. When the inflammation occurs, the middle ear lining begins producing extra mucus which stagnates, and the bacteria move in and pus collects behind the eardrum. Otitis media frequently follows a cold when bacteria get into the nose and move up the closed eustachian tube into the middle ear (292).

Earache is a common occurrence in childhood. Otitis media occurs most often in 6 to 24 month old infants, and then peaks at four to eight years of age, when the child enters day care, kindergarden, or school, then gradually declines. Boys seem more likely to suffer it than girls. Black children seem to have otitis media less frequently than do white children, probably because fewer black children drink milk as they are more likely to be sensitive to it, due to lactase deficiency. This condition protects them against middle ear infection. There is often a family history of ear infections. Permanent hearing loss probably never occurs, even in children with recurrent attacks. Once eardrums become inflamed they may require six weeks to return to normal, and hearing may be decreased during that time.

Glue ear has been called catarrhal otitis media in the past and typically was left alone to resolve spontaneously. Giving generous amounts of water and leaving off all concentrated foods will help this to clear. Propping the head of the bed up about four inches will turn the eustachian tube downward, encouraging drainage. Gargles with hot saline assist in opening the eustachian tube.

Acute earache, difficulty hearing, and fever are typical symptoms but are not always present. The pain is due to the fluid pressing on the eardrum. Removal of this fluid brings relief of pain.

Acute otitis media, also called suppurative or purulent otitis media, may be associated with fever of 101 to 102 degrees F., ear pain, difficulty hearing, and nasal discharge. Young children, who are unable to verbally express the pain, may continually tug at the ear, and be irritable or restless. Examination of the ear will reveal a bulging red, yellow or blue ear drum. (Ear drums in crying infants may be red without infection.) The drum may look thick and dull; the normal drum appears thin, and deflects light shown on it. See the chapter on the physical examination for instructions on how to examine a child's ears.

Fluid may remain in the middle ear for several months following an infection. This is called "effusion" by physicians. It has been estimated that as many as 70 percent of children may have middle ear fluid following a bout of otitis media, especially if they have been given antibiotics and antihistamines which dry the ear secretions. It may persist for a month in about 40 percent of children; for two months in about 20 percent of children, and four months or longer in about 5 percent of children. It causes the child no pain and many feel that watchful waiting is the treatment of choice.

Children with ear infections generally have one of three types of fluid which accumulates in the ears. Doctors call a thin, watery fluid "serous;" yellow fluid which looks like pus is called "purulent;" and a thick, mucus-like, sticky fluid is called "mucoid."

Treatment

Repeated studies have demonstrated that 70 to 80 percent of all cases of earache which are untreated will resolve within three days (292). Simply applying a warm towel to the ear to relieve the discomfort may be adequate treatment for most cases.

Heat may be applied in a number of ways. A heating pad, hot water bottle wrapped in a towel, or a towel wrung from hot water may be applied to the painful ear. Care must be taken to avoid burning the child. A common desk lamp held close to the ear is often soothing but this should not be done without supervision with small children as they may burn themselves. A salt compress may be made by heating one-half cup of table salt in a frying pan, then placing it in a clean cloth, tying loosely, and applying to the ear. The salt may be reheated as it cools (293).

Some children receive greater relief from cold applications. Cold applications may be very helpful in reducing swelling. If there is no drainage and the ear drum is not ruptured, a few drops of ice water may be dropped into the ear for pain relief.

Steam inhalations under an improvised sheet tent or in the form of a hot bath or shower, are helpful to some.

Hot foot baths will draw blood from the head, decreasing congestion. Place the child's feet in a foot tub of water as hot as he can tolerate without burning himself. Keep it as hot as the child can tolerate for 20 to 30 minutes by adding more hot water as the water cools. The head should be kept cold by a cloth wrung from ice water. At the conclusion of the foot bath, remove the feet from the hot water and pour the ice water used for the head compress over the feet. Dry the feet quickly, and cover them to prevent any chilling. The child should be placed in bed until perspiration ceases.

A throat gargle may be helpful in children old enough to carry out the procedure. Use plain hot water and continue gargling for ten minutes. A greater astringent action can be obtained from goldenseal tea used as the gargle solution. A charcoal slurry (one tablespoon of charcoal in a glass of water) will often open up the eustachian tube after a ten minute gargle.

Hot baths should be given daily, using as hot a temperature as the child can tolerate. The bath should be continued for three minutes for a child three years of age or under, with one additional minute for each year of age over three. Finish off the bath with a cold water pour over the entire body and a brisk rub with a dry towel. The child should be placed in bed immediately after the bath, and will usually sleep following this treatment.

A charcoal poultice molded over the ear and jaw may be helpful, especially when combined with a steady source of heat. See treatment section for directions.

If the child has a cold, alternating hot and cold compresses (three minutes for the hot, 30 seconds for the cold) may be applied over the face and sinuses to decongest the head.

The incidence of children suffering chronic middle ear disease has increased since the advent of antibiotics. Antibiotics have been shown to be capable of producing conditions favorable for fluid retention in the ear, which prevents healing (292). The use of antibiotics should be carefully considered, as they are certainly not without risk. Antibiotics do not go just to the ear when they are given for earache. They go throughout the body and may produce numerous unwanted effects, such as diarrhea. Bacteria become resistant to antibiotics over a period of time and may rapidly and allow multiply. Some antibiotics also reduce the number of white blood cells, which are the body's method of fighting disease. Do not insist that your physician prescribe antibiotics for your child just so you can feel that something is being done. Several antibiotic ear drops have been shown to produce marked inflammation of the ear drum (294, 295).

Antihistamines and decongestants are routinely given in cases of earache but neither of these medications has been proven effective (296, 297). However, they may damage the tiny hairs which line the nasal passages.

Nose drops are often prescribed but these may produce a worsening of symptoms. Normal saline nose drops, made by adding one-half teaspoon of salt to one cup of water, may be used if the child has nasal stuffiness. Nose drops must be instilled in such a way that they reach the area where the eustachian tube and throat meet to be most effective. A young infant may be placed on his back on your lap with his head hanging off the edge of your lap. An assistant may be required to restrain uncooperative children. Older children may lie on their back on the bed with their head hanging over the edge. Insert two drops of the saline solution into each side, then roll the child's head gently from side-to-side. If the child coughs, or reports that he tastes the nose drops, you will know you have gotten them to the right spot.

Breast feeding protects children from otitis media; the longer the child is breast fed the fewer episodes of earache he is likely to have (292).

A child may develop otitis media from inhaled allergens such as pollens, molds, musty odor, tobacco smoke, and house dust. Exposure to these substances should be minimized in sensitive children. Pets should not be permitted in the home, and stuffed toys, carpets, and fluffy bedspreads, sheets and pillows should be removed from the child's bedroom. The heater filter should be cleaned frequently (292). See the section on asthma for instructions on allergen control in the home.

Food allergens are also common factors in otitis media (298, 299). Milk and dairy products are the most commonly involved foods. If the child has chronic runny nose, sneezing, wheezing, puffy eyes, itching nose, headache, irritability, moodiness, or listlessness, one should suspect allergies.

Earache often follows a cold. The parent may decrease the chance of earache by assisting the child to keep the eustachian tube open. Young children may require frequent suctioning of the nasal passages (see cold section for discussion of procedure), and all children may benefit from the use of vaporizer. However, care must be taken to prevent a humid, moist situation which encourages mold growth (292). If the child develops chest congestion he may be taken into the bathroom and the hot water turned on to steam up the bathroom. After about fifteen minutes of steam inhalation the child may be placed face down and the parent may gently pat his back with cupped hands to help loosen the mucus. Children with colds should not blow their noses forcefully as this may force secretions into the middle ear. They should be taught to blow one side at a time, holding the tissue loosely over the nose (300).

Sugar decreases the body's ability to fight infection and should be eliminated.

A myringotomy is a small incision made in the eardrum which allows the fluid behind the eardrum to escape. While myringotomy may relieve pain drainage, which reduces pressure on the ear drum, it does not cure the infection (292).

Tubes are often placed in the ears to assist in drainage. Side effects from tubes include sometimes a permanent hole in the eardrum, plugged tubes which do not function and are therefore of no help, and tubes that either fall out shortly after surgery or become permanently stuck in place and must be surgically removed (292). Some feel that bacteria may gain entrance to the middle ear through these tubes. Some children seem to have allergic reactions to the tubes and have chronic drainage requiring removal of the tubes. A permanent scar may occur on the eardrum (301). Some people feel that tube insertion benefits the physician's bank account more than the child. Ear tube insertion was not a common practice twenty years ago, but there are no adults today who have hearing problems from otitis media. This seems to indicate to us that the tubes do not assist the child appreciably, if at all. Others point out that children from higher socioeconomic levels are more likely to have tubes inserted than are children from poorer classes.

A 15-year study of children aged four to ten years, who underwent insertion of a tube in one ear provides another interesting insight to ear tubes. Examination 15 years later revealed tympanic membrane abnormalities in 70 percent of the tube ears, while over half of the ears not operated on were normal. There were no significant differences in hearing in the two groups. Another study revealed that 12 months after the insertion of tubes there was no difference in symptoms in those who had been treated with tubes and those who had not.

Adenotonsillectomy has also not been proven effective in reducing the incidence of otitis media (302).

Young children may be soothed by a wintergreen and rosemary oil rub (340). Combine one-quarter teaspoon of wintergreen oil, one-quarter teaspoon of rosemary oil, and two-and-a-half teaspoons of pure olive oil in a small container. Stir to mix thoroughly. Warm slightly before applying around the ear, rubbing gently until all of the oil is absorbed. This may be repeated twice daily.

Ear drops may be made using olive oil and garlic (303). Peel four garlic cloves and mash. Add the garlic to one-fourth cup of pure olive oil and allow to stand for one to three days. Carefully strain out all of the garlic pieces. Warm slightly before dropping into the child's ears. To instill drops in the ear of a child under three years of age, pull his ear down and back to straighten the ear canal; in children over three years of age the ear should be pulled up and back. Have the child lie quietly for two to three minutes to allow the drops to run down into the ear. Cotton balls may be inserted into the ears to keep the oil in. The drops may be applied twice a day. If the child reports increased pain with the drops discontinue them immediately. Be certain that the ear drum is not ruptured before any type of ear drops are used. The oil may be stored for up to six months in a tightly closed jar.

Children in day care centers are exposed to a wide variety of germs carried by other children (292). Their immature immune systems are unable to resist the disease, so they become ill. Having a cold or other respiratory infection increases the risk that the child will develop otitis media.

Children who are exposed to cigarette smoke from their smoking parents, or other caregivers, are at increased risk of developing otitis media. Smokers should not be permitted around children.

Habitual breathing through the mouth is felt by physicians to be a factor in one-third of all cases of otitis media with effusion (304). We believe these children have chronically stuffy nose due to an allergy. Since dairy products account for 60% of all food allergies, we could therefore expect dairy products to be the most likely culprit. Indeed, the simple dietary measure of removing dairy products from the diet often bring to a halt the earaches suffered by many families.

It is well known that an infant who is bottle-fed is at increased risk of developing otitis media (305, 306).

Children who live in poorly ventilated homes are at increased risk of otitis media (307). Airing out the house reduces the incidence of colds. Keeping the extremities properly clothed, giving the child a daily tepid-water bath, and plenty of outdoor activities, all improve the resistance against colds and earache.

Children who have repeated episodes of otitis media may benefit by activities designed to open the eustachian tube frequently. A pacifier or teething toy will encourage the child to swallow more frequently (292). Older children may be taught to swallow while the parent holds the nose closed. Blowing up a balloon four or five times a day may also be helpful. Older children may perform what is known as the Valsalva maneuver, by closing the lips tightly, pinching the nose closed, and forcibly blowing (308). The same thing can be accomplished while trying with all the might to lift one end of a car or piano. This will often pop the ears. This should be done ten to twelve times a day.

The child who is prone to earaches should be protected from chilling. The ears should never be exposed to cold or drafts.

Some have felt that otitis media associated hearing loss led to developmental delays in children but recent studies indicate that while the child's development may be slowed during the acute illness, as soon as the fluid clears and hearing becomes normal again the child quickly catches up with his peer group (309, 310).

ECZEMA (ATOPIC DERMATITIS)

Infantile eczema is a fairly common skin problem. It usually appears between two months and two years of age. This is the commonest, and often the earliest, manifestation of allergy. Many of these children have, or will develop, asthma or hay fever. There is often a family history of allergy.

It rarely occurs before the child is two months of age, but appears before five years of age in 85 percent of children who develop it. Onset in infancy is generally a red, very itchy rash on the sides of the cheeks with the arms and legs becoming involved as the child matures. There may be oozing and crusting. There may be fissures behind the ears and dryness and scaling of the skin of the arms and legs (311).

At about four or five years of age, the distribution of the rash changes, with the area behind the knees and front of the elbows involved. There may be eczema behind the ears, and on the side of the neck.

Treatment

Aloe vera gel may be applied to inflamed areas (312).

Oatmeal baths may be quite soothing (313). Alkaline or soda baths may be very helpful. Add one cup of baking soda or two cups of cornstarch to a tub of water at approximately 94 to 98 degrees. The child should sit in the tub while the parent dips water up over the body parts not covered by the water. After the bath the child should stand for a few moments to allow water to drip off. Blot the skin dry; do not rub. Epsom salts, chamomile tea, and comfrey tea baths are also reported helpful. Oil may be applied to assist in retaining moisture in the skin. Carefully avoid chilling the child during the bath.

A mixture of olive oil and lime water shaken together in a tightly sealed bottle may be very helpful for itching. Apply as needed to control itching (314).

Soaps are often irritating and should be avoided or used very sparingly. Never use bubble bath (311).

Because food allergy is a common cause of eczema a trial of avoiding the most common food allergens may be very helpful. Eliminate all the foods on the list (see Appendix 1) for a week, then introduce one food at a time, with a new food every three to five days. If the disease worsens with the addition of a food, it should be avoided. The most common offenders are cow's milk, eggs, chocolate, citrus, and wheat; these foods should be returned to the diet last. Chicken, tartrazine and artificial colorings, and benzoate preservatives, peanut, fish, soybean, string beans, shrimp, and pork are also common causes of eczema (314).

Inhaled allergens such as house dust, pollens, or animal danders may also cause eczema. Vapors from cooking eggs may induce eczema in sensitive children. Children who have pollen sensitivity should not be allowed to lie on the grass during pollen season.

A soft cloth may be used to apply olive oil to dry and crusted skin areas.

Avoid contact with nylon, suede, or wool materials. Silk or cotton clothing should be worn next to the skin. Synthetic fabrics also retain moisture and heat. New clothing should be washed before it is worn (315). Clothing should be thoroughly rinsed after laundering. Rough bed linen should not be used.

Sudden temperature changes and extremes in temperature may worsen symptoms and should be avoided. Air conditioning is helpful for some; but worsens symptoms in others. A humidifier in the child's bedroom may be helpful (311).

Itching is a common problem. A "vaseline milk" may soothe itching and encourage healing. Immediately after washing, and while the skin is still wet, rub a bit of petrolatum into the water still adhering to the skin. This forms a milky fluid, which should be gently soothed over the affected skin.

White cotton socks may be placed over the hands of young children to prevent scratching, which may worsen itching (313). The fingernails should be kept short, and the hands washed frequently. Itching is often most intense during the evening and night hours.

Red clover and goldenseal tea may be applied as cold compresses for 20 minutes four times a day. The tea may also be drunk. Comfrey tea may be used as a compress, but should not be drunk, as it has been associated with some cancers. Normal saline solution may also make a very effective compress.

Many researchers feel that eczema may be prevented by breastfeeding infants for at least four months. A 1981 study revealed that children with allergic parents given solid food within four months after birth, had two-and-a-half times the rate of eczema of children with non-allergic parents and not given solid foods within four months of birth. The rate of eczema increased in almost direct proportion to the number of different kinds of food eaten (316, 317).

Several studies have shown that breast-fed infants may develop eczema from foods eaten by their mothers. Eggs, milk, and soybeans eaten by some breastfeeding mothers have all been shown to produce eczema in their infants (316).

Sunlight is beneficial to most patients; but some have a worsening of the inflammatory process with sun exposure. Sunburn should be guarded against.

Charcoal baths may be helpful. Add one-half to one cup of powdered charcoal to a tub of lukewarm warm. Soak once or twice daily for thirty minutes. Finish with a tepid shower to remove the charcoal, and pat dry. For a small child this procedure is best done in a laundry tub out of doors, to avoid cleaning the bathtub.

Evening primrose oil, applied to the inflamed skin areas after a bath, has been reported very effective. It may also be taken internally.

Chlorinated water is felt to cause allergic reactions in some children with eczema (311). These children may need bottled water.

Many children with eczema develop chronic Staphylococcus aureus infections (313). These may be effectively treated by bathing the child in a solution of two tablespoons of household bleach to a gallon of water. This solution may also be used as a compress for application to small areas of the body. This solution is drying to the skin and lubricant should be applied at the conclusion of the bath.

A salt-free diet has been reported helpful for some (318). A trial of it may be worthwhile. Sugar consumption has also been reported higher in children who developed eczema, than in normal controls (319).

ENCOPRESIS

Encopresis is passage of the stool, formed or liquid, in inappropriate places. This may occur several times daily or monthly. The child may pass only a small amount or may have a full bowel movement in his clothing. It rarely occurs during the night, and is more frequent at home than at school. It is more common in afternoon and evening hours. It has often been attributed to conflicts between mother and child over toilet training, but constipation is almost always the cause (320). These children do not empty their rectum entirely. Painful stool passage from anal fissure or fistula, diaper rash, or other inflammatory processes in the rectum or surrounding area may cause the child to attempt to retain his stool. Stress and personality may also contribute. These children often have behavior disturbances, or developmental delays. Bedwetting is often a problem, and these children were often chronically constipated as infants.

Encopresis is considered to be either primary or secondary. In primary encopresis the child has never gained bowel control, even though past the age (about 4 years of age) this would ordinarily be expected. In secondary encopresis the child loses bowel control after having developed it. This type often occurs after some stressful incident--moving, parental divorce, birth of a sibling, starting school, or the death or loss of a person close to the child.

Treatment

Because these children typically have a fecal impaction treatment must begin with bowel-cleansing procedures. Enemas may be given (see treatment section) to clear the impaction, or, more sure and more simple, is to insert a finger (wearing a surgeon's or food handler's glove well-lubricated with lotion or petroleum jelly) into the rectum and pull out the impacted stool.

The goal of treatment is to establish regular bowel habits. Retained fecal material may have permanently distended the colon, causing weakness of the colon muscles (320). Treatment must be continued for five or six months, to allow the colon to regain normal bowel tone.

Children are often shunned by classmates and adults because of the fecal odor. Parents may humiliate the child or treat him with scorn or rejection because of his problem. The child, in turn, may appear to be unconcerned about the problem and may attempt to hide his soiled clothing to prevent parental disapproval (321). These children may not feel the need the defecate because the rectum is chronically distended. They feel inadequate and guilty. If a child is old enough, self-cleaning and clothing change after each episode should be taught. Parents should not ridicule or scold the child. Many of these children have no control over the problem and criticism is useless. They would control it if they could. They may be unaware of the passage of stool. Neither parents nor child should feel responsible for the problem, but they must work in cooperation to resolve it.

These children have no regular bowel habit; establishing one is an essential part of the treatment (321). The child should be placed on the potty or toilet at the same time every day (324). The bathroom should be comfortably warm, a stool should be used if the child's feet do not touch the floor and the child should be given privacy if he desires (322).

Regular out-of-doors exercise should be encouraged as it promotes bowel function (322).

The diet should be high in fruits, vegetables, and whole grains. Bran (no more than one tablespoon at a meal) and prunes may be added to the diet (320). Refined foods, junk foods, milk and dairy products, meats, eggs and sugar should be eliminated from the diet, as all of them promote constipation. Food should be thoroughly chewed. Meals should be taken on a regular schedule (324). Eating between meals should be prohibited.

Adequate fluid intake is essential for proper bowel function. The child should consume enough water to keep his urine pale in color at all times. Thirst is not an adequate guide to sufficient hydration.

Three percent of children are estimated to be encopretic (325). About one percent of children still soil their panties at seven years of age, but this problem usually resolves by 16 years of age, even without treatment (322).

Boys suffer it more than girls. Parental anxiety often worsens the problem.

FEVER (FEBRILE) CONVULSIONS

Febrile convulsions are frightening experiences for parents, but we now understand that there is very little risk of permanent damage from them. Febrile seizures are the most common type of childhood convulsion. There are two classifications of febrile seizures: simple and complex. Our discussion will be limited to the simple type, which are less than 15 minutes in duration, occur only once, and are not associated with other neurological disorders. The complex type lasts longer, may be repeated multiple times, and have associated neurological abnormalities (326).

The trend in the past has been to place children who have had a febrile seizure on medication to prevent further seizures, but recent studies demonstrate that the risk of recurrent seizure is very little, and that these medications have adverse effects which are far out of proportion to the possibility of benefit from medication (327). Only a small percentage of children who have one febrile seizure will ever have a second, and the risk of more than two seizures is even smaller. Giving medication to prevent seizures does not decrease the risk of later development of epilepsy, and 40 percent of children given these medications have at least one adverse effect (328). Some say that the medication is given to the child to treat the parent.

Febrile seizures are most common between six months and six years of age, with peak incidences in the group from 18 months to three years of age. They are felt to occur in two to four percent of children at some time during their early childhood (329) and there is often a family history of them. Children with allergies or cerebral trauma at birth are more inclined to febrile seizures. Of children who have a second febrile seizure half of them will occur during the six month period following the initial seizure, and 90 percent will occur within the first three months following the initial seizure. Children with a family history of epilepsy, developmental or neurological abnormality, seizure before the age of 12 months, and prolonged, complex seizures are at greater risk of manifesting complications such as epilepsy after a febrile seizure.

These seizures often occur as the temperature is rising rather than after a long period of fever. They seem to occur more frequently in association with a rapid rise in temperature, whereas a slower rise, even to a higher degree, is less likely to induce them. The seizure is due to abnormal brain activity, although the actual trigger that sets off the seizure is not understood; but it is probably not the temperature elevation itself, as an "artificial fever" with hot air or hot water never causes a seizure in a normal child. It is very likely the quality of the toxin causing the fever.

At the onset of the febrile seizure the child may hold his arms and legs stiffly for a few seconds. This is quickly followed by twitching of the arms and legs, and sometimes the face. The eyes may become dilated, and skin color may change. The child may fall to the ground if he is upright, his eyes will jerk and roll back in his head, and he will jerk and twitch uncontrollably. He may foam at the mouth. He may lose control of his bowel or bladder, and may vomit. The child may have a high-pitched scream at the beginning, due to the contraction of the diaphragm squeezing air from the lungs out past a contracted larynx. This is harmless. He will stop breathing for a few seconds, but resumes breathing in a short time. The stiff and jerking part of the seizure may pass in just a few seconds, and always less than three minutes. Then the child sleeps. The child is unaware of what is happening during the seizure and has no memory of anything until he awakens. Seizures that last longer than 15 minutes may be due to factors other than a fever.

Treatment

The first step is for the parent to calm herself. Panic often prevents rational thinking, and the parent must be cool headed in order to properly deal with the situation. The parent should stay with the child at all times; if help is needed someone else should be sent.

The child should be protected from hurting himself as he has the seizure. Young children can be held in the parent's lap, as shown in the illustration. Notice that the body is on the side and the head is turned down with the chin pulled forward by the parent's hand. This is to keep the airway open, and prevent the child from inhaling any vomitus. Once the seizure is over the child may be placed in the face down position with the head turned to the side until he awakens from the sleep portion of the seizure. Older children may be placed in this position during the sei-

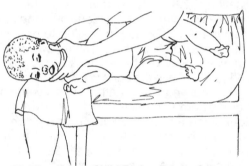

Holding Young Child During Febrile Seizure

zure, but the parent should watch to be certain the airway remains open (330). It may be necessary to remove vomitus from a small child's nose and mouth with a rubber tipped syringe, or even your finger.

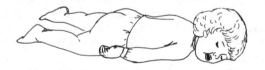

Rest Position After Febrile Seizure

Frequent fluid intake in small amounts has been shown to increase peripheral perfusion and encourage heat loss. Encourage the frequent intake of fluids any time your child has a fever (328).

Febrile seizures have been associated with pertussis immunization.

Do not give aspirin to reduce the fever, as it has been associated with the development of Reye's syndrome.

Try to prevent the child from falling at the onset of the seizure. If you can catch him as he falls ease him gently to the floor. Loosen tight clothing. Move any nearby furniture or objects he may strike as he convulses. Do not attempt to force anything between his teeth even if he is biting his tongue, for one minute, repeated four times, and done four times a day for two days, and do not attempt to give him food or fluids during the seizure.

At the conclusion of the seizure allow the child to rest quietly. Noise and much activity should be avoided. They will fall asleep after the convulsion and awake acting entirely normal.

FEVER BLISTERS, COLD SORES (HERPES SIMPLEX)

Cold sores are common in both children and adults. Recovery is usually complete in a week to ten days. Early symptoms are itching, burning, or a tingling sensation in the border of the lip with the skin. The lesions crust over in about 48 hours. They often recur in susceptible individuals. The virus which causes them, **Herpes simplex**, may remain inactive in the body throughout the person's lifetime. Most people who suffer cold sores have their first episode before the age of five.

Cold sores are small, very painful blisters, which typically occur around the mouth, but may be found on the genitals or in the eye. They sometimes develop in clusters which fill with fluid, then slowly dry up and disappear. They are spread by person-to-person contact with saliva, urine, discharge from the ulcer, or stool. They are more common in children who have eczema, after periods of emotional stress, after illness with associated decreased resistance to infection, or fever. Excessive sun exposure may induce them, as may the use of some drugs, menstrual changes, irritation from friction, and dental procedures which stretch the mouth.

Treatment

An ice cube should be applied to the lesion for 90 minutes at the first indication of development. This will usually abort the blister formation. Treatment must be instituted within 24 hours of the onset of symptoms to be effective, and preferably within the first 20 minutes. Try not to shorten the duration of the treatment, but it will be somewhat helpful if even 30 minutes of icing is done.

Cool liquids and frozen ices may be used to reduce pain when blisters are present. The person should be careful not to rub or scratch the eyes during the disease, to prevent spread to the eyes. The hands should be washed often.

Care should be taken to avoid sunburn, as that often triggers the onset.

Aspirin should not be used for pain because of the association with Reye's syndrome.

Some individuals develop fever blisters after eating foods they are allergic to. Chocolate is a common cause of fever blisters.

Regular out-of-doors exercise is helpful in increasing the body's ability to fight infection, and also reduces stress.

Lesions may be treated with 70 percent alcohol to hasten drying. This will sting at the time of application, but will often decrease the swelling. Goldenseal powder may be applied to the blister by wetting the end of a toothpick and using it as an applicator. This may be repeated as often as necessary.

Do not apply ointments to the blisters, as air exposure hastens drying and healing. Hot compresses for six minutes, followed by ice cold compresses will help dry up the blisters.

Some have found a tincture of capsicum to be helpful. Apply enough to cause a slight burning sensation, once or twice a day, especially at night. Put one tablespoon of cayenne in two ounces of alcohol, shake occasionally for three days before pouring off the liquid. Apply liberally.

FIRE ANT BITES

Fire ants belong to the same insect order as bees, wasps, yellow jackets, and hornets. They are most commonly found in the Southern states.

A sterile pustule develops within 24 hours after the bite, and then subsides over the next few days. Plunge the part which has been stung into very hot water for 20 to 30 minutes to inactivate the venom. Ice, witch hazel, alcohol, baking soda, a mixture of vinegar and lemon juice, or a cut potato may provide pain relief. Apply a charcoal compress for eight to ten hours after the first aid has been finished.

Seek medical attention if the child manifests such allergy symptoms as breathing difficulties, hives, severe swelling, shock, or dizziness.

FLATFEET (PES PLANUS)

Flatfoot is a common finding in young children. One study showed 97 percent of infants aged 0-18 months had "flatfeet," but by 10 years of age only 4 percent still had flatfeet. This is most often what is called flexible or physiological flatfoot. Many of these children have "fat" feet instead of "flat" feet (331). They have a fat pad which makes the foot appear flat, but as the child begins to walk the fat pad disappears and a normal arch appears. This physiological flatfoot tends to run in fami-

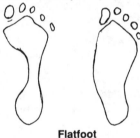

Flatfoot
A. Normal   B. Flatfoot

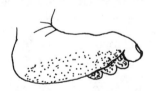

"Fatfoot" Appears to be Flatfoot

lies, and is more common in black people and Jews (332). The appearance of flatfoot is normal in young children. Examination of the foot while the child is sitting, or standing on tip-toe, demonstrates a normal arch, and free movement of the foot. Another simple test is called the "toe-raising test of Jack." The parent observes appearance of an arch as the big toe is lifted. On the basis of these simple examinations the parent may be assured that his child will most likely eventually develop a normal arch.

Diagnosis of True Flatfoot

Parents often bring their child to the physician complaining that their child

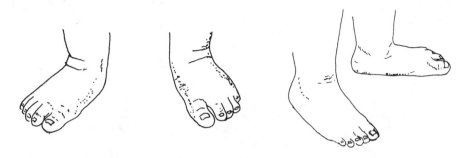

Normal Foot Appearance in Young Children

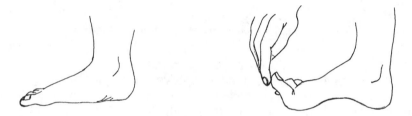

Toe-Raising Test

has flatfeet. Many of these parents were themselves treated as youngsters, so they feel that they must provide treatment for their child. It is difficult to convince many of them that benign neglect may be the treatment of choice, and that their child's "flatfoot" is normal. The child with true flatfeet walks on the inside of his feet, and wears down the inner edges of his shoe soles and heels. He may complain of pain in his feet after little activity. If the child wears down the inside of his shoes, is unable to flex his feet freely, and cannot flex his foot upward normally he may require professional evaluation.

Treatment

Flatfoot persisting in older children is sometimes treated by various exercises such as picking up marbles with the toes, walking on the outsides of the feet, or toe curls, but these exercises are probably useless, and are certainly tedious to the child. The child may benefit from being bare footed out-of-doors, or on a thick indoor carpet. A few children, who have flatfoot due to contraction of the muscles which flex the foot, may benefit from stretching exercises (333). These exercises may be done by the parent or the child. When exercises are carried out by the parent, the knee should be kept straight, and the heel turned slightly inward. The parent should flex the foot as far as possible in the manner illustrated, and hold it for a count of ten, then relax, and repeat for 20 times at each of three daily sessions. The child should remain relaxed during the exercise. The older child may do his own exercises by standing with toes turned inward, heels flat on the floor, and knees straight as he leans into a wall about 12-18 inches away.

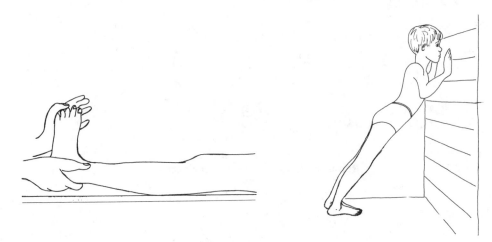

Stretching Technique for Flat Foot Done by Parent

Corrective Shoes

Although widely recommended, corrective shoes have not been proven effective in the treatment of flatfeet. Many pediatric orthopedists consider them an unjustified expense to the parent, and a source of unnecessary emotional distress for both parent and child. A number of studies demonstrate that most children who go barefoot, or wear the cheapest available shoe, will develop normal arches by four years of age (334, 335). One study revealed that 72 percent of pediatricians and pediatric orthopedists (who probably have more experience with flatfooted children) recommend no treatment at all for flexible flatfoot. Podiatrists, however, were likely to recommend special shoes, heels or wedges. Shoe salesmen are also likely to recommend special shoes or lifts.

Children who have painful flatfeet may obtain pain relief from alternating hot and cold foot baths. Fill two deep basins with water--one hot and one cold. Place both feet in the hot water for one minute, then in the cold water for one minute, alternating back and forth for ten minutes, twice a day.

FROSTBITE

Frostbite occurs most often in the fingers, tip of the nose, earlobes, cheeks or toes. The skin becomes numb or tingly, white and cold. If the skin is wet at the time of cold exposure the symptoms are often worse. Frostbite may occur when a cold metal surface, such as a car, is touched with the bare hands.

Treatment

Treatment involves warming the frostbitten skin. The area may be placed in very warm water or covered with warm, wet compresses. The water should not be so hot that the area is burned; frostbitten skin is readily burned. Heat application to the area should continue until color returns to the area, often at least 30 minutes. Some frostbite victims report pain during the last phase of warming (336).

Warm fluids may be given during the warming procedure.

The child's entire body should be kept warm during the rewarming process.

Do not massage the area with snow. The massage may damage tissues.

Electric heaters or heat lamps may cause burning, and should not be used to thaw the area. The temperature can be controlled much easier with water than with electrical devices.

GASTROENTERITIS

Gastroenteritis is an inflammation of the lining of the stomach and intestine (342). It may be caused by viruses, bacteria, chemical irritation (foods, concentrated nutrients, drugs, contaminants), or allergy. Symptoms include vomiting, diarrhea, sometimes fever, and dehydration if the diarrhea and vomiting become prolonged. Gastroenteritis is said to occur in approximately 10 percent of infants under one year of age in the United States (343), and probably in every child during childhood at least once. It is far more common in countries with poor hygienic standards. It is readily transmitted by contaminated foods such as milk and other dairy products, meat or eggs. The introduction of new foods may produce gastroenteritis if the child is allergic to them. Overfeeding the child or giving an excess of fat or sugar may cause diarrhea (344).

Diarrhea is defined as an increase in the number of stools or a thinning of their consistency. A parent is probably the best judge of how severe the child's diarrhea is as she is acquainted with what is normal for the child. The stools are often watery, green from bile, and may even contain pus or blood.

The child should be given nothing for 4 to 6 hours, then given water for 12 hours to allow the gastrointestinal tract to rest. Ice chips may be given to a child old enough to avoid choking on them. Clear diluted (half-strength) herb teas such as red clover, catnip and peppermint may be given frequently in small amounts. Some recommend one to two ounces every hour. Fluids should be given at room temperature as bowel motion is increased by cold temperatures. If the child is taking ice chips they should be held in the mouth until thoroughly melted. As the diarrhea slows, the fluids may be decreased and given only as needed to prevent dry lips or other signs of dehydration. Neither sugar nor honey should be added--the tea should be plain. After that time diluted fruit juices (avoid citrus fruit juices) may be added, and if well tolerated the child may be given such easily digested foods as dry toast, well-cooked rice, whole-grain cereals, applesauce, mashed ripe bananas and baked potato may be added as the symptoms improve. Use only one food at a time to test for sensitivities. Avoid crackers made with baking powder as it interferes with calcium balance. The introduction of food may produce a mild increase in stools, but this should resolve spontaneously. Milk and all milk products should be strictly avoided as lactose intolerance often occurs after bouts of diarrhea.

Sometimes fluids or food taken immediately after a vomiting episode will be retained, as the vomiting reflex will be in the refractory phase.

Infants being breast-fed are less likely to develop gastroenteritis, but if they do so the breast feeding may be continued. Additional water may be given as needed. The mother should simplify her diet, removing milk, onions, garlic, spices, and any known irritant.

Cow's milk is capable of causing inflammation of the intestine, and should always be suspected as a cause of nausea and vomiting. Gastroenteritis may be due to cow's milk intolerance. A two to four week trial of a milk free diet may be quite helpful, particularly in children with symptoms such as recurrent respiratory tract infections, feeding problems, eczema, diaper rash, and "colic," all of which may suggest allergy.

Charcoal, obtained from the drug store or health food store, may be very useful in the treatment of diarrhea. Powdered charcoal may be mixed in water and drunk, or tablets or capsules taken. Pureed pumpkin (345) or carrots are said to be soothing to the gastrointestinal tract, as well as pureed apple. Raw fruits and vegetables should be avoided for several days.

Adequate water intake should be encouraged as the appetite improves.

The parent should watch carefully for signs of acute dehydration. Sinking of the fontanelles (see physical examination section) and the eyeballs indicates dehydration, as do dry skin, dry lips, very little saliva and scanty tears. The child may become increasingly irritable and the arms and legs may become blue and chilled. Even though the child takes fluids eagerly he may lose them as vomiting or diarrhea. Skin turgor may be checked by the parent by pinching up a large skin fold on the child's abdomen. If the skin quickly resumes its normal position skin turgor is normal; in a dehydrated child the skin fold will remain elevated after the parent turns loose. This indicates dehydration. Decreased urine output may also indicate dehydration. The child should wet at least six diapers in any 24 hour period, and a dry diaper for more than four hours may indicate dehydration in an infant (346). The younger the child the greater the risk of severe dehydration.

Small retention enemas of lukewarm normal saline may be useful in those who cannot retain any fluids given by mouth. Add one level teaspoon of salt to a quart of water. Use a small rubber bulb syringe to inject one or two ounces of fluid into the rectum and hold the buttocks together for several minutes. Repeat every one to two hours until the child is able to take fluids by mouth. Do not over-hydrate, but you may be certain you can give as many ounces of saline by rectum as the child is losing in diarrhea.

These children may find great comfort in sucking and should be given their pacifier if they use one, or allowed to suck their thumb if it comforts them.

Infants in diapers should be changed promptly after an episode of diarrhea. The skin may quickly become irritated by the acidic stools if not cleaned promptly. The area should be thoroughly but gently cleaned using a mild soap, and air dried if possible. A fan or heat lamp kept a safe distance from the child may hasten resolution of any irritation. Petroleum jelly may be applied over the area to prevent irritation, or cornstarch applied after cleansing. Cornstarch is both soothing and drying (346).

The parent should carefully wash the hands after changing diapers or being in contact with a patient with gastroenteritis to prevent spread (346).

Antidiarrheal medications and medications to stop vomiting have potential serious side effects, which may worsen the condition. It is better to manage the disease without these, using copious quantities of charcoal, the treatment of choice in gastroenteritis.

If the child becomes weak or listless, or fails to improve after 24 hours of treatment your health care provider should be consulted immediately.

GASTROESOPHAGEAL REFLUX

Gastroesophageal reflux is the return of the stomach contents back into the esophagus (347), the tube that runs between the mouth and stomach. Parents should be aware that this may occur in very healthy infants and is not necessarily a sign of illness or abnormality. Many children grow and develop normally despite spitting up their food from time to time. In very young children gastroesophageal reflux is often due to chalasia, a malfunction of the lower esophageal sphincter, which normally functions to prevent food from returning to the esophagus. This malfunction is considered by some to be simply an indication of immaturity of the sphincter, which in a few weeks or months, begins to function as it does in adulthood. Most children who demonstrate gastroesophageal reflux before they reach the age of three months may be expected to be symptom free by the time they reach two years of age (348). Symptoms persist in some children until four years of age. By the time the child reaches 12 months of age he is spending most of his time in the upright position and even those whose sphincters are slower in development may expect improvement in symptoms with the change in position (349).

Gastroesophageal reflux can also be caused by hiatal hernia, but this is more common in older children than in the young age group most likely to suffer chalasia.

Symptoms include vomiting, failure to gain weight, irritability, refusal to eat, blood in the stools, and anemia (350). Vomiting is the main symptom in about two-thirds of all infants with gastroesophageal reflux. Onset may be at the time of birth or six weeks later. The vomiting may be mild, a sort of spitting up, or may be projectile, shooting out of the child's mouth. Children may be hungry immediately after vomiting and wish to eat again (351).

The repeated return of food and hydrochloric acid into the esophagus may cause irritation or even esophagitis, making it painful for the child to eat. If the irritation becomes severe the esophagus may bleed, and blood may pass through the digestive system and be eliminated with or in the stool, or the child may vomit fresh blood. The continued blood loss may lead to anemia (352).

About one-third of these children fail to grow properly because of inadequate nutrition, but once successful treatment is begun they grow normally.

Some children have episodes of cessation of breathing. There may be associated respiratory problems, such as cough or asthma, because of inhalation of the refluxed material. Cow's milk placed in the trachea of some very young laboratory animals causes cessation of breathing (350). For this reason it may be well to avoid giving cow's milk to children with gastroesophageal reflux. Older children who suffer gastroesophageal reflux, for whatever reason, may have heartburn.

Most of these children will rapidly outgrow gastroesophageal reflux. The treatment is controversial, but we will discuss both sides, and if one method does not work the other is worth a trial. Both sides claim high success rates.

For decades gastroesophageal reflux has been treated by keeping the child upright at about a 60 degree angle in an infant seat to enable gravity to assist in keeping the food in the stomach. However, some observers point out that children slump in the infant seat, increasing pressure on the abdomen, which encourages the food to reflux upward (347). These people claim that the proper position for the child is lying face down on a board slanted upward at a 30 degree angle. This may be done by the use of a board with a brace, or a harness attached to the head of the bed. This position is felt to encourage stomach emptying. The child should be kept in this position constantly during the treatment program, which should last at least six weeks. After this period of time the child may be taken off the board for short periods of time, gradually increasing the time if symptoms do not recur. During the treatment time the child should be removed from the slant board for bathing and diaper changes before feedings, and held up to the shoulder or placed back on the board immediately after feedings. He should never be placed flat after a feeding.

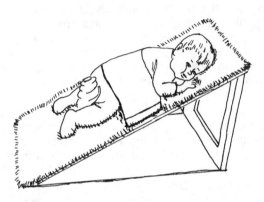

Resting Position for Gastroesophageal Reflux

Older children who have gastroesophageal reflux should have the head of their bed raised, and should not go to bed for several hours after eating. Foods high in fat and chocolate should be eliminated from the diet as these are known to decrease the lower esophageal sphincter pressure.

Some children develop stiff neck while on the slant board. The parents should turn the head from one side to the other frequently to prevent this. Sometimes the position causes the child's legs to swell from fluid accumulation. Simply lifting the legs up for a few minutes will often be effective in resolving this (347).

Until at least six months of age infants should receive only breast milk. For the older infant feedings should be thick, as thick material is less likely to reflux. Whole grain rice cereal boiled gently for three hours or blended with expressed breast milk or fruit juice may be spoon-fed in small amounts every four hours, or at regular feeding times; or the child may be fed rice cereal prior to nursing. If the child is receiving formula it may be necessary to enlarge the nipple hole to allow the food to flow freely. Symptoms may worsen if the child swallows air in an attempt to get his food. He should be burped frequently. Many children on thickened feedings show improvement within about two weeks, but the feeding schedule demands cooperation on the part of all family members.

The child should be kept upright after every feeding, and as quiet as possible. Excessive activity, crying, and flat positions cause reflux in some children.

Infants who are kept in infant seats may benefit from the use of a pacifier, but those who are kept in the face down position will probably have an increase in the gastroesophageal reflux if given a pacifier. Crying may increase gastroesophageal reflux, and attempts should be made to keep the infant's crying to a minimum. Symptoms persist so long or are so severe in some children that surgery is required, but every attempt should be made to manage the child without surgery if at all possible. As long as the child grows and gains weight normally the treatment program should be continued.

GEOGRAPHIC TONGUE

Geographic tongue is a harmless process found in 10 to 15 percent of children (353). Smooth, bright red patches appear on the tongue, and may change size, shape or location over several hours or days. There may be one patch or many and patches may enlarge to grow together and form large patches. Sometimes they spread to involve the floor of the mouth, the buccal mucosa, tonsils, edge or bottom of the tongue. The name comes from the resemblance of oceans and land masses on a map. The condition may clear up in a few days or persist for years and may recur after disappearing. There is no scarring or sign of abnormality after the lesions clear. There is usually no pain, although some have reported sensitivity to spicy, hot, or cold foods. The cause is not understood, but it may be a manifestation of allergy. Many of these children have family histories of hay fever, eczema, asthma, or other allergic diseases.

Children with low grade fever, as with colds, may develop red patches on the tongue very similar to geographic tongue. Treatment is unnecessary (354).

Deep furrows of the tongue, called fissures, are sometimes associated with geographic tongue (355). These too are generally considered harmless symptoms.

Treatment is neither necessary nor effective. The child should be treated for any allergic condition which may co-exist.

GERMAN OR THREE-DAY MEASLES (RUBELLA)

Rubella is an infection acquired by droplet spread via the respiratory system (356). It is a form of measles that is generally mild. Its greatest importance lies in the fact that women who are exposed to the virus in the first five months of pregnancy are at increased risk of having an infant with a birth defect (357).

Peak occurrence is during the summer months. The incubation period is 14 to 21 days from exposure to the onset of the rash. In many, symptoms of fever, cough, sneezing, nasal congestion, swelling of the lymph glands, and conjunctivitis are present seven to fourteen days after exposure. The child may initially complain of stiffness of the back of his neck. A rash follows which begins on the face, and spreads over the body. The rash, which does not occur in all children, is light pink and may spread to run together. It may last up to five days, or be present for only a few hours. Often there is the appearance of distinctive enlargement of pea-sized lymph nodes on the mastoid processes, the bony prominences just behind the ears. In older children, particularly females, there may be arthritis-like pain in the joints and arthralgia, which often occurs on about the third day of the illness. Fever may be as high as 102 to 103 degrees F., or may be absent. It usually subsides on the second day of illness.

The disease is usually very mild, and drug medication is contraindicated and should be avoided.

Treatment

Fluid intake should be liberal and the diet should be light, without fats or sugars.

A hot half bath may be given every two hours for fever or itching (see treatment section).

Saline compresses over the eyes may be soothing, as may a darkened room.

Salt water or plain hot water gargles may be used for irritated or sore throat.

Steam inhalations are helpful for cough.

Itching is relatively uncommon, but if present, may be treated by adding one cup of corn starch to about four inches of water in a bathtub (358). Have the child sit in the tub for 20 to 30 minutes. Use a cup to pour the water over body parts not covered by the water. Pat dry after the bath, leaving as much starch as possible on the skin.

Ice bags may be applied to swollen lymph glands for 5 to 15 minutes every hour for severe discomfort.

Catnip tea may be given for irritability or itching.

GIGGLE MICTURITION

These big words refer to the leakage of urine while laughing. It is more common in girls, and often disappears as the child matures. The greatest risk of this syndrome is the possibility that the child will be subjected to urological evaluation unnecessarily. It is common, but its exact frequency is difficult to determine, as most people do not report it to their physician. A 1975 study suggests that about 25% of children suffer from it, and 10% of them still have some trace of the problem after they reach the age of 20. It tends to run in families (359).

These children may suffer social isolation because of the odor.

Some children wet their underwear only slightly; others are unable to regain bladder control, and voiding continues until the bladder is entirely empty.

Treatment is reassurance that the child will most likely outgrow it. Some are helped by sitting down while laughing (360, 361).

GINGIVITIS

Gingivitis is an inflammation of the gums of the mouth. It is due to the collection of plaque on the teeth. Mild gingivitis is common in children. Symptoms include bleeding, bad breath, red, swollen and soft gums, and sometimes fever (362).

If other parts of the mouth lining become involved the process is called stomatitis; and if all the mouth becomes inflamed it is called gingivostomatitis. Acute necrotizing ulcerative gingivitis, a more severe form of gingivitis, with swollen, painful gums, ulcerations, bad breath, a gray coating over the gums, and easy bleeding, is not common in young children. People with acute necrotizing ulcerative gingivitis often report a metallic taste, sensitivity of teeth, and sometimes associated headache, low-grade fever, swelling of the lymph glands, and generally feeling bad. It is felt that poor oral hygiene, stress, smoking, fatigue, and poor nutrition may be contributing factors.

Poor nutrition, inadequate cleansing of the mouth, some medications, and some diseases encourage gingivitis. There may be a mild gingivitis with the eruption of a new tooth.

Prevention should be stressed by teaching the child to carefully brush and floss his teeth. The diet should be low in sugar, and the child should have regular dental care.

Treatment

The teeth should be cleaned after every intake of food, using a soft tooth brush. The bristles should be placed at the gum line, and rotated gently downward (362).

A saline solution made by adding one teaspoon of salt to one pint of water or a dilute solution of hydrogen peroxide may be used as a mouthwash if gingivitis develops. The mouth should be vigorously rinsed several times daily, or may be irrigated with the use of a Water Pik (363).

Charcoal powder made into a thick paste the consistency of very thick peanut butter can be spread on a gauze, molded over the teeth and gums, and left there for two hours. This process can be repeated constantly with a fresh gauze compress. The charcoal paste may be put directly on the gums and swallowed as it dissolves in saliva. This treatment is a very good one for acute gingivitis or stomatitis.

GROWING PAINS

Growing pains are apparently harmless aches and pains which typically occur in the legs at night after the child goes to bed. In some children there is arm or lower back pain. The pain may awaken the child from a sound sleep or may appear before he goes to sleep. The pain may be severe enough to cause crying (364). The pain may persist for only a few minutes, or half an hour, and is entirely gone by morning. The child may appear normal during the day and have pain again in the evening. The pain is generalized throughout the area and is located in muscle masses rather than in joints. The incidence of growing pains is unknown as not all children who suffer them are brought to medical attention. They may occur in half of all children.

Episodes come and go, sometimes appearing several nights in a row, then disappearing for weeks or months, only to recur.

The name "growing pains" does not identify the cause, as episodes are most common during periods of slow growth (365). There appear to be two peaks of highest incidence, three to nine years of age, and during adolescence.

Examination of the area reveals no abnormalities. If the parent sees redness, swelling, heat, or incomplete range of motion the child should be evaluated for a disease process (366). Children with growing pains have no skin or joint abnormalities. The pain does not persist into the next day.

Treatment

Heat applications in the form of a heating pad or towels wrung out of hot water and covered with plastic to retain the heat may be useful. Hot water bottles are generally not large enough to cover the entire involved area. Hot baths may be used.

Gentle massage is often very effective in relieving the pain. Children who object to massage should be examined for some disease process. Inflamed joints or bones are very tender, and a child who objects to massage most likely has something other than growing pains.

Food allergy is a common cause of growing pains (367). Milk elimination may be the only treatment required. If this is unsuccessful other common food allergens should be eliminated on a trial basis. Many children who have growing pains also suffer headaches or abdominal pain, both of which may be signs of allergy.

Leg elevation may also be helpful.

Stretching exercises may speed resolution of symptoms. Exercises to stretch the calf, hamstring, and quadriceps muscles are performed twice a day for ten minutes. Each stretch position should be held for 15-20 seconds, with each stretch performed 10 to 20 times on alternating legs.

Exercise 1A: With patient lying face down, the parent flexes the leg to 90 degrees, and pulls down on the front of the foot to stretch the leg muscles.

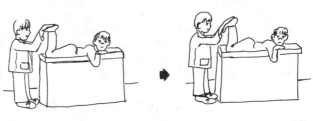

Exercise 1A

Exercise 1B: The child turns over on his back, and the parent pushes up on the top of the foot.

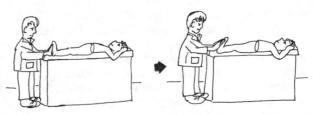

Exercise 1B

Exercise 2: With the child still on his back the parent lifts the leg by the heel. The leg is lifted straight up, keeping the knee straight. The hip is flexed to stretch the hamstring muscle.

Exercise 3: With the child lying face down, the heel is pushed up on the hip, lifting the thigh off the table.

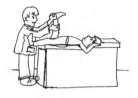

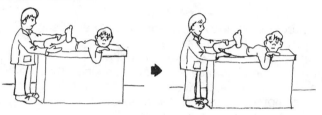

Exercise 3

HAY FEVER (ALLERGIC RHINITIS)

Hay fever, contrary to its name, is not due to hay, nor does it always cause a fever (368). It is an allergic reaction to substances the sufferer comes in contact with. While most people think of pollen as a cause of hay fever many other substances may be just as guilty of producing symptoms: dust, mold, many foods, and pets are common causes. It has been estimated that about 10 percent of people suffer some sort of nasal allergy (368). There is often a family history of allergic disease. For some not yet understood reason, children born in the months of March and April seem to have a higher than average incidence of hay fever. The severity of symptoms is related to the extent and duration of exposure to the allergen. Symptoms vary throughout the day, and are usually worse in the morning and evening hours.

Symptoms include episodes of sneezing, stuffy nose, red, itchy eyes, ears, nose, palate, and throat, nasal drainage, tearing of the eyes, headache, loss of appetite, irritability, difficulty sleeping, and sometimes sore throat. The child may become a mouth breather because of a constantly stuffy nose. There may be hearing loss due to swelling in the ear canals. A child who has had hay fever for several years may manifest "allergic shiners," (dark areas around the eye), or a crease on the bridge of the nose from the "allergic salute." There may be chronic cough or throat clearing. The child may

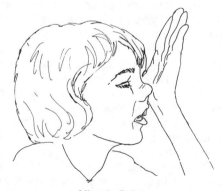

Allergic Salute

have an associated history of frequent colds, otitis media, or nosebleeds. The child may pick his nose in an attempt to clear it, and may cause bleeding. Itching is a useful symptom to distinguish hay fever from the common cold (369).

Some feel that the predominant symptom is a clue to the allergen. Eye irritation and itching suggest a mold allergy; pollen allergy is suggested by nasal itching, while itching of the palate and throat suggest food allergy. This guide may not be effective, as there may be a number of precipitating factors.

Treatment

Treatment is best directed toward avoiding the precipitating allergens and a program to improve the general health.

A humidifier or vaporizer may be used during the winter months to ease nasal stuffiness. The child may sniff normal saline drops up his nose to relieve nasal dryness. Over 90% of hay fever sufferers reported improvement in their symptoms with the use of saline drops made by adding 1 teaspoon of salt to 1 pint (2 cups) of water (370).

The child should have abundant sleep, with a regular sleep schedule regardless of weekends, holidays and vacations.

The diet should be free of the most common food allergens (see appendix). Common foods demonstrated capable of causing hay fever include milk, eggs, wheat, spices, meats, fish, shellfish, cheese, asparagus, tomatoes, potatoes, peanuts, lentils, soybeans, corn, Chinese cabbage, peaches, apples, onions, various berries, grapefruit, pineapple, nuts, pepper, sage, horseradish, chili powder, Worcestershire sauce, mustard, cereals, melons, cantaloupe, string beans, bananas, cocoa, tea, coffee, chocolate and vanilla. Most children react to more than one food, making it rather difficult to determine the culprit. Milk is especially suspect, as it has been shown to contain pollen in an unchanged state. Parents should keep a food diary to determine what foods the child eats prior to onset of hay fever symptoms, even if the principle suspect is pollen, not food. The pollen sensitivity is made much better by eliminating the food which also causes allergy. Food allergy tests are generally ineffective in determining the dietary causes of hay fever.

Meal time should be regular, and eating between meals should be forbidden. Wheat, rice, oatmeal, and other grains eaten as cereals should be boiled gently for three hours, having first heated the grains while stirring constantly to lightly toast them. This step will prevent mushiness from the long cooking. Adequate cooking makes grains lose some of their allergenic quality. Long cooking is especially important for babies. Even instant cereals should be cooked for three hours. Emphasis should be placed on raw fruits and vegetables, as they contain vitamin C, a natural antihistamine.

These children are often more susceptible to respiratory tract infections, and keeping them away from crowds may decrease their risk of acquiring such diseases.

It is often helpful to keep children sensitive to pollen inside early in the morning, in the evening, and on windy days, when pollen is most likely to be circulating.

Air conditioning, especially with an anti-allergy air filter, is often helpful in symptom relief. However, some people report worsening of their symptoms with air conditioning.

A cool bath every morning followed by skin stimulation with a brush or rough washcloth are useful. Alternating hot and cold showers are also helpful as a general health measure.

Hair sprays, fumes from gas stoves, cigarette smoke, paint fumes, and other odors should be eliminated from the home as much as possible.

Antihistamines are advocated for the use of hay fever, but considering the side-effects (drowsiness, dizziness, ringing in the ears, blurred vision, confusion, nausea, vomiting, diarrhea or constipation, stomach distress, incoordination, nervousness, heart tremors, dry mouth, fast heart rate, skin problems, asthma, and increased risk of cancer) the treatment may be more dangerous than the disease.

Nasal sprays may induce a rebound phenomenon, with symptoms worse than before treatment, or cause inflammation of the nasal mucosa.

Exercise improves air flow through the nasal passages. Blood vessels tend to relax when the body is inactive (371). Three minutes of vigorous exercise has been shown to reverse nasal congestion. Children should be encouraged in activities which they enjoy. During times of high pollen count the child may need to participate in activities which can be done indoors, such as jumping rope, aerobic exercises, or even stair climbing.

A hot foot bath is often very effective in relieving nasal congestion. (See treatment section for procedure.)

Hot fluids help open nasal passages. Herbal teas, such as goldenseal, red clover, or nettles, without additives, provide extra fluids and increase the ease of breathing. (Goldenseal should not be taken by pregnant women as it may induce uterine contractions.)

Apple water (for those not allergic to apple) may be made by pouring boiling water over freshly sliced apples, allowing the fruit to soak for 15-20 minutes, and then the fluid drained off and drunk still warm. Onion water may be made in the same manner, soaking fresh onion slices. Onions are known to have natural antibiotic properties.

One doctor has reported relieving his symptoms of hay fever by applying a thin coat of petroleum jelly to the nasal membranes (372). It is important to avoid sleeping in a position that petrolatum (or any other oily material) could slide around the corner high in the nose and get into the trachea and finally into the lungs to cause lipid pneumonia. Make the thin coating of petrolatum just that--thin.

Some children develop hay fever after swimming in a lake which is heavily infested with algae. Others are aggravated by swimming in heavily chlorinated swimming pools.

Cold applications to the forehead and face have been reported successful in curing even very severe hay fever (373). Wring the compress out of ice water, and freshen them as soon as they begin to warm up. The treatment should be continued for three or four hours, although relief may be expected within one hour.

The child's bedroom should be made as dust free as possible. Remove all carpets, heavy rugs, drapes and upholstered furniture, as these collect dust and are difficult to clean. Wet mop the floors daily, and keep the floor well waxed. Wipe the bed frame and springs with a damp cloth regularly. Put plastic covers over all mattresses and pillows. Wash bed clothing frequently. If a throw rug is used on the floor it should be washed weekly. Curtains should be made of plastic, and wiped daily. Use cotton sheets, and blankets made of synthetic fibers. Avoid chenille bedspreads, comforters and quilts. Keep all pets out of the bedroom. Do not allow the child to keep stuffed animals. There should be no smoking in the house. Indoor plants may collect mold spores.

Older children may be taught Gaonkar's maneuver. The child takes normal saline water into his mouth, tips his head back as if to swallow it, and attempts to gargle it out through the nose. The ears should be stopped up with the fingers, the mouth closed, and an attempt made to cough while flexing the head to bring the face downward. This maneuver should force water into the nasal passageway. This should be done three or four times daily (374).

The child should not be permitted to become excessively tired, although he should not be treated as an invalid. The motto should be "moderation in all things." Daily exercise is beneficial, but children who have very heavy schedules may need a midday nap or rest period.

The largest meal of the day should be taken at breakfast, with a hearty meal at dinner, and a very light supper. The child should go to sleep with an empty stomach. Fatty foods, spices and condiments, sweets, cola drinks, coffee, tea, pickles, and pork should be strictly eliminated from the diet.

The child should be properly clothed to prevent the least chilling of the limbs. A draft is a current of air that causes chilling of the skin; drafts must be avoided. The bedroom should be well ventilated. Chilling constricts the blood vessels of the skin, driving blood into other parts of the body, including the nasal mucosa (375). The accompanying swelling may worsen symptoms. House dust may be a chronic problem in houses with central heating systems.

If the child has been out-of-doors during hours of high pollen count he should shower thoroughly when he comes indoors. At the very least he should shower before bedtime. He should avoid contact with pets that have been out of doors. The face and eyelids should be carefully cleansed to remove all traces of pollen. Cold compresses may be applied to the eyelids if they feel irritated.

Inhalations of hot, humid air often bring great relief in hay fever (376). Three 30 minute inhalation treatments in a single day may bring improvement within 24 hours. Symptom relief may last for two or three days. There are inexpensive devices now on the market that provide heated air at approximately 100 degrees F. They may give excellent symptomatic relief. Do not use the proprietary medications that come with it; use only the heated air.

HEADACHE

Headaches are fairly common in children. By the age of seven almost half of all children have had at least one headache. The incidence of headache increases as the child matures, and in older children headaches are more common in girls than in boys. Headaches more commonly occur in the afternoon and early evening (377). They are generally not long lasting. One study showed that children who had high physical education grades had decreased headache incidence (377). This may suggest that physical fitness is a factor in prevention of headaches. A very small percentage of headaches in children are caused by poor vision or eyestrain.

Headache may be caused by many factors including injury, migraine, allergy, infection, noise, poor lighting, excessive television watching, poor ventilation, excessive heat, tension, or other miscellaneous factors.

Headaches which are present on awakening in the morning may be due to inadequate ventilation in the bedroom during the night. "Turtle" headaches occur in people who sleep with the covers over their head.

Monday morning headaches may be due to an irregular schedule over the weekend. The child's bed time and rising time should be same every day. Some people report headaches after sleeping late in the morning.

Girls often have headaches in association with their menstrual period.

Snow or sun glare may produce headache.

Teeth grinding (see section) may produce headache.

Tension Headaches

Tension is probably the most common cause of headache in children. Stress, excitement, or long periods of intense concentration may be sufficient to produce headache. Tension headaches present with a dull, constant pain, typically in the forehead and neck muscles.

Tension headaches are very common, and may last for hours. They may occur on a daily basis. They are often related to depression, stress, or anxiety. There is sometimes associated nausea and vomiting.

Migraine Headache

Migraine headaches occur in about four to five percent of school age children (378). Onset of migraines is most common at about age 12, although they may develop in younger or older children. In young children migraines are more common in males, but in adolescence girls suffer migraines more frequently (379). Migraine headaches tend to run in families, and if both parents suffer migraine the child has a 70% chance of having them. With only one affected parent the child has about a 45% chance of having the problem. Onset is before 15 years of age in about five percent of children.

Fatigue, stress, illness, menstrual periods, and medication may induce migraine.

Migraine may occur once or twice a month, or four times a week. It is often in the afternoon, and may be preceded by paleness and irritability. Some children have vision changes such as wavy lines or a sensation of flashing lights prior to the headache. During the headache the child may have abdominal pain, nausea and vomiting.

The pounding or throbbing pain is sometimes limited to one side of the head. Relief may come from a few hours of sleep.

Childhood-onset migraine often resolves as the child matures. Half of all patients have a decrease in the frequency of their headaches within six months of diagnosis, and over the next few years another 30 to 50 percent of children will have remission (380).

Sinus Headache

Sinus headaches generally occur at the same time of the day. Fever may be present. The child has a history of upper respiratory allergies, postnasal drip, recurrent ear infections or cough. They come on slowly, and build up in intensity over a period of time. The pain may vary with change in position.

The sinuses are not well developed in young children, and before the age of five years sinus headache pain is generally confined to the face or midfrontal region.

Febrile Headache

Headaches often occur in association with fever or other illness. These headaches resolve as the illness subsides (381).

Treatment

Cold compresses have been used for headache relief for many years. A study conducted at the Chicago College of Osteopathic Medicine revealed that about half of patients who used a cold pack received immediate pain relief. Interestingly, migraine patients had the greatest relief (382). A simple cool washcloth applied to the forehead is sometimes helpful (383).

A hot foot bath is a very effective headache treatment. (See treatment section.) Some like to add a tablespoon of mustard to the foot bath water. A towel may be dipped in cool water, wrung dry enough to prevent dripping, and placed around the neck while the feet are in the foot bath.

Food allergies are known to produce headache. Foods containing tyramine (cheese, and other dairy products, wine) milk, seafood, onions, citrus fruits, coffee, tea, chocolate, or pork are all capable of inducing headache (378). Foods containing nitrites (preserved luncheon meats, salami, bacon, hot dogs) are also suspect, and should be eliminated. Sugar should also be avoided. Octopamine, found in citrus and some beans, may produce headaches in some (384). Unfortunately, food allergies are difficult to determine by tests. The search for a food allergen should begin with elimination of the foods the child eats in large amounts for a month. He may even crave the very food to which he is allergic. At the end of the time, one food at a time should be reintroduced, and the child observed for return of symptoms.

Tension headaches may be helped by heat which relaxes the muscles of the back of the head, neck and scalp. A hot shower, heating pad, or hot water bottle may be used.

Massage is also useful. If the child complains of tenderness on massage, rub more gently, but consider this a clue that the headache is indeed a tension headache.

Children who suffer allergen-induced sinus headaches may obtain relief from sleeping in a bed with the head elevated on blocks. The sinuses are enabled to drain more readily.

A humidifier during the night may also assist sinus headache sufferers.

Sage, peppermint, or catnip tea may be helpful.

Sometimes a period of rest in a quiet, cool, darkened room will permit the child to sleep, and awaken without a headache.

A shower, with warm water sprayed over the back of neck, is often helpful in tension headaches.

Constipation may cause headache.

HEADBANGING (JACTATIO CAPITUS)

Headbanging is a rhythmic banging of the head against a hard object such as a wall, crib walls or headboard, or the floor. The child may assume a position on his hands and knees and bang his forehead against the object. Other children sit and bang the back of their head. Less commonly, the child may be in a face down or standing position during the banging episodes.

Onset is typically from ages 6 to 12 months, but may occur earlier or later. There may have been previous episodes of rhythmic movement such as body rocking or head rolling (385). The child typically outgrows

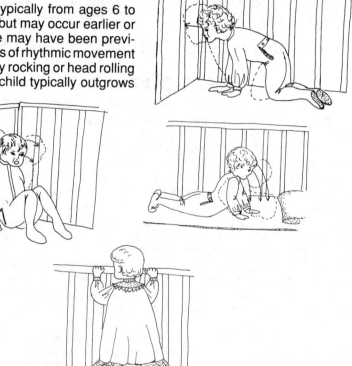

Headbanging Positions

this behavior by two to four years of age. Individual banging episodes may last 15 minutes to four hours. The episodes are most commonly associated with bedtime, but also occur at nap time. The banging may continue even after the child falls asleep. In some children there are episodes at other times during the day. Headbanging is estimated to occur in up to 20% of children, and is three to four times more common in males than in females.

The cause of headbanging has not been determined, but some parents have reported an increase in headbanging episodes during times of illness such as earache, or teething (386), or when the child is overly tired. Some feel that these children are musically inclined (387) and enjoy rhythmic activities. They may be encouraged in such rhythmic activities as hobbyhorses, swings, or see-saws during the day (388).

Most researchers consider headbanging a harmless behavior pattern in children with no other neurological, developmental, or psychological abnormalities. Some have claimed that headbanging is indication of mental or neurological abnormality, because many retarded children bang their heads, but EEG studies of headbangers without other symptoms show no abnormality. The child may have bruising or form a callus from his headbanging, but no cases of brain injury have been brought to our attention. The parent may wish to pad the area where the child bangs, but no other action is necessary (389). The parent should not attempt to force the child to stop headbanging as this often reinforces the behavior (390).

HEART MURMUR, SEE MURMUR

INFECTIOUS HEPATITIS

Hepatitis is an inflammation of the liver. Viruses, bacteria, or toxic substances are all capable of causing liver inflammation, but our discussion will be mainly limited to viral hepatitis.

Adolescent girls seem to have the highest incidence of viral hepatitis. It ranks among the top four infectious diseases reported in the United States.

Hepatitis is typically divided into three groups: A, B, and non-A/Non-B. Hepatitis A is the milder type. Contaminated milk, food, such as shellfish, or water may spread the virus, or it may be caught from animals. The virus may be acquired by swimming in infected water. Once it occurs in a family member, it frequently spreads to others. The incubation period is 14 to 40 days, and onset is usually abrupt, with fever. Peak incidence is autumn and winter, and it occurs most frequently in children and young adults. The virus is found in the stools from two to three weeks before the onset of symptoms, and until about a week after the appearance of jaundice (yellowing of the skin and whites of the eyes). Many cases of hepatitis never manifest jaundice.

Type B hepatitis does not have a seasonal pattern, has no age preference, and may be slower in onset, with little or no fever.

Non A/Non B hepatitis is responsible for about 90% of transfusion transmitted hepatitis.

Symptoms of jaundice, fever, headache, chilliness, malaise, itching, fatigue, mild upper respiratory tract infection symptoms, lack of appetite, vomiting, diarrhea or constipation, dark urine, upper abdominal pain, and joint pains may appear four to five days before the onset of jaundice (391). With the onset of jaundice the fever may disappear. Stools become pale cream or "clay" colored. There may be a skin rash.

The jaundice may last two to six weeks, and resolve slowly. It may be followed by four to eight weeks of fatigue and malaise. The liver is often tender and enlarged; the spleen is enlarged in about 15% of cases.

Infants may have a mild form of hepatitis without jaundice. Symptoms include vomiting, diarrhea and anorexia. Infectious hepatitis is usually mild in children, and is self-limiting. Treatment is symptomatic.

Recurrences are common, and are considered benign.

Recent outbreaks of Hepatitis A have occurred in day care centers. Caretakers who do not wash their hands carefully between diaper changes carry the virus from one child to another. Young children often have minimal symptoms with hepatitis, and the disease often goes unrecognized. Day care centers who accept only toilet-trained children have much lower incidences of hepatitis.

Treatment

Rest and supportive care are the keystones of treatment for hepatitis. For many years bedrest was considered essential, but now it is generally felt that the hepatitis sufferer may participate in activities up to the limitations of their fatigue (392). They should be careful not to become overly tired.

The appetite is generally poor, and sometimes even the smell of cooking food is sufficient to induce nausea. Appetites tend to be best in the morning, so efforts should be directed toward making breakfast as nutritious as possible (393). The diet should be simple and free of fried foods and animal fat. The liver is unable to handle fats as well as it does when healthy. Low-fat foods are easier to digest (394), and a totally vegetarian diet is ideal. Very hot or very cold foods are often not taken well.

Constipation should be avoided, as toxic substances are eliminated from the body with the stool. This lightens the work load of the inflamed liver.

Fluid intake should be encouraged, to allow the urine to flush toxins from the body.

The patient should wash his hands frequently to prevent spread of infection. If possible it is best for him to use separate toilet facilities from other family members. He should not be allowed to participate in family food preparation, and his eating utensils, if not disposable, should be washed separately from those of other family members. His clothing and bedding should be laundered separately (394). A 1:10 solution of household bleach and water may be used to clean soiled surfaces (395).

Many drugs are toxic to the liver, and all drugs should be avoided. No antibiotics are effective in the treatment of hepatitis (394). Such over the counter medications as Tylenol (acetaminophen) and iron supplements are known to be very toxic to the liver (395). Children given large doses of aspirin to treat rheumatic fever may suffer hepatitis, even at salicylate levels that have been considered nontoxic in the past. The hepatitis may occur as early as the second week of therapy (396).

Very hot fomentations over the liver area for 15 minutes may be carried out daily. A hot half bath may be given to raise the body temperature, assisting the body to fight the virus by strengthening the immune system. Be sure to give the patient plenty of fluids while in the bath, as perspiration will lead to the loss of fluids.

Goldenseal root tea may be taken one to three times a day.

Tepid baths may be used for itching.

Hot and cold compresses may be used for joint pains.

Fever may be treated by hot half baths.

Activities should be restricted for several months after the jaundice has passed. Strenuous sports should be avoided.

If a virus is not the cause of the hepatitis, always consider next a drug or poison in food as in the 16-year-old Colorado boy who was admitted to the hospital and diagnosed as having toxic hepatitis. It was learned that he had consumed milk from cows given nitrofurantoin, a frequently prescribed antibiotic. The cows had been given the medication for one week without apparent adverse effects (397).

HICCUPS (SINGULTUS)

Hiccups are involuntary jerking contractions of the diaphragm, the flat strip of muscle located between the chest cavity and the abdomen. The sound is produced when the inflow of air is abruptly stopped. They usually occur four to ten times per minute, the rate varying with individuals. They are persistent in men more often than in women. Sometimes they stop during sleep, only to recur when the person awakens.

Hiccups are sometimes due to overdistention of the stomach. Carbonated beverages, eating too rapidly, or overeating may produce hiccup-producing distention. Nursing infants who swallow air during feedings may suffer hiccups. Irregular eating habits may produce hiccups. Inflammation of the stomach, due to fermentation, was recognized as a cause of hiccups centuries ago. Stress or other excitement, chilling of the skin, lack of activity, intake of very hot or very cold beverages, cold showers, sudden environmental temperature changes, smoking, and alcohol ingestion are all known to cause hiccups.

Hiccups in an unborn child are apparently rather common. Mothers may think that the child is kicking, but the rhythm is a clue that the movements are really hiccups. Some believe that these are a manifestation of allergy in the child (398). Some mothers report that eating specific foods, such as milk, nuts, watermelon, or chocolate, induces hiccups in the infant. Sometimes the hiccups cease when the mother leans forward or changes position (399). The hiccups usually persist after birth.

Treatment

Traditional treatments for hiccups include breathing into a paper bag, having someone frighten you, drinking water, and holding the breath. Young children may be unable to cooperate with these methods. The parent may use a cotton-tipped swab to massage the roof of the mouth, in the area where the hard palate and soft palate join, for about a minute (400). The child may use the thumb to reach back and rub the soft palate.

Lifting the uvula, the small fleshy appendage hanging down in the back of the mouth, is often helpful. Use a spoon, your finger (for infants), or a ballpoint pen to press upward, instructing the child to breath slowly and shallowly during the procedure, and for several minutes afterward (401).

A sneeze or vomiting will sometimes relieve hiccups.

Stretching the diaphragm is said to relieve hiccups. A child may lie on his back with his head, shoulders, and arms hanging over the edge of a bed. He should take a deep breath and hold it as long as possible (402).

The hiccup sufferer may stretch the diaphragm by pulling the knees up to the chest, or leaning forward, and holding the position for a few minutes.

Other breathing treatments include breathing deeply and slowly for five minutes.

Ice packs to the sides of the neck are said to relieve hiccups.

A hot bath may be helpful.

A small child may stop hiccuping if placed on his left side for 10 to 15 minutes.

Grasping the tongue with your fingers and pulling it outward for a few minutes may be effective (403).

Older children may benefit from chewing on ice.

Variations on the drinking water treatment include bending over the glass to drink from the far side of a full glass of water (404), plugging the ears with the fingers while drinking, and drinking from a glass with a metal object such as a fork or spoon in the glass and pressing against the temple.

Older children may bend over at the waist to place his head lower than his diaphragm, then drinking a glass of cold water through a straw. He should remain in this head-down position for several minutes after drinking the water.

Children who suffer repeated episodes of hiccup may be helped by hot fomentations over the stomach two or three times a day and an abdominal bandage at night. Stomach massage is sometimes helpful.

Hiccups in nursing infants may be treated with a few teaspoons of hot water or diluted lemon juice (405). Anise or peppermint tea may also be used (406).

Pulling a young child up by the hands is often successful, but should be done gently, so as not to dislocate the arms (406).

Charcoal may be used to treat hiccups due to air in the stomach (407). Older children can be instructed to chew two tablets once an hour.

Hiccups in small infants may be cured by rectal massage (408). Lubricate a gloved finger, insert it gently into the rectum, and massage with a slow movement around the circumference of the rectum. Pressure may be applied to the pit of the stomach, below the breast bone, with the flat of the hand (409).

Foot massages are said to be helpful.

CONGENITAL DISLOCATION OF THE HIP

Some infants suffer dislocation of the hip joint before, during or shortly after birth. It is the displacement of the infant's thigh bone (femur) so that the hip socket does not form correctly.

Several factors are felt to contribute to this problem. Some feel that it is due to the infant's position in the womb before birth. It tends to run in families, is more common in girls, and is most common in the first born child. A breech birth, (hips presenting first instead of the head at the time of birth) is also felt to increase the risk of congenital hip dislocation (410), as may cesarean delivery. It is more common in premature than in full term infants. Shorter mothers are more likely than tall mothers to have infants with congenital hip dislocation, probably due to crowding of the infant in the smaller womb (411). Infants born during the winter months seem to be slightly more likely to suffer congenital dislocation of the hip (412). Some feel this is because the child is kept tightly wrapped in an attempt to keep him warm. Populations who swaddle their infants have a high incidence of congenital hip dislocation while it is said to rarely occur in populations where mothers carry their infants on the hip or back, with the legs straddling the mother's body (412).

Congenital hip dislocation is estimated to occur in one or two of every one thousand children (412), but the exact incidence is difficult to determine, as diagnosis rates vary with the skill of the examiner. Any examination should be carried out gently, and the examiner's hands should be warm. The child should be relaxed. It is felt that hormones secreted by the mother during late pregnancy to relax the mother's ligaments during the birth process to allow easier passage of the infant may affect the infant, decreasing the ability of his hip ligaments to hold the femur in place. Female infants, who have similar hormones of their own, are probably more dramatically affected by the mother's hormones (412). However, proponents of this theory are unable to explain why only one hip is dislocated in many children.

The left hip is involved about three times more often than the right. About half of cases have dislocations of both hips.

About 20 percent of infants with congenital hip dislocation come from families with other members who had the same condition (412). The child of a parent who had congenital hip dislocation has about a one in seven chance of being affected. It rarely occurs in black infants.

Diagnosis

Examinations should be done gently, as some recent research indicates that overly vigorous examination for congenital hip dislocation may actually cause it in a normal child (413).

The parent can do an examination for hip dislocation. Place the infant on his stomach, and look at the skin folds around the hips. They should be equal on both sides. If one side has more folds than the other this may suggest hip dislocation. The parent may feel a click in the hip during diaper changes.

Place the child on his back, flex his knees to 90 degrees, and see if the knee level is the same in both legs. Separate the knees and press the legs outward down toward the bed to see if the legs go down equal distances. They should almost touch the mattress on each side. Listen for a click with the maneuver.

Unequal Gluteal (Hip) Folds in Congenital Hip Dislocation

Another maneuver, called Barlow's method, is done by placing the thumbs on the inside of the infant's thighs with the fingers on the hips. The knees are brought together and pushed backwards. The examiner may feel a click or clunk in the hip, indicating dislocation. The legs are then separated and pressed down toward the mattress or examination table, with the thumbs and fingers positioned over the hip joint.

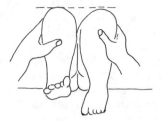

**Unequal Knee Height in
Congenital Hip Dislocation**

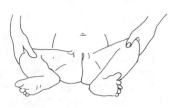

**Difference in Hip Abduction in
Congenital Hip Dislocation**

Treatment

Some feel that over half of infants whose examination suggests a dislocated hip will undergo spontaneous "cure" within the first week of life. For this reason examination should be repeated before treatment is initiated. One study of 548 hips considered to be dislocated revealed that approximately 90% need not have undergone treatment of any type. However, distinguishing those who do not require treatment from those who do is impossible, and for this reason most physicians treat all children.

A young infant may be treated by simply applying three or more cloth diapers to hold the legs in proper "frog-leg" position. Some feel that merely keeping the child resting on his stomach provides sufficient positioning to treat mild cases (414). Severe cases may require bracing, casting, traction, or even surgery.

Treatment itself is not without risk as it may produce avascular necrosis (breaking down) of the femoral head, a complication which may lead to permanent deformities of the femur.

HIVES (URTICARIA)

Hives, or urticaria, are manifest by a very itchy rash and raised pink or red spots of various sizes with pale centers. The shape and location of the spots may vary during the course of the process. They may resolve in a few minutes, or persist for several hours before disappearing. They generally last no more than 12 hours. They are an allergic reaction to some substance the child has contacted. Foods, drugs, insect bites, or viral diseases are common causes of hives. It is estimated that at least ten percent of children develop hives at some time, although most of them have them only once.

Treatment

Cool baths are often soothing (415). Two cups of baking soda or epsom salts may be added to a tub of tepid water. Pat dry after the bath. Rubbing may stimulate itching. Cold compresses are often helpful in relieving itching. Compresses made with a baking soda solution (1 teaspoon baking soda to four ounces of water) may be soothing.

A hive ointment may be made by melting three-quarters of a cup of petroleum jelly in a cast-iron skillet. When the petroleum is entirely liquid add 1 1/2 ounces of dried chickweed, and simmer gently for about ten minutes. Do not allow it to burn. Strain the mixture through a cheesecloth, pour into a jar, and cover tightly. This ointment may be applied liberally over hives. A muslin covering may be applied to prevent the ointment getting on clothing and furniture. This ointment is said to keep for about six months (416).

If the allergic reaction is felt to be due to a food the child has eaten a laxative may be given to hasten removal of the food from the body. Nuts, eggs, fish, lobster, strawberries, citrus fruits, and yeasts are common causes of food-allergy induced hives. Rather large amounts of charcoal taken in water may help to adsorb offending agents and toxins.

Drugs are also a frequent cause of hives in children. Almost any drug may be the offender. Penicillin may be found in milk from treatment of infected cows. Even tiny amounts of penicillin in milk may induce hives. Aspirin is a common offender.

Inhalants such as pollen, animal danders, plant products, mold spores and aerosols may cause hives. Wash the skin thoroughly to remove any allergenic substances from the skin.

Insect bites and stings may induce hives in sensitive children. Bees, wasps, fleas, spiders, mites, bedbugs, mosquitos, scorpions, and jellyfish may cause hives.

Scratching should be discouraged. The fingernails should be kept short and the hands kept clean.

If the child develops difficulty swallowing or breathing, a swollen tongue, abdominal pain or acts very sick he should be evaluated immediately by your health care provider.

HYPERACTIVE CHILD

Hyperactivity is a very common childhood problem today and causes major difficulties in many American homes. It is undoubtedly a major stress in many families, and may even lead to child abuse. About five to ten percent of American children are estimated to be hyperactive. The term "attention deficit disorder" is gradually replacing the term "hyperactivity." Almost all children display overactive behavior at one time or another during their lifetime.

Some have reported that blue-eyed blonds are more likely to be hyperactive. The hyperactive child squirms and fidgets, cannot remain seated for any period of time, runs instead of walks, and constantly goes from one thing to another. They must grab, poke, feel, and touch everything about them. Many hyperactive children never stop talking and they talk loudly. They make many sounds, including whistles, and clicks. Their attention span is short, they act before thinking, are impulsive, easily distracted, and forget easily. Noises, people and lights distract them. They start many projects which are never completed. They are often unable to follow a series of instructions and have a low frustration level. They are often moody, irritated, easily upset, and have difficulty concentrating. They do not understand why their parents are upset with their behavior, and may demonstrate an attitude of indifference when disciplined. They are clumsy, and have problems throwing a ball, buttoning their shirts, skipping, or even walking. Once they decide they want to do something it is difficult, if not impossible, to stop them. They often have dark circles under their eyes, leg aches, glassy eyes, and fatigue, all suggestive of allergy.

Some cases of hyperactivity are due to emotional problems or to intelligence levels. Some are due to inadequate, inconsistent, or ineffective discipline in the home. Parents often yield to the child's wishes to avoid a confrontation. Children who are often disciplined by screaming parents soon stop listening and become uncontrollable. Parents must control their own behaviors in order to have control of their children.

Spoiled children have greater control of home situations than do their parents. When such a child enters school, where controls are placed on their behavior, he or she (but more often he) may manifest overactive behavior in an attempt to control this environment as well. Parents must remember that children require consistent discipline.

A developmental deviation or lag accounts for one type of hyperactivity. These children are unable to control their behavior, as their "control center" does not develop as rapidly as does the motor division of the body. Controls catch up with motor activity by puberty, and the level of activity decreases; concentration and attention span improve.

Learning disabilities are often observed in hyperactive children. These learning disabilities are also due to developmental lags and may be outgrown with time. This type of child may be able to repair his own bike or assemble complicated models, but unable to learn to read. Many educators are now suggesting that children not be sent to school until they are eight to ten years of age, to allow time for fine muscle coordination to develop and for the brain centers to mature sufficiently to enable the child to cooperate with proper discipline. Boys suffer from learning disabilities more frequently than girls, because until puberty, their development is slower. Any child with a developmental lag, a learning disability, or hyperactivity, should have out of home schooling delayed until these clear properly, or the child may acquire a personality defect which may last a lifetime--inferiority, goody good, defeatism, delinquency, etc.

Overstimulation from television, competitive games, etc., may lead to hyperactivity. Some psychiatrists feel that the constant change of visual frames seen in television shows, as well as the content of violence in many programs, has a simulating effect on sensitive children. With the frequent change of scenes the child is trained to a short attention span. Children with overtaxed nervous systems often indulge in unfocused activity and irritability. This probably explains why a guided exercise program directed toward the large muscles of the body has been shown effective in calming hyperactive children. Gardening, yard work, and similar activities carried out with the parents will be very beneficial to the hyperactive child.

A child is three times more likely to be hyperactive if his mother smoked 23 or more cigarettes per day during the pregnancy than if she did not smoke at all. The reasons for this are not clearly understood, but it may be that the decrease in blood flow to the placenta which occurs in smokers may retard the development of the fetus.

Lead poisoning may produce hyperactivity (417).

Dr. John Ott believes that certain types of fluorescent lights are stimulating, and he cites studies in which a group of students in a classroom demonstrated behavior improvement when the type of lighting in their classroom was changed. However, this theory needs further study before it can be definitely cited as a cause of hyperactivity. Some families may wish to leave fluorescent lights off.

Some hyperactive children are easily identified, even as infants. They may have difficulty sleeping or eating (they often have colic), and they frequently crawl out of their cribs. When they begin crawling these children seem to keep their parents constantly on the run trying to keep them out of things. They may get up during the night and get into things. They may show reactions to medication the opposite of what one would expect; medications given to calm other children may keep these children up all night. They manifest peer problems as they mature. They may play well with one child, but with more than one playmate arguments break out. They usually try to control their playmates. This is cited as another reason to delay the school enrollment and instruct these children at home, especially boys.

A major effort to correct hyperactivity and out-of-control children should be made early in life since a high percentage of these children grow up to be troubled teenagers with serious problems--drugs, dropouts, depressions, crimes, etc.

Undoubtedly, the majority of cases of hyperactivity are due to nutritional factors, as discussed later.

Treatment

Regardless of the reason for their hyperactivity, overactive children respond favorably to a structured and predictable environment. The more consistency in the environment the greater the decrease in overactivity.

Consistency is the key in the management of hyperactive children. For child management to be effective the child must know that the parent means what he says. Threats like "If you do that one more time I will break both your arms," obviously will not be carried out, and the child, knowing that the parent will not actually do as he says, finds it easy to believe that he will not carry out other disciplinary measures. Overstatements train the child to disobedience, because he knows that the parent doesn't mean what he says.

Changing one's mind after giving instructions to a child leads to a fluid, unstable environment. A mother telling her child to go take his bath may be met with such resistance from the child that she decides to let him go to bed without his bath. The child learns that he can force the parent to change his or her mind.

The parent of an overactive child must check to be certain that the child has actually done what the parent instructed. A child who knows the parents will not check to see if instructions were followed may tell the parents that they were followed.

The best book in print on the subject of child management is a book called *Child Guidance* by E. G. White; Review and Herald Publishers, Washington D. C.

Another reason to check whether or not the child has carried out instructions is that this type of child is easily distracted and forgets what he was supposed to do. The child must be trained to remember.

Parents must present a united front to their child. They must have set rules and expectations. When one parent undermines the other, confusion and unpredictability result, which may be expected to increase overactivity in the child. Additionally, the child is able to play one parent against the other to get his own way.

There is a strong impression, though definite studies may be lacking, that children from broken homes are more likely to have behavioral problems such as hyperactivity.

Physical exercise may help the hyperactive child expend some of his energy which would otherwise be spent in random behavior. One study suggested that a jogging program was as effective as low dose medications in the treatment of hyperactive children. Children in the study demonstrated lower levels of aggressive behaviors on days they jogged than on days they did not (418).

A regular schedule is vital in the management of hyperactive children (419). Rising time, meals, and bedtime should be at a set time 365 days a year. A child who is accustomed to going to bed at a set time will resist less than a child who has an irregular bedtime. Established routines make the environment more stable.

When setting rules for children, parents should also state the punishment if the rule is broken. This enables the child to know what the consequences of misbehavior will be. If the child knows that the parent will enforce the rule he comes to understand that he is responsible for his own behavior, and that the things that result from it--good or bad--are caused by him.

Some children misbehave to gain attention. In many homes the only time a child's behavior is noticed is when he is misbehaving. Parents often pay more attention to mistakes, shortcomings, and failures than to successes and achievements. Not reacting to misbehavior is an effective method of discipline if properly used. Behavior that disturbs others or may produce damage to people or property cannot be safely ignored, but temper tantrums, pouting, and whining are often best ignored. Often when a child observes that the parent is ignoring his behavior he will intensify it, but this increase should not last more than five days at the most. As the child sees that the parent will not react to even this increase in inappropriate behavior he will give it up.

Recognizing a child's good behavior tends to reinforce it. If the child cleans his room, runs an errand without complaining, etc., he should be commended for it. Do not fall into the trap of paying the child or giving rewards for good behavior. However, you may remove things for misbehavior.

A study done at Ohio State University College of Medicine revealed that activities that involved spinning, such as swinging and merry-go-rounds, and playing ring-around-the-rosey helped hyperactive children to coordinate their senses, improved balance and motor coordination, calms and relaxes children, and increases alertness and attention span (420).

The physical environment of the child should be calming. Busy curtains, wallpapers and drapes should be avoided (421). Color schemes should be restful and not stimulating. The household should be kept as quiet as possible, without radios, record players, televisions or stereos playing in the background.

Diet

Recent reports have incriminated milk and dairy products, eggs, wheat, corn, citrus, peanuts and chocolate as common causes of hyperactivity.

The Feingold diet has been useful in many cases of hyperactivity. This diet eliminates all foods containing salicylates. (See Appendix 3.)

Foods containing BHT, artificial colors and flavors must also be eliminated. If after four to six weeks, the child shows a favorable response to the diet by less hyperactivity, the discontinued foods may be reintroduced to the diet, one at a time. If no increase in activity is noted after three or five days of using the food, another food may be added. Test all foods in this fashion.

A study carried out at George Washington University School of Medicine revealed that a carbohydrate and sugar rich breakfast lead to increases in hyperactive behavior, but a protein food eaten with the sugar decreases hyperactivity. It was felt by the researchers that the combination of carbohydrate and sugar produces increases in serotonin levels (a neurotransmitter) in the brain, which produces unwanted biochemical changes (422).

The diet must be strictly followed. Even a slight breakover may nullify the benefits of the diet.

Dr. Feingold suggests that the entire family go on the diet at the same time. This makes it easier for the mother and child. Food allergy is felt by many researchers to be a frequent cause of hyperactivity. Sugar and milk are considered the chief offenders, but eggs, corn, wheat, citrus, beef and pork are all frequent causes of allergic reaction. Foods that irritate the stomach or inflame the nerves must be removed from the child's dietary. That would include coffee, tea, colas, and chocolate, any vinegar products, cheese, sauerkraut, soy sauce, miso and any fermented food, baking soda and baking powder products; and most foods having very strong or pungent flavors such as spices. Sweets and highly refined carbohydrates should be strictly prohibited. They can be replaced by natural foods such as the whole grain products, both breads and cereals; vegetables and fresh fruits (fruits canned without sugar are generally acceptable); with beans, and other legumes. These foods provide an abundance of the nerve-calming B-vitamins and minerals, whereas highly refined "junk foods" not only tend to be deficient in these essential nutrients but also require more of them in order to be metabolized. It can readily be appreciated that the diet must involve a thorough reformation of the kitchen and management of spending money. A superficial attempt at dietary management is doomed to failure and has led many to believe that diet is uninvolved in hyperactivity, whereas in truth it is a principal factor.

Allergy to chemicals in the environment, such as tobacco, perfumes, formaldehyde, varnish or paint may produce an allergic reaction leading to hyperactivity.

Medications:

A 1988 issue of the Journal of the American Medical Association questions the extent of the current use of medications to treat hyperactivity (423). A 16-year study showed that every four to seven years the number of children receiving medication for hyperactivity was doubling, and in 1986 six percent of all children in public elementary schools were receiving these medications. They projected that by the early 1990s over one million children would be given these medications. They point out that studies to date do not demonstrate long-term gains, even though the medications may produce short-term apparent improvement in behavior. One must wonder if the temporary benefit outweighs the associated risks. Medications commonly given for hyperactivity may produce loss of appetite, muscle stiffness, shaking, trembling, dizziness, constipation, insomnia, headaches, stomach aches, and increased nervous behaviors such as nail biting. Some children develop allergies. There are studies suggesting that these medications also produce growth suppression. One study showed that four years of Ritalin treatment caused up to an inch of loss in expected height (424). Parents are now organizing to fight against the abuse of such medications as Ritalin. Many feel that medications should be used for hyperactivity only as last resort. They take from the child the responsibility for his own behavior, and serve as a crutch.

IMPETIGO CONTAGIOSA

Impetigo contagiosa is a common childhood skin disease. It occurs more frequently in warm climates and during warm months of the year. Peak incidence is in the two-to eight-year-old group.

Minor skin injury, such as cuts, abrasions, or insect bites allow entrance of the bacteria which cause impetigo. A red patch, often with tiny red bumps, appears followed by a blister-like lesion. If these lesions are not scratched they will often break down over a period of four to six days, to form a honey-colored lesion which heals slowly. The skin under the blister may lose its color and remain pale for several months after the blister is gone. The face and extremities are the body parts most frequently involved in the disease.

Itching is common, but scratching should be avoided, as it may spread the infection.

Treatment

Crust removal leads to a more rapid clearance of symptoms (425). The child may be bathed in soapy water every four hours during the day, or warm compresses may be applied if the disease is confined to a small area. Stubborn scabs may require a solution of one teaspoon of bleach to one quart of water to loosen them. A small amount of dishwashing detergent added to the bleach solution is felt to improve penetration of the solution. Hot and cold compresses may be used after the crusts are removed. Use water at 110 to 115 degrees for hot compresses for three minutes at a time, alternating with cold compresses wrung from ice water for 30 seconds, with five changes with each treatment. Be careful not to burn the child.

Fever therapy is said to be helpful, particularly in cases severe enough that the lymph glands are involved. Use a series of hot baths to raise the body temperature. The child one to three years of age may be put in a hot tub of water (be careful not to burn the child) for three minutes; older children may remain in the tub for one additional minute for each year of age over three. (See Table 1 in Treatment section.) Be accurate with the time, as overheating may be quite uncomfortable. Keep the head cool with the use of a fan or washcloths dipped in ice water.

Starch or charcoal poultices may be applied to the lesions. Camomile tea may be cooled and used to wash the lesions (426). Pat dry gently afterwards. The medical literature contains at least one report of the use of adhesive tape in the treatment of impetigo. Adhesive tape was applied over the lesions, removed, and the lesions cleansed each day and new tape applied. They reported that the treatment required four to six days (427).

The fingernails should be kept short and the hands should be kept clean, to decrease the risk of spread. Scratching should be strictly prohibited.

The hair may need to be cut short if the scalp is involved.

Pillowcases and bed linens should be washed daily. The patient's clothing, towel, washcloth, and bedding should be laundered separately from those of the rest of the family (428). They should be boiled for ten minutes before laundering. Add bleach or Lysol to the wash water.

Air and sun exposure are quite helpful. Sunlight is known to have antibacterial properties.

The diet should be simple, and free from sugars and free fats.

INFECTIOUS MONONUCLEOSIS

Infectious mononucleosis ("mono," "kissing disease") is caused by the Epstein-Barr virus, a very common virus, with 90 percent of the American population exposed by the age of 21. Once the Epstein-Barr virus invades the body it remains there throughout life, with intermittent episodes of activity which permit spread of the virus in the saliva (429).

Symptoms of infectious mononucleosis are often flu-like with sore throat, headache, fatigue, fever, achiness, depression, lymph node enlargement and, in some cases, liver involvement and spleen enlargement. Lymph glands in the neck, under the arms, and in the groin are most often involved. There may be a loss of appetite, a measles-like rash, or yellowing of the skin. The disease is benign, with improvement over a course of weeks, although some patients feel fatigue for months after the illness. Spleen enlargement may persist after other symptoms have resolved. The rare instances of mortality in infectious mononucleosis are nearly always due to internal hemorrhage from a ruptured spleen. Fever may reach 103 to 104 degrees F. and may persist for one to two weeks. There may be chills. Sore throat may make eating difficult for several weeks.

When young children develop infectious mononucleosis, symptoms are often very mild. The parents often think that the child has a cold which clears up in a few days. Older children and teenagers have more severe and longer lasting symptoms. Some children, however, have such mild symptoms that the disease is never recognized.

Spread is by sneezing, coughing, and, of course, kissing. This is how it acquired the name of "kissing disease." However, it is not highly contagious, and brothers and sisters of infected children do not generally become ill. Nonetheless, the sick child should be kept away from others to decrease the risk of spread. The incubation period is estimated to be from two to eight weeks. It is most common during the teen and early adulthood years.

Tincture of time is the best treatment for infectious mononucleosis. Complete recovery takes several weeks, but the restriction of activity is often difficult for a young person to tolerate.

Luella Doub, who practiced hydrotherapy for many years, stated that 30 minutes of fever therapy daily for three days, maintaining the body temperature at 102 to 103 degrees F., was adequate to treat even the most advanced cases of infectious mononucleosis (431). In our experience, the hot bath fever therapy has produced almost as dramatic results as the use of corticosteroids, with none of their drawbacks.

Corticosteroids have been given in the past but these medications impair immunologic function (436).

Adequate fluid intake must be ensured (432), with six to eight glasses of water per day. Cool drinks are generally soothing to the sore throat but some prefer hot drinks. Salt water gargles may be used (433). Avoid acid juices such as citrus.

The diet should be light, well balanced and free of sugars and fats. A soft diet may be better tolerated if the child has severe sore throat.

Headaches may be treated with a hot foot bath (see treatment section).

No known antibiotic is helpful in treating this infection (434), and they may produce an allergic rash or other complications; they are contraindicated in this disease.

Bed rest has been recommended in the past, but it is now felt that mild activity does not have an adverse effect on recovery. Excessive activity may lead to a relapse and should be guarded against.

Physical activities should be restricted as long as the spleen is enlarged to decrease the risk of injury to this organ (435). Six to eight weeks may be required. Children will probably restrict their activities themselves due to fatigue, but vigorous and contact sports should be guarded against by the parents.

Constipation should be avoided, as some feel that straining at the stool may cause injury to the spleen (433).

Isolation of the child is not necessary, but glasses, cups and drinking straws should not be used by others.

INFLUENZA

Influenza, or flu, is a viral disease which affects sinuses, ears, nose, throat, bronchial tubes and lungs. A number of different viruses are capable of producing the disease.

Symptoms appear 24-48 hours after exposure to the disease (437). There is usually sudden onset of symptoms including muscle aches and pain, headache, runny nose, lack of appetite, sweating, sneezing, hoarseness, cough, sore throat, chills, fever, and fatigue. Sometimes diarrhea or abdominal pain are present. Muscle aches, pain, and fever generally subside over two or three days.

Spread is by direct contact with an infected person, or droplets on objects.

Treatment

There is no specific treatment for influenza (438). Antibiotics are useless in the treatment of the "flu bug." Treatment should be directed toward making the child as comfortable as possible.

Fluid intake should be encouraged. The fluid will help thin secretions, making them easier for the body to handle. Milk, however, should be avoided (438).

The diet should be light; do not urge the child to eat if he does not wish to, as long as fluid intake is adequate. Use a sugar-free, low-fat diet if the child is willing to eat.

Care should be taken with the child's eating utensils. Disposables which are discarded after use are often preferred.

A cool mist vaporizer should be used to humidify the air. Steam inhalations are often helpful (439).

Over-the-counter nosedrops should be avoided. Use saline nosedrops (see cold section for instructions on how to prepare them). It is often helpful to have the child blow his nose gently, instill the nose drops, wait three minutes, then have the child blow his nose again. The procedure may be repeated if the nose is not clear. Parents should suction the nasal passages of young infants who have not learned to blow the nose. (see common cold section for procedure).

Avoid the use of aspirin as it has been associated with Reye's syndrome (437), a serious condition that may cause death or severe central nervous system disability. Muscle aches may be treated with warm baths and massage. The room should be cool, but the child should be protected from drafts. Particular care should be taken to keep the arms and legs warm.

A hot half bath, fomentations to the chest and back, followed by cold mitten friction, or a neutral bath (see treatment section) may be used for fever control (440).

A hot foot bath may be used for headache and nasal congestion. Salt water gargles are helpful for the sore throat. This may be carried out for ten minutes every one to four hours. The child may find a soft diet easier to swallow.

Backrubs are often soothing to the child, and are felt to stimulate the immune system to fight disease. Be careful to avoid chilling during the procedure.

An enema may be given at the first symptom of the flu. The bowels should be kept open during the illness.

INGUINAL HERNIA

An inguinal hernia is the protrusion of some of the abdominal structures into the inguinal or scrotal area. It is about nine times more common in males than in females, and occurs on the right side more often than on the left. They occur bilaterally about 20 percent of the time (441). There is often a history of inguinal hernia in other family members. It is estimated that about 40 percent of all inguinal hernias appear before the age of six months, and half appear between one and five years of age (442).

In premature infants inguinal hernias are more common in girls, and are more often bilateral.

Inguinal hernia may be present at birth but may not be observed until the child is three or four months of age. The parent may notice a bulging when the child coughs, strains or cries (442). The bulge may subside spontaneously, or may resolve with gentle pressure over the area. An ice pack may be applied over the area and the child placed in a position with the hips above the head if the hernia does not resolve with gentle pressure. There are usually no symptoms other than the bulge as long as the hernia remains easily reducible. However, in some cases the neck of the sac closes about the protruded abdominal structures, trapping them in the sac and producing what is called a strangulated or incarcerated hernia, which may require emergency surgery. The child may cry with pain, vomit, have abdominal enlargement, redness and swelling of the area, or bloody stools with an incarcerated hernia.

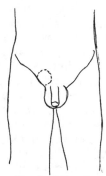

Inguinal Hernia

The only permanent solution to inguinal hernia is corrective surgery, which can be done simply and easily by a skilled surgeon.

ITCHING

Itching may be due to a number of conditions. We will discuss general principles of treatment, which should be adapted to the condition being treated.

Dry skin often causes itching (443). Baths should be short and cool, with avoidance of the use of harsh soaps. Liquid castile soaps made with olive oil are not strongly alkaline, and are usually well tolerated. Baby or mineral oil may be applied to the skin after getting out of the tub. Moisture is trapped under the oily layer and serves as an effective moisturizer.

The application of heat in the form of very hot water can be an effective measure in the treatment of itching. Some individuals with insect bites, poison ivy, or other skin conditions obtain immediate and complete relief, which lasts for several hours, with the application of very hot water (about 110 to 115 degrees F.). This hot water treatment is most suitable for small areas of itching; if large areas require treatment the water should be applied to only a small area at a time. Brief applications with a wash cloth or running water may be effective if the water is sufficiently hot. Care should be taken not to burn the child during the treatment. Diabetics and others with decreased blood flow are readily burned (444).

Ice applications are often soothing in itching (445). Cool compresses or ice packs may be used. Use heat or cold, depending on which seems the most effective.

Itching skin may be soothed by wetting the area with water, dipping the fingers in water, then in salt, and rubbing the involved area with the salt sticking to the fingers. The writing physician reports that initially there is a sensation of burning, which is followed by a feeling of coolness with disappearance of the itching (446). Salt applications should not be used in conditions which would be worsened by the abrasive action.

A slippery elm ointment may be helpful in the treatment of itch. Combine one-half cup of olive oil and three tablespoons of powdered slippery elm bark in a cast-iron skillet. Fry gently for about five minutes, being careful not to let it burn. Add two tablespoons of cocoa butter, and when it is completely melted continue cooking the mixture for about ten minutes. Strain the mixture through a cheesecloth. Pour the liquid into a jar which can be tightly closed, and refrigerate until the ointment becomes firm. The ointment keeps for about two months (447).

A sage leaf tea bath is often helpful in itchy skin diseases. Combine four ounces of dried sage leaves to two quarts of water, and simmer gently for five minutes. Remove from heat and allow the leaves to steep for 15 minutes. Strain out the leaves, and pour the tea into the bathwater. Allow the child to soak for about 20 minutes in the tub, remove, and pat dry. The bath may be repeated daily until the condition improves.

Another bath solution may be made by combining one-half cup of rolled oats, one-half cup of pearled barley, and two quarts of water in a pot, and simmering for 20 minutes. Strain the liquid, and add to the bathwater.

KNOCK-KNEES (GENU VALGUM)

Knock-knees are common in the two-to-six-year-old child (448). It has been estimated that 22 percent of children between the ages of three and three-and-a-half years have knock-knees, but only one to two percent of seven year olds still demonstrate it.

The inside of the child's knees seem to almost touch when he is standing straight. Knock-knees seem to develop as the child outgrows his bowlegs, at around two years of age. In most children this is a normal developmental pattern, but professional evaluation may be required if the change in one leg is more marked than in the other, if there is more than three-and-one-half inches of distance between the insides of the ankles when the child stands with his knees touching, if the child does not seem to be growing properly, or if there may be some metabolic abnormality in the child.

LARYNGITIS

Laryngitis is an inflammation of the lining of the voice box (larynx). This may be caused by a cold or other infection, allergies, smoking, or overuse of the voice.

Symptoms include hoarseness or complete loss of the voice, and sometimes cough. There may be fever, scratchy throat, loss of appetite, and a general feeling of illness. Symptoms may last for up to two weeks.

The child should be instructed not to talk (or even whisper) until his voice returns (449). Children old enough to write may use notes to communicate. He may be given a bell to ring if he needs attention, and he should be provided with book, toys, and games for quiet entertainment.

Hot compresses may be applied to the throat every three hours.

A heating compress may be applied to both the throat and chest at bedtime, and between treatments during the day (see treatment section).

Steam inhalations for ten to fifteen minutes are said to be helpful (450). A steamy, hot shower may provide the same effect.

A hot foot bath is excellent for the voice.

An ice bag may be applied to the throat (27). Cold compresses may be wrung from ice water and applied to the throat (452).

Extra rest may be called for, and over-fatigue should be avoided.

Extra water should be taken to assist the body in the elimination of toxins. Some find cool fluids soothing; others prefer hot.

White oak bark tea is one of the finest treatments to restore the voice. Use one teaspoon of white oak bark from a health food store to one cup of boiling water. Let it set for twenty minutes, then strain. Give four to six times a day. Children up to three years of age should be given one tablespoonful; from three to seven years of age give one-fourth cupful; from eight to twelve or thirteen years of age the child should be given one-half cupful; and teenagers and adults can take a full cup.

Water is a good cough medicine. Encourage the child to drink water with every coughing episode.

Gargling with warm salt water may relieve the itchy sensation in the throat (453).

LICE

Three types of lice commonly infect man--Pediculosis capitis (head louse), P. corporis (body louse), and P. pubis (crab louse).

Head lice are usually found on the scalp and hair at the back of the head and behind the ears. Children and people with long hair are most frequently infested. The tiny nits (eggs) are laid at the base of a hair shaft; as the hair grows the firmly attached egg moves away from the scalp. Itching and the appearance of lice and eggs are the most common symptoms. The tiny nits may look like dandruff to the casual observer, but the nits are not readily combed out.

Head lice may be spread by coats hung together, caps, scarves (454), carpets, upholstered furniture, bedding, coat hooks, earphones, pets, combs and brushes.

Adult lice live about 30 days. The female may lay about ten eggs per day, producing hundreds of offspring.

Body lice live mainly in the clothing, chiefly in the seams. They migrate onto the body for their twice a day feedings.

Crab lice are transmitted chiefly by sexual contact and are generally localized to the genital region. The chief symptom is itching. Inspection reveals tiny black or rust-colored dots clinging to the base of the hairs. The lice may spread to infest the hairs of the chest, beard, and eyelashes.

Because lice are extremely contagious the entire family should be inspected for infestation. Many recommend treating the entire family even if they show no signs of lice. Use a magnifying glass to check all hairy parts of the body.

Many feel that lice are a sign of lack of cleanliness but this is not necessarily the case.

Since simple measures are effective in eradicating lice, there is little justification for using toxic pharmacologic agents. Lindane (Kwell) and pyrethrins (RID) are the two most widely used treatments for lice. Lindane has been reported to induce convulsions (455). The Environmental Protection Agency has suggested that lindane (Kwell) be banned as it is reported to cause cancer, birth defects, nerve damage and aplastic anemia. Pyrethrins (RID) are also toxic, irritating to the mucous membranes and eyes. Allergic reactions have been reported. It is especially harmful to those sensitive to ragweed pollen.

Treatment

Body lice may be eradicated by laundering the clothing and bedding in hot water. A 30 minute very warm soaking bath with soap will kill any lice which may be on the body. The lice are generally on the body only for feedings, then return to the clothing. Body lice will leave a person with a fever, or one overheated by exercise.

Sprays are sometimes recommended for use on carpets and furniture, but they are no more effective than vacuuming.

Combs and brushes may be soaked for an hour in 2 percent Lysol, heated in water to a temperature of about 66 degrees C (151 F.) for five to ten minutes, or frozen for about 30 minutes.

Bedding and clothing should be washed and dried in the hot cycle of the washer and dryer. Unwashable items may be deloused by sealing in a plastic bag for ten days, as the lice will hatch out and die in that period.

Dousing the hair with kerosene and wrapping it in a towel is an old remedy for head lice. Equal parts of olive oil and kerosene or vinegar and kerosene, or vinegar and rubbing alcohol may be applied to the scalp to get rid of the eggs. Allow the solution to remain on the hair for a couple of hours, shampoo thoroughly and inspect the head for lice. Remaining lice should be combed out.

Toilet seats should be wiped frequently, and carpets and upholstered furniture vacuumed frequently.

Flowers of sulfur compresses may be made by mixing with water to make a paste. Work the paste into the hair and scalp. An alternative method is to simply cake the dry flower of sulphur on the scalp. Either way, a towel is then wrapped around the head and worn all night. Cover pillows, as the sulfur is a bit hard to wash out.

Garlic compresses applied directly to the scalp and worn for two hours are smelly, but effective. Blend several garlic cloves with water in a blender; work the solution into the hair and onto the scalp. Wrap with a towel.

Hot vinegar applied to the hair may loosen eggs and allow them to be combed from the hair with a fine-tooth comb or picked off with tweezers.

A 1:1 vinegar-water rinse followed by vigorous combing with a fine-toothed comb will assist in nit removal (456).

Lice of the eyebrows may be treated with petrolatum applied thickly twice daily for eight days, followed by combing with a fine-tooth comb.

Pennyroyal oil mixed with an equal amount of alcohol may be dabbed on the scalp of the patient. Rub it into the scalp thoroughly, especially about the hairline and ears; allow it to remain ten minutes, then shampoo thoroughly.

Eight grams (2 1/2 tablespoons) of rue (*Ruta graveolens*) may be boiled in 200 gm. (1 cup) of water and used to treat lice.

Itching may be soothed by a warm baking soda bath (457).

Citronella oil may be applied to the hair and the head covered with a bathing cap or hat to slow evaporation (458). Shampoo the hair after eight hours. Comb or pick out nits. The odor will disappear in a few hours. (Some people are allergic to citronella oil-- if itching, burning, or other adverse effects occur, immediately wash the citronella from the hair.) Citronella is available in many drugstores.

MEASLES (RUBEOLA)

Measles is another of the common childhood diseases and occurs even in immunized populations.

The peak incidence is in preschool or early school years (459). It is readily spread in groups. Measles outbreaks occur most often in temperate parts of the world in the winter and early spring months.

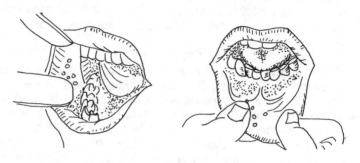

Koplik's Spots with Measles

Symptoms begin ten to twelve days after exposure as typical cold symptoms of dry, barking, hoarse cough, sore throat, fever, sneezing, fatigue, runny nose, and red, irritated eyes. The eye irritation may progress to conjunctivitis. Lymph glands often become enlarged. These symptoms worsen over three to five days. Koplik's spots appear about a day before the rash begins (460). These bluish-white bumps that look like salt grains surrounded by

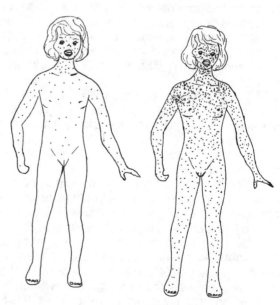

Typical Measles Rash
A. First Day   **B. Third Day**

a red circle typically begin on the lining of the mouth beside the lower molars and spread, then disappear as the rash progresses. They are most readily seen in bright daylight.

The rash begins to appear on the fourth to sixth day after onset of the initial symptoms. It is a blotchy, flat, pink rash which typically begins on the temples, scalp, hairline, behind the ears and on the face and neck, and spreads down to the feet over the next two or three days. The rash usually blanches under pressure early in the course of the disease but becomes darker as it progresses. The rash may enlarge to run together in patches. The skin may swell and become edematous. There may be slight itching associated with the rash. The child is most uncomfortable on the fourth or fifth day of the illness (second or third day after the rash begins). The fever drops as the rash begins to subside. The child may also complain of abdominal pain, muscle aches, vomiting and diarrhea. Chills may accompany the fever.

Treatment

The diet should be light, but the child often has little or no appetite. Do not be concerned if he refuses solid food. Adequate fluid intake is essential, particularly during fever. The child should be kept quiet, but not necessarily in bed if he is not very ill. If the temperature exceeds 101 F. the child may be sponged with cool water (461). Be careful not to irritate the skin while sponging (462). A patting motion rather than rubbing is recommended. A hot bath (see treatment section) of one minute's duration for each year of age may be repeated every two hours. Aspirin should not be given for fever as it has been associated with Reye's syndrome. Dress the child lightly and avoid overheating. The room should be well ventilated but the child should be protected from drafts. (A draft is a current of air that chills the skin.)

If itching does occur the older child can be taught to press the area rather than to scratch. The fingernails should be kept short and the hands washed frequently to decrease risk of infection. Cold baths are sometimes helpful in relieving itching. Cornstarch or oatmeal baths (see treatment section) may be used.

The child may be sensitive to light and more comfortable in a darkened room or wearing sunglasses. If he is not light-sensitive, light will not damage his eyes. Wipe the eyes frequently with a clean, wet cotton ball (460). Inflammation of the eyes may be treated with hot fomentations over the eyes and forehead for 15-20 minutes. Charcoal poultices (see treatment section) may also be used.

The cold-like symptoms are not helped by decongestants. The continuously running nose may cause irritation between the nose and upper lip. The application of a thin layer of petroleum jelly may protect the skin. Fomentations to the chest, with a hot foot bath (see treatment section), twice a day, may be used for cough. Use a heating compress (see treatment section) overnight. Cough medications are usually ineffective. A humidifier may be used for the cough (461). Water is a good treatment for cough. Drink some with every episode of coughing. Salt water gargles and rinses are helpful for sore throat and mouth, as are mouth washes of goldenseal tea. A heating compress (see treatment section) may be used for sore throat.

Headaches may be treated with hot foot baths (see treatment section), or hot and cold compresses (see treatment section) to the head.

Antibiotics are useless in the treatment of measles. They are sometimes given in the hope of preventing complications but may cause them. Proper care and previous good nutrition will go far in preventing the development of complications. Complications are more frequent in children who suffer from chronic malnutrition. No one with a cold or sore throat should be allowed near a child with measles, as this increases the chances of complications.

A young child developing otitis media (ear infection) may be unable to vocalize his complaint. Watch for ear pulling and irritability. Ice may be applied to the throat on the affected side. See the section on otitis media for other treatments.

Measles encephalitis probably occurs in 1 of every 10,000 to 100,000 cases of measles. A rising fever, vomiting, headache, drowsiness, stiff neck, pain on straightening the leg after it has flexed up on the abdomen, convulsions and coma call for examination by your health care provider.

Measles is contagious from three to five days before the rash occurs, and continues to be contagious until the rash is gone. Nose and throat secretions, droplets sprayed by coughing or sneezing, or direct contact with freshly soiled articles are sufficient to spread the infection. Complications of pneumonia, eye infection, or ear infection are fairly common, and should be watched for and treated at the first sign.

The Measles Vaccine

This is a highly controversial immunization. Adverse effects include encephalopathy, hardening of the brain, paralysis of eye muscles, arthritis, hyperactivity, learning disabilities, incoordination of muscle movements, mental retardation, one-sided paralysis, painful joints, meningitis, seizures, and perhaps, encephalitis, multiple sclerosis, allergic shock, Reye's syndrome, Hodgkin's disease, cancer, diabetes, Guillain-Barre syndrome, and blood clotting abnormalities, among others.

Ironically, the vaccine has not been shown to be effective. Over 80% of measles cases in some outbreaks occurred in people who had received the measles vaccine! While vaccine manufacturers claim that the decreasing incidence of measles is due to their product, Dr. Robert Mendelsohn pointed out that in 1962, the year before the vaccine was developed, the annual number of cases in the United States dropped by 300,000 cases from 1958. A 30 state survey conducted in 1978 revealed that more than half of the measles cases occurred in fully vaccinated individuals. Meanwhile, a World Health Organization study revealed that those who have been vaccinated are 15 times more likely to catch measles than those who are unvaccinated!

MENSTRUAL PAIN (DYSMENORRHEA)

Menstrual discomfort is said to occur in at least half of all adolescent females, but it is possible that the incidence is much higher than 50 percent, as many girls consider it normal and do not seek a remedy. Dysmenorrhea is the leading cause of school absence in adolescents. It is felt to be due to uterine muscle spasms. Dysmenorrhea does not generally occur for six months or a year after menstruation begins, when ovulation normally begins. Symptoms include abdominal pain and cramping, backache, leg pains, headache, mood changes, nausea and vomiting, diarrhea or constipation, fatigue, fluid retention, and sometimes fainting. Symptoms usually begin a few hours before the bleeding begins and subside within a day or two. Symptoms vary in nature and intensity from girl to girl, and even from one period to another in the same girl.

Dysmenorrhea is classified in two divisions: primary and secondary. Primary dysmenorrhea is menstrual discomfort for which no physical cause can be found. This is the most common type and our discussion will be directed toward this type. Secondary dysmenorrhea occurs in association with such diseases as endometriosis or pelvic inflammatory disease.

Treatment

The knee-chest position is helpful for some (463). (See anal fissure for illustration).

The diet should be light and simple, and should consist largely of fresh fruits and vegetables. Overeating encourages abdominal congestion. Girls who suffer edema (water retention) with their periods may benefit greatly from using a low salt diet, beginning a week prior to the onset of the period (464). See Appendix 3 for a low salt diet. Remember that all dairy products are high in salt!

A heating pad or hot water bottle to the abdomen or back is often soothing (465). The best relief experienced by two young ladies came from applying a heating pad to the back from the waist to the end of the spine, beginning an hour before the expected onset of pain (with the first discomfort or show of bleeding). Keep the heat as high as can be tolerated for one hour. Often this brings complete relief. Others prefer warm baths.

Some girls report greater pain relief with the use of an ice pack over the abdomen (466).

The girl should indulge in regular out-of-doors physical activity on a daily basis. Activity should be continued to tolerance during menstrual periods. It has been shown that women who are physically fit have less discomfort with their menstrual periods (467). Waist-bending exercises are felt to be the exercise of choice, along with leg exercises. Walking up 100 steps every day and back down again will help approximately 80 percent of women.

Overweight women have higher rates of dysmenorrhea than women of normal weight (467). Reduce your weight to normal or slightly below normal if you are overweight.

Regularity in rising time and bed time to assure adequate rest is essential in the treatment of painful menstruation.

Good posture will assist in pain relief. An exercise for improving posture is as follows: The patient stands about 18 inches from a wall with the heels and toes together, and the side of the body toward the wall. The elbow is placed against the wall at shoulder height, and the forearm and hand rested against the wall. With the shoulders perpendicular to the wall and the knees straight, contract the abdominal and hip muscles and shift the hips toward the wall, attempting to touch the wall. The exercise should be done three times a day, a total of nine stretchings per day. One study reported that mild cases reported relief after about one month of exercises, moderately severe cases after about two months, and severe cases after three or more months.

Dr. L. J. Golub reported success with a twisting and bending exercise. The girl stands with the feet parallel and about 15 inches apart. The arms are outstretched to the side, at shoulder height. Keeping the knees straight, the girl twists the trunk to the left, bending down and touching the floor (or merely stretching toward the floor) with the right hand in front of the left foot. She returns to the starting position and repeats the exercise on the other side. The first week the exercise should be done four times daily. During successive weeks the exercises should be increased by two each week, until a total of ten repetitions per side are performed daily. Some patients reported relief with the next period but most people required several months before relief occurred (468). The author cautions that the exercises should not be started during a period, as they may worsen the pain.

Painful menstruation may be due to food allergy (469). D. R. Smith, M.D., reported 12 cases of painful menstruation, vaginal discharge and irregular menstrual periods, who were tested for allergies. The foods they demonstrated sensitivity to were eliminated from their diets, beginning one week prior to the expected menstrual period. Eight of the twelve in the study received complete relief of their symptoms: the remaining four had partial relief. Milk, eggs, wheat, nuts, chocolate, fish, beans, cauliflower, cabbage and pepper were common allergens in this study, but other foods may be involved. (See list of most common food allergens in Appendix 1.)

One physician who has studied dysmenorrhea says that women who have diaphragmatic (abdominal) breathing have no dysmenorrhea. Constriction of the breathing movements by tight clothing induces rib breathing, reducing the use of the abdominal muscles and diaphragm, and causing pelvic congestion. She recommends the following exercise: The girl should remove all clothing and lie on her back on a flat surface. She should flex the knees and place the arms at the sides to assist in relaxation of the abdominal muscles. One hand is placed on the abdomen to assist in evaluating the amount of movement of the abdomen. The woman attempts to raise the hand as high as possible by lifting the abdominal wall, and then see how far she can lower the abdominal wall. The exercise should be repeated ten times morning and evening in a well-ventilated room. Jerky movements should be avoided, and a smooth respiration sought for. Initially this deep breathing may induce some dizziness, but with repetitions she will be able to complete the exercise without discomfort.

A four-minute back massage to the area an inch to the right of the spine in the lumbar ("small of the back") area may bring relief of menstruation associated pain. The person doing the massage stands over the patient, and with the heel of the hand puts as much pressure as the patient can bear to the right of the waist and rotates three to four times. Move the hand an inch downward and repeat, continuing to the end of the spine, and back up again several times for the full four minutes.

Some receive considerable relief from the use of a hot sitz bath (105 to 115 degrees F.) with a hot foot bath (110 to 117 degrees F.) for three to ten minutes. Some have had good results with a cold sitz bath (55 to 75 degrees F.) for two to ten minutes, with friction (470).

Because toxic shock occurs most frequently during the menstrual period, the girl who uses tampons should change them every three to four hours during the day and use pads during the night (465).

Brief rest periods, with the feet elevated may be helpful (464).

Some girls are comforted by hot herbal teas such as alfalfa, red raspberry leaf, catnip, peppermint, or chamomile. Coffee and tea should be avoided (471).

Constipation should be avoided. See the section on this topic for further information.

MITRAL VALVE PROLAPSE

Mitral valve prolapse is the most common heart abnormality in children and adolescents (472). Estimates of its incidence range from 5 percent to 20 percent of the population. It occurs in males and females in about equal distribution. The variant is generally first noticed in mid-childhood. There

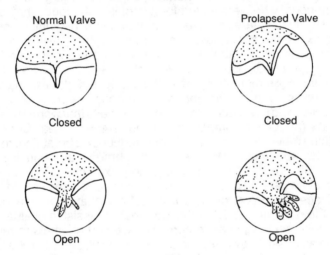

Normal Valve   Prolapsed Valve

Closed   Closed

Open   Open

Normal Mitral Valve

appears to be an associated family history (473). Some say that it is more common in thin young women, but others dispute this observation. Emotional stress may increase the intensity of the abnormal heart sounds heard (513).

Diagnosis can be made with the stethoscope in most cases and does not require extensive medical testing (474). The physician will hear an abnormal heart sound, described as a click. This is produced as the mitral valve (the valve which allows blood to flow from the left atrium of the heart into the left ventricle) flops closed. Some valves are thinned and do not close tightly; in these cases the physician will hear a murmur as blood leaks backward in the heart. This backflow is generally not sufficient to cause any problem for the heart.

There may be symptoms of palpitations or chest pain in some children, but most cases of mitral valve prolapse are discovered incidentally during a routine physical examination or at the time of some other medical problem.

A study of over 200 people revealed that chest pain, shortness of breath, and fainting did not occur more often in those with mitral valve prolapse than in those who did not have it, suggesting that associated physical symptoms may be due to causes other than the mitral valve prolapse. Mitral valve prolapse is generally a benign disease, although it has not been considered so in the past. Thousands of children have had their physical activity restricted, and even become "cardiac cripples" because of the fear of heart problems. We now understand that in most cases this is a normal variant in healthy children. Unfortunately, many parents (and children) become overly concerned over their health when they learn that they have a mitral valve prolapse. Physicians have subjected many children to unnecessary diagnostic procedures and to repeated follow-up for a harmless condition (475).

Only 3.6 percent of a group of children with mitral valve prolapse were shown to have any other medical problems.

The child should be permitted to engage in physical activities and should be encouraged to achieve and maintain a high level of physical fitness with daily out-of-doors exercise.

Deep breathing exercises, breathing in slowly and deeply with expansion of the abdomen, followed by slowly releasing the inhaled air is helpful in relieving stress.

Like everyone else, children with mitral valve prolapse should eat for a healthy heart. The diet should be low in salt and fat. Overeating should be guarded against. Overweight should be avoided. Extra pounds require the heart to work harder to pump blood through additional tissue. Caffeine should be avoided, as it is known to induce palpitations.

MUMPS (EPIDEMIC PAROTITIS)

Mumps is another of the common childhood diseases whose incidence has decreased in recent decades. It is most common between the ages of

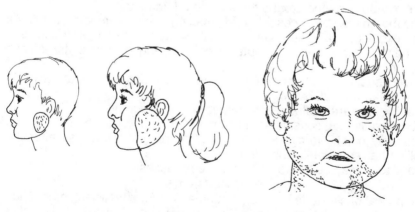

Parotid Gland
A. Normal Gland   B. Gland in Mumps   **Mumps**

5 and 15, and rarely occurs before the age of three. Spread of infection is by airborne droplets or direct contact with contaminated objects, and may occur 48 hours before the onset of swelling and for nine days afterward. Epidemics most often occur in the later winter and early spring months. The incubation period ranges from 12 to 22 days, but is typically 16 to 18 days. It is felt that 20 to 40 percent of mumps cases are not recognized as such because of the lack of swelling (473). These people may never know that they had mumps.

Typical symptoms include swelling of the parotid gland, fever, lack of appetite, abdominal pain, and headache in older patients. There may be pain on eating, opening the mouth, or talking. Parotid swelling may occur on one side or both; the opposite side often becomes involved two or three days after the initial swelling. It is said that 70 percent of children have bilateral swelling (474). Swelling usually reaches the maximum on the third day, and then begins to subside slowly. The amount of swelling is indicative of the severity of the disease.

The fever usually subsides in three to four days, and swelling and pain usually disappear within seven days (474).

Treatment

Fever may be treated by cool sponging or hot half baths (see treatment section). A 20-minute neutral bath twice a day will be helpful in reducing fever, as may a cold mitten friction or cold towel rub. See treatment section for procedure.

The diet should be light and fluids should be encouraged (473). Some have jaw pain with acid or sour foods, and should not be given citrus, pickles, tomatoes or highly seasoned foods (476). Foods should require minimal chewing (474).

Because the pancreas may become inflamed during mumps some recommend the use of a low fat diet during mumps.

Cold compresses may be applied to the swollen area for pain relief (474). Some benefit from the use of an ice collar. Others report greater pain relief with warm compresses, hot water bottles, or hot towel applications. A large scarf may be wrapped around the neck to retain heat.

The mouth may be excessively dry, making oral care important. Others report excessive salivation. Saline mouth washes and careful cleansing of the mouth after eating contribute to comfort and decrease risk of oral infection.

Fever usually ranges from 100 to 104 degrees F. It may be treated by cool sponging, or hot half baths.

Medications are ineffective in the treatment of mumps.

Bed rest is not considered essential, but the child should be kept reasonably quiet. Normal activities may be resumed one day after the swelling has completely subsided.

Headache may be treated with cool compresses.

Complications

Complications include orchitis (inflammation of the testicles), more common in males 15 to 29 years of age. Symptoms usually appear 3-8 days after onset of the mumps. Initial symptoms of orchitis are often rapid in onset with lower abdominal pain, fever elevation, headache, chills, nausea and vomiting. The scrotum swells and becomes red. The testis becomes enlarged and bluish in color. Symptoms usually begin to resolve in four days. Tenderness may persist after the swelling subsides. Support of the testes by an athletic supporter or a towel under the scrotum and ice applications (473) are said to be helpful, although some prefer the use of heat. Some suggest the use of tight-fitting pants or a stretch bathing suit to provide warmth and support. Antibiotics are ineffective. There is no evidence that keeping the child in bed reduces the incidence of orchitis, which may occur in 30 to 40 percent of post-pubertal males. Infertility as a result of mumps orchitis is rare. Typically only one testes is involved in the inflammatory process.

Pancreatitis (inflammation of the pancreas), mastitis (inflammation of the breast), and oophoritis (inflammation of an ovary) are occasional complications. Mastitis may occur in one-third of females over 15 years of age. Vomiting, fever, and lower abdominal pain may be indicative of oophoritis. Meningitis (inflammation of the brain or spinal cord membrane), neuritis (inflammation of a nerve), myelitis (inflammation of the bone marrow or spinal cord), deafness, and encephalitis (inflammation of the brain) are also reported complications. Hearing loss may be regained over the course of a few weeks, but permanent deafness may also result.

If you child develops stiff neck, confusion, sudden increase in fever, drowsiness, convulsions, very severe headache, or acute abdominal pain a physician should be consulted.

Vaccination

Mumps epidemics occur in immunized populations. Allergic reactions include bruising, rash, itching, febrile seizures, nerve deafness, and encephalitis.

MURMUR, INNOCENT

An innocent murmur is a heart murmur unassociated with heart disease or abnormality. It has been estimated that 90 percent of children referred for cardiac evaluation are referred for an innocent, or functional, murmur (477). Probably every child has an innocent murmur at one time or other (478), and the possibility of proper diagnosis varies considerably with the skill and experience of the physician examining him. Most general practice physicians, who will take the time, can determine by simple listening that a murmur is indeed harmless.

There are four or five different variants of the innocent murmur, and a child may have more than one type at a time, or at various times (479).

Parents need to be aware that an innocent murmur has no significance whatsoever, and when told that his child has an innocent murmur the parent should react in the same manner he would if the doctor announced that the child had two arms. It is now understood to be a normal part of growing up. In the past many children were restricted in their activities because of these murmurs, creating a disease from a normal condition. Long term studies following children with innocent murmurs reveal no increased incidence of heart problems in adulthood, when compared to those without innocent murmurs.

These murmurs are felt to be due to vibration of the heart muscle or to the pattern of blood flow, which is easily heard in children because of their thin chest wall. The murmur may be present in adulthood but the thicker chest wall may prevent the physician from hearing it. Murmurs tend to be louder in anemic children, or children with fever. Anxiety, excitement, or exercise may also make murmurs louder (480).

Most innocent murmurs disappear by the time a child is in his mid-teens, but even if it does not, it is not a matter of concern. The child should not be restricted in his activities, nor have periodic follow-up for the murmur once it is determined that it is a benign murmur. It has been said that more children have lived restricted lives because of innocent, harmless murmurs, than have children with actual heart disease. Physicians debate whether or not the parent or child should even be told of the murmur, because of the acute anxiety that this news often produces (481).

NEONATAL JAUNDICE

Neonatal jaundice is yellowing of the skin and whites of the eyes which appears shortly after birth. It is estimated that 80 percent of newborns demonstrate some degree of jaundice, but only five percent have jaundice which requires treatment (482).

Neonatal jaundice appears to be more common in children born at high altitudes, in males, in infants born to diabetics, in infants whose mothers had hypertension of pregnancy, in those who have siblings who had neonatal jaundice, in children delivered by cesarean section, forceps or vacuum extraction, in children whose mothers had epidural anesthesia during delivery, in premature or low birth weight children, in the first born child, in children of older mothers, in mothers with blood type O, and in those who lose large amounts of weight immediately after birth (483). American Indian infants and Orientals have higher levels of bilirubin than do blacks or whites.

Red blood cells are very fragile in the newborn and are rapidly broken down. The liver converts these broken down cells into bilirubin, which is usually passed by the gall bladder into the bowel and out of the body with the stools. The liver becomes overwhelmed by the great amount of red blood cells destroyed, and the bilirubin which cannot be excreted is absorbed into the skin, causing yellowing.

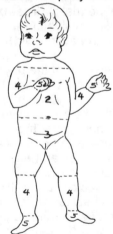

Neonatal Jaundice

The parent should watch the newborn for jaundice. The skin should be examined carefully, using natural light. If jaundice develops, the amount may be estimated using the accompanying illustration. The yellowing typically begins with the head and spreads downward as levels increase. Jaundice involving only the head suggests a level of 5-8 mg. of bilirubin/100 ml; if both head and chest are jaundiced the level is approximately 6-12 mg/100 ml., jaundice reaching to the knees suggests a level of 8-16 mg/100 ml., jaundice involving the arms and lower legs is often associated with levels of 10-18 mg/100 ml, and if the hands and feet are yellow, levels may be expected to be 15 or more mg/100 ml. (484) Some have felt that treatment should be started when levels reach 15 mg/100 ml, but others feel that waiting until levels reach 20 mg/100 ml. is entirely safe. We suggest starting at 15.

There are three main types of neonatal jaundice: physiological, breast-milk, and blood group incompatibility (ABO or Rh problems).

Physiological jaundice is present in about fifty percent of all babies. It is felt to be due to the immaturity of the liver, which is not yet able to handle bilirubin processing as quickly as it is broken down. This type of jaundice generally appears when the child is two to four days old, and resolves within the first two weeks of life. Physiologic jaundice is not dangerous in an otherwise healthy infant.

Breast milk jaundice occurs in one to two percent of breast-fed infants. It first appears when the infant is about five days of age and tends to run a prolonged course, sometimes persisting for twelve weeks. In the past breast feeding was temporarily discontinued, but more and more physicians now are continuing breast feeding, feeling that the advantages far outweigh the possible disadvantages, and it may be that mild jaundice stimulates nerve cell growth. Babies who are breast-fed are often allowed to remain in the hospital nursery overnight without being taken to their mothers, and may be given bottles of formula or water during the night (485). Children born at home may be fed frequently, rather than as convenient for hospital routine.

Blood group incompatibility occurs if mother and infant have different blood types so the mother's antibodies destroy the baby's red blood cells, leading to high bilirubin levels. This jaundice often appears within 24 hours of birth. They should be treated from birth with charcoal slurry and sunbaths if the incompatibility is known ahead of time, but certainly with the onset of jaundice. These mothers are usually given Rho GAM to prevent similar problems in subsequent children.

Treatment

Frequent breast-feeding, begun immediately after birth, stimulates bowel function. Small, frequent feedings may be very helpful in the elimination of bilirubin. In one study infants fed eight or more times per day had lower bilirubin levels than those fed less frequently (482). Dr. William Gartner, professor and chairman of the department of pediatrics at Pritzker School of Medicine at the University of Chicago, states that feedings every two hours reduce bilirubin levels. Infants who are given glucose solution have higher bilirubin levels (514), probably because they do not accept breast milk so readily, and bilirubin accumulates in the bowel as bowel movements are not stimulated. Parents should not permit nursing personnel to give their child glucose water to drink.

Adequate caloric intake is felt important in bilirubin excretion (486). One study suggested that infants who received less than 90 calories/kg/24 hours had higher bilirubin levels than those who received more calories. This may be a significant factor in breast-milk jaundice, as breast milk contains fewer calories than cow's milk. Another study demonstrated an association between weight loss after delivery and high bilirubin levels. Bilirubin is excreted with the bowel movement. A Florida State University report indicated that taking the infant's temperature by the rectum stimulated the passage of stool, and decreased bilirubin levels in newborn infants, as the bowel does not reabsorb the bilirubin into the blood stream (487). Great care should be taken to avoid injury to the rectum during the procedure. The thermometer should be inserted gently and slowly. Your lubricated little finger may also be used to stimulate the bowel action.

The North American Indians treated neonatal jaundice by exposing the infant to the sun (488). This procedure works just as well today. Commercially available light units may be purchased and are typically used in hospitals, but natural sunlight is probably just as effective. The child may be entirely undressed and placed on a blanket in the yard while the parent sits nearby. The child's eyes should be protected from light exposure and sunburn should be avoided. Change the child's position frequently, to expose all skin areas.

Some question the safety of bilirubin lights. Associated adverse effects include eye damage, growth retardation, diarrhea, hemorrhage, respiratory distress syndrome, dehydration, feeding problems, and irritability (489). Bilirubin lights have not been used long enough to convince us that they are entirely without risk.

Neonatal jaundice of any type may be prevented in some children by the administration of powdered charcoal. Charcoal adsorbs the bilirubin and carries it out of the body (490). Charcoal administration should begin early; best results are seen when it is begun at four hours of age. The charcoal may be stirred in water and given from a baby bottle. Two to three heaping teaspoons of charcoal per day are probably adequate to bind almost all bilirubin from the duodenum.

Induction of labor may contribute to neonatal jaundice and the procedure should not be entered into without careful consideration. Epidural anesthesia and some medications given during labor have been associated with increased risk of neonatal jaundice. The mother should avoid the use of as many medications as possible during the pregnancy and during labor and delivery. Even the glucose solution often given intravenously during labor is felt to increase neonatal jaundice (491). Medications given during labor and delivery may reach the infant, and cause them to be sluggish, and less vigorous suckers.

Some have reported that giving the child agar, an extract of seaweed, increases stool frequency, hastening removal of bilirubin (492).

NIGHT TERRORS (PAVOR NOCTURNUS)

Night terrors occur in about 3 percent of children between the ages of one and twelve. They are different from nightmares, in which the child may be awakened. It is a harmless disorder which is generally outgrown. They are episodes of partial awakening from sleep. They may occur several times a week and numerous times during a month, but usually subside spontaneously over a period of a few months. The child awakens a few hours after falling asleep, thrashing and screaming, and may run frantically about the room. His eyes are generally open but he does not recognize his parents or siblings. He has rapid heart rate, perspiration and rapid breathing. Attempts to comfort the child are ineffective; the child often pushes away the parents' attempt to touch him, all the while crying for Mom or Dad. Attempts to awaken him are not successful and should not be made (493). The parent should protect the child from injury by removing sharp or breakable items and locking doors or windows. Attempts at physical restraint should not be made. If successful the child

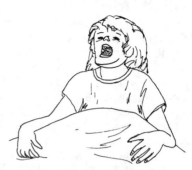

Night Terrors

will be confused and frightened and have difficulty getting back to sleep. The episode subsides as suddenly as it begins, and the child goes back to sleep. He will have no recollection of the event in the morning. Night terrors have been reported to occur during naps (494).

Night terrors occur more often when the child has a fever, when he is excessively tired, has been frightened by a bedtime story, television program, or movie, or is having irregular sleep patterns. A heavy meal before bed may cause them. Some say guilt from masturbation may produce them. They are not due to psychological problems. These children are often imaginative, articulate, sensitive and above average in intelligence (494).

Treatment

The event is more disturbing to the parents and siblings than to the child himself. Parents should remain calm during the attack and not mention it to the child who will not remember it the next morning.

The child should have either no supper at all, or only a light supper several hours before bedtime (495).

He should not be allowed to watch frightening movies or television programs. Young children cannot distinguish real from unreal concepts.

His sleep schedule should be regular with an established bedtime (496), even on weekends. If he is unusually active physically he may need a nap during the day. Sleep deprivation may increase the incidence of night terrors.

Parents are often tempted to bring the child into their bed for the remainder of the night. This should not be done as the child may wish to make it a regular habit.

In children with frequent episodes parents should keep a record of when the child's night terrors occur, and awaken the child 10-15 minutes before the expected episode. After about five minutes the child may be allowed to return to sleep. In a study group of 19 children, the night terrors ceased within one week. In some children they recurred several months later, but subsided when the parents again began awakening them. The treatment can be discontinued after the night terrors cease, generally within a week (497).

NIGHTMARES

Nightmares are very bad dreams. The child suddenly cries out in his sleep, and awakens with physical signs of acute anxiety, including rapid breathing, perspiration, and an expression of fear on his face. His pupils may be unusually large, and some children complain of chest pain or tightness, which is due to hyperventilation (overbreathing). They may occur as early as two years of age, and sometimes occur in association with illness, excessive fatigue, or stress. A sudden loud noise may induce them, and some medications are known to be capable of causing nightmares. Television of any kind can cause nightmares, as can a frightening experience. It has been estimated that children between the age of two and five spend about 30 percent of their sleep time in dreams, in contrast to the 15 percent found in adults. Nightmares differ from night terrors, in that the child can be awakened and can often recall the dream when he awakens (515).

Treatment

The parent should comfort the child in his own bed. Stay calm and speak quietly and reassuringly, telling the child that you are there to protect him. Assure him that his nightmare is not real. Make-believe attempts to "kill the monster" only make it more real to the young child, who has not yet fully developed the ability to tell the real from fantasy (498).

A regular bedtime routine should be established and carefully performed every night (499). This may include a 20 minute warm or neutral (99 degree) bath (500), story time, bedtime prayers, and tucking in by the parent. This provides a sense of security at bedtime.

Evening activities should be quiet and non-stimulatory. Exciting television programs, stimulating bedtime stories, and vigorous physical activity all induce tension which the child takes to bed with him.

If the family situation has recently changed, children may experience stress, which may increase nightmares. A new baby in the family, marital problems or divorce, a death in the family, or moving to a new home may produce stresses which the child is unable to cope with. The parents should spend time with the child, assuring him that he is still loved.

The child should have vigorous out-of-doors activities every day. This will help discharge much of the child's stress.

Some say that sleeping on the back increases nightmares. Try teaching the child to sleep on his stomach or side. A sponge ball sewed into the night clothes in the back may help the child to sleep on one side or the other.

Some nightmares are felt to be due to undigested food. The child should not be fed for about three hours before bedtime, to permit digestion to be well underway before the digestive system is slowed by sleep (501).

NOSEBLEED (EPISTAXIS)

Nosebleed is rare in infants but frequent in children. It is estimated that from birth to five years of age 30 percent of children suffer at least one nosebleed (502). More than half of children six to ten years of age suffer nosebleed. After puberty the incidence of nosebleed decreases.

Nosebleeds may be due to sneezing, nose picking, injury (such as a blow to the nose), high altitudes, and drying of the nasal membranes. They may occur spontaneously in sleep. Allergic rhinitis (hay fever) is a common cause of nosebleed in children. Nosebleed may also be due to sinusitis. Increased blood flow in the nose, as with allergy, hay fever, or a common cold, increases the risk of nose bleed.

Nosebleeds often follow upper respiratory tract infections. One study found that 62 percent of children treated for nosebleeds had suffered an upper respiratory tract infection the week before. The lining of the nose may have suffered injury during the cold-associated blowing and wiping.

Most nosebleeds stop on their own, but in most cases treatment is easily carried out by the parent. The child should be placed in a chair and instructed to lean forward over a basin. He should spit out any blood which drains into the throat. Instruct the child to breath through his mouth. The parent should firmly, but gently, pinch the soft parts of the nose, holding it for ten minutes without releasing the pressure. If the child becomes frightened the parent should assure him that they can stop the bleeding. If bleeding persists after ten minutes a gauze covered with petroleum jelly may be inserted into the nose, and the nose again pinched for ten minutes. The gauze should be allowed to remain in place for an additional ten minutes.

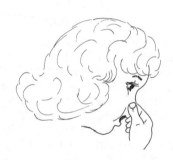

Technique for Stopping Nosebleed

The child should not lie down while he is suffering nosebleed as he may swallow or inhale blood. Vomiting may restart the bleeding. Swallowed blood may be vomited up, or may be passed in the bowel movement and cause concern for intestinal bleeding. If the child suddenly develops black stools the parent should suspect that the child has swallowed blood which has passed through the digestive system. Vomited blood will often look like coffee grounds.

In cases where the pinching has not effectively stopped the bleeding apply a cold compress or ice pack over the forehead and bridge of the nose (504).

Stubborn nosebleeds may be stopped by placing the child's hands and feet in water as hot as he can tolerate without burning (505). An alternative treatment is to place the hands and feet in a tub or pan of ice water for four to six minutes.

A clean gauze pad may be packed into the nose if bleeding is persistent. Do not use cotton, and leave enough of the pad sticking out of the nose that it can be easily removed.

Some say that raising both arms over the head will stop a nosebleed. A cold pack to the back of the neck at the hairline will stop many nosebleeds.

Do not allow the child to pick or rub the nose after a nosebleed. This may dislodge the clot which has formed.

About an hour after the nosebleed is stopped apply a thin layer of petrolatum to the lining of the nose.

Dried and cracked nasal membranes are a common cause of nosebleeds, particularly during the winter months. Indoor heating lowers air humidity. A humidifier may be used to increase humidity, or containers of water may be placed on heaters throughout the house (504). Petroleum jelly may be applied to the nasal membranes twice a day to prevent drying. A nasal saline spray made by adding one teaspoon of ordinary table salt to one pint of water may be used at bedtime.

Noseblowing during a cold should be done gently. Nasal sprays and drops used to treat cold symptoms may irritate or injure the lining of the nose, making it more likely to bleed.

Aspirin increases bleeding and should not be given to children.

Some report that a wad of cotton placed under the upper lip will constrict the labial artery and stop nosebleed.

NURSEMAID'S ELBOW

Nursemaid's elbow is also called pulled elbow and subluxation of the radial head. It is common between one and five years of age, with the greatest incidence in the 15-30 month old group (506). It is probably the most common musculoskeletal injury suffered by young children. Boys suffer it more often than girls, and the left arm is involved more often than the right (507). It occurs when the child is pulled by his forearm or wrist. The child may stumble on the steps or fall off the curb while an adult is holding his arm. The child may pull against the parent's grasp, in an attempt to go in an opposite direction. The child may fall on his outstretched arm (508). The child immediately holds his arm against his body and generally refuses to let anyone touch it.

The elbow pain is generally relieved with a simple maneuver. When the child is taken for x-ray the radiologist often replaces this dislocation (reduction) while trying to get x-rays.

If the parent is certain that the child has

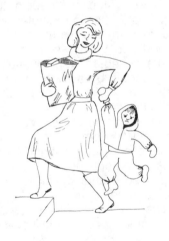

Nursemaid's Elbow

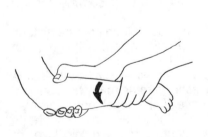

Technique of Reducation of Nursemaid's Elbow

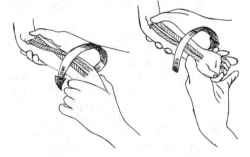

Another Reducation Technique for Nursemaid's Elbow

not suffered any other injury it is relatively easy to reduce the injury. The elbow should be flexed 90 degrees and one hand placed over the elbow as illustrated. With the other hand the forearm is rotated from a palm down position to a palm up position. As the reduction occurs a click in the elbow will be felt by the examiner. The child may cry during the procedure and for a few moments afterward, but is generally using the arm normally within 10 to 15 minutes.

About 10 percent of reduction attempts are at first not successful. If the dislocation is not reduced it is suggested that the maneuver be repeated more than two hours after the injury (506). Most reduction failures occur in fresh injuries. It may be that swelling which occurs over a period of time after the injury may make reduction easier. One case required six reduction attempts before success was achieved.

Reduction may occur spontaneously while the child sleeps, or when he supinates his forearm during activities (504).

Parents are often embarrassed or humiliated at having caused injury to the child (506). They should understand that it is a common occurrence and not an indication of child abuse.

Some children have repeated episodes of nursemaid's elbow but generally outgrow them as the child matures.

OBESITY (OVERWEIGHT)

One of four American children is overweight. There are more than 12 million overweight children in the United States alone. Overweight is the most common form of malnutrition in the United States. While obesity has not been considered unhealthy in the past, it is now understood that four of five overweight children become overweight adults. Overweight in childhood is associated with poorer school performance (probably because of poor self-image), diabetes, high blood pressure, kidney problems, increased accident rate, and more frequent respiratory problems; obesity in adulthood is associated with an increased risk of heart disease, diabetes, high blood pressure, stroke, cancer, liver and gallbladder disease, arthritis, back problems, varicose veins and premature aging. Overweight adults between 20 and 39 years of age have three times the incidence of high blood pressure of normal weight people (509).

Overweight has psychological as well as physiological implications. The typical overweight child does not think highly of himself. He feels inadequate, even disgusting, and is often self-defeating and self-depreciating. His life is often a search for love and acceptance, with a fear of rejection.

It requires the intake of 3,500 more calories than we burn to gain a pound of weight. Children and adults store accumulated fat differently, resulting in two different kinds of obesity (510). An adult stores excess fat in his fat cells. The typical adult has 30 to 40 billion fat cells, which are made bigger by the excess fat. When he diets his body takes fat from the fat cells. It is believed by many, however, that children create new fat cells rather than storing fat in preexisting cells. Excess caloric intake probably results in the production of new fat cells until a child is in his mid-teens. At maturity the number of fat cells is fixed. If the child develops excess fat cells he will have them the rest of his life. Adults who became overweight during childhood may have 90 to

120 billion fat cells and may be fat due to too many cells which they are unable to eliminate. To achieve normal weight these individuals must force their fat cells to become even smaller than normal cells. These individuals are able only with much effort to maintain any significant weight loss over a prolonged period. To further complicate matters, when these cells become smaller than their normal size they shift their metabolism into a more efficient mode, to make more complete use of what calories are available, thus slowing weight loss further.

The three months immediately before birth, the first three years after birth, and in early adolescence (about eleven to sixteen years of age) children are particularly prone to obesity.

Overweight women often give birth to heavier children. These children have already accumulated more fat cells than a smaller baby. The child absorbs more nourishment than required because of the excess on the mother's part. One study showed that infants born weighing eight pounds or more are likely to be overweight when they reach the age of six or seven years than are those who weighed seven pounds or less at birth. Thus, a child can be set for a lifetime battle with fat before he takes his first bite of food.

Overfeeding is the most common cause of overweight after birth. Breast-fed babies are much less likely to become overweight than are bottle-fed infants. Mothers who bottle feed feel that the child must finish the bottle, but a breast-feeding mother cannot see the remaining milk and allows the child to decide when he has had sufficient. In the past it has been felt that an overweight child was a healthy child. Mothers urged their children to eat a few more bites, to clean their plates, and offered food as rewards for good behavior or as comfort when the child was unhappy. The continual overeating destroyed the natural satiety level children are born with. Wise mothers realize that some days children are hungrier than other days, and allow the child to determine his own needs. Meal time may become battle time as the mother tries to convince the child to eat more. Artificially overriding this satiety signal will eventually destroy it and the individual will never regain it.

Sugar and Obesity

Sugar is responsible for much childhood obesity. The typical American eats 95 pounds of sugar per year. Seventy-one pounds of it come from commercially prepared food; only 24 pounds are sugars added to foods by the cook or at the table. Everyone knows that cake, cookies, ice cream, candy, and soft drinks contain sugar, but many are not aware that almost any food available in a can, package or bottle contains some sugar. If you doubt this read the labels on the foods you buy. Corn syrup, in reality a liquid sugar, is not counted in the 95 pounds listed above, but the typical American consumes 33 pounds of it a year.

Soft drink manufacturers account for one-quarter of the sugar added to foods. The average American is said to drink 350 twelve-ounce bottles or cans of soft drink a year. You can count on at least one-half teaspoonful of sugar per ounce of soft drink; and most have more than that.

The 95 pounds of sugar eaten annually in the United States provides us with 157,000 calories. A person who obtained adequate calories from a diet excluding sugar could gain 45 pounds per year if he consumed that many additional calories. In the United States sugar calories account for about 20 percent of the total caloric intake.

Salted snack foods such as corn or potato chips are about 40 percent fat. Furthermore, most of these snacks are consumed between meals, not only adding calories, but replacing more nutritious and less caloric foods. There are some studies suggesting that a high salt intake leads to an increased sugar intake.

Some authorities feel that merely stopping the intake of sugar will be adequate to prevent or treat obesity in a child. Refined sugar is not a natural food, and contains no food value other than calories. There are no vitamins, minerals, fiber or protein in sugar. Unfortunately, the average American is a "sugar junky." The formula for sugar is very similar to the formula for cocaine. Once the taste for sugar is acquired it may be very difficult to overcome it. We apparently become as easily addicted to sugar as to cocaine.

Never giving a child sugar is the easiest way to prevent sugar addiction. A child who is not given sugar until late in adolescence will not have the craving for it manifested by those who are given sugar from infancy. Mothers may breast feed their children, and prepare their own baby food when it is time to begin solid foods.

Parents will have to take the responsibility for preventing and controlling a young child's overweight. They must teach the child proper eating habits, just as they teach him to tie his shoes or wash behind his ears. The younger the child the easier it is to control his diet--the teenager is often impossible to control, and unless he takes responsibility for the diet he will not lose weight. Children should be trained from the first day of life to proper eating habits. Children are like blank pages in a book when they come into the world, and everything they know they learn from someone else. Eating habits are learned from parents. If parents eat between meals, use a lot of sweets, and have a bedtime snack the child will do likewise. The key to prevention of overweight in a child is proper eating habits on the part of the parents.

As soon as obesity is noticed its treatment should be started. Many people claim that overweight "runs in my family," implying that it is genetically based. They don't stop to think that one cannot make fat out of air; calories must be taken in to make fat.

The treatment of obesity requires a two-part approach: diet and exercise. A combination of too many calories and too little exercise leads to obesity.

By the time a child is old enough to have some say in his eating habits parents may have difficulty in obtaining a child's cooperation in a drastic dietary change. It may be more effective to introduce gradual changes with little fanfare with these children. Stop buying sweets, baked goods, and unhealthful foods; replace them with fresh fruits and vegetables. Always keep in mind that your goal is not merely to diet, but to change eating habits for the rest of your life.

Do not rush your child onto solid food. Children do perfectly well on breast milk until at least six months of age and at the turn of the century were not given solid food until they were about one year of age. Some obesity researchers feel that an infant's satiety level is based on the volume of food eaten. Filling the allotted volume with high caloric (sugared) ready-prepared baby foods increases caloric intake.

Some mothers feel that getting their child to take solid food before the neighbor's child is a sign that she is a better mother. They may feel that this is a sign of early development of their child, and this becomes part of the subtle competition that goes on between mothers when they discuss the age at which Johnny said his first word, took his first step, became toilet trained, or any of a few dozen other developmental skills.

To make your own baby food, puree simply prepared foods without added salt or sugar, blend and freeze in ice cube trays. After they are frozen they may be popped out of the individual compartments and wrapped in plastic or a plastic bag. You may remove one of the pieces and thaw it at mealtime. Many mothers feel that they are depriving their child if they do not add salt or sugar to their diet, but they should remember that the child knows nothing about these foods and unless they are trained to like them they will never miss them.

Typical babies double their birth weight in five or six months. They often gain about two pounds per month during the first three months; by six months of age the weight gain slows to about a pound a month. Four to six pounds of annual weight gain may be expected in a two to six year old child. Children who do not exceed these rough guidelines are not likely to become overweight.

The years before a child reaches six years of age are the most important in determining whether or not a child will become obese. Fortunately for the parent, these are the years that it easiest to control the child's diet and to teach him proper eating habits. The child should never be allowed to eat between meals, and by one year of age he should be on a regular, three meal a day schedule. If the child is not hungry at mealtime he should not be forced to eat, but should be calmly and quietly told that he will have to wait until the next regularly scheduled meal if he does not choose to eat this meal. Many children will refuse to eat what is set before them because they know that if they complain of being hungry an hour or so after the meal they will be given a cookie or other snack food. Then they are not hungry for the next meal and the cycle continues.

Television and Obesity

Television is a significant contributor to childhood obesity. Children see advertisements for highly sugared breakfast cereals and other snack foods and demand that their parents buy the foods for them. These foods are very low in nutritional value, but high in caloric value.

Television also encourages obesity by discouraging physical activity. The obese child often prefers television to playmates because playmates make fun of their obesity. Furthermore, they are often more clumsy than their slimmer counterparts and do not do as well in sports and physical activities. They tire more readily than non-obese children. A 1982 study revealed that United States children aged six to twelve years spent 24 hours a week watching television. A Boston study revealed that obesity increases two percent for every additional hour of television viewed each day in the 12 to 17 year old group (511).

Snacking and television watching often go together. The types of foods eaten while viewing television are typically the kind the child sees advertised--high in sugar, fat, and salt.

Some parents, without realizing it, give their children television instead of attention. It is easy for a parent to sit his young child in front of the television set to keep him entertained while the parent goes about other activities. This type of "babysitting" results in not only flabby bodies but also flabby minds. If parents were to encourage physical activity such as bike riding, walking, or going to the beach, the child's body and mind would both be improved and the child would enjoy quality time with his parents.

Behavioral Methods of Weight Control

The first step in weight control is getting an adequate breakfast. A child who does not eat breakfast wants a midmorning snack, decreasing appetite for lunch. Oftentimes those who skip breakfast feel that they have a caloric allowance which they can use on other foods (generally snack foods high in fat and sugar). A University of California study showed that overweight teenagers were usually breakfast skippers. Meals should be eaten sitting at the table--not running about the house, in front of the television, or even standing in front of the refrigerator. Eating episodes should not be associated with any other activity--no television, reading, or listening to music. Giving attention to the eating process will assist the body in feeling satisfied.

Exercise

Dr. Jean Mayer very wryly states that "The best diet is exercise." Exercise not only burns calories, but assists in appetite control. Vigorous exercise has been shown to decrease the appetite. A University of Pittsburgh School of Medicine study revealed that increasing physical activity by 40 to 50 percent above normal before lunch caused the children to eat 20 percent less at lunchtime (512). Non-competitive sports are preferable, not only because of the psychological stress associated with competition, but because overweight children are often not graceful or well-coordinated and are embarrassed to perform at a lower standard than their counterparts. This embarrassment will discourage physical activity. Non-competitive activities such as walking, bicycling, helping with house and yard duties, and swimming are preferred. Exercise replaces fat with muscle, making the child look stronger and healthier. It also improves his self-image, something overweight children usually have problems with.

For young children a chart listing the forms of physical exercise and the associated energy expenditure may enable the child to select a wide variety of exercise. If the child understands that if he burns 3,500 calories more than he takes in he will lose one pound. he can determine how long a specific type of exercise must be carried out to lose one pound. Some have found that walking is accepted more readily by youngsters, and performed more faithfully than other types of exercise. Some weight control programs actually go so far as to give the child a pedometer to measure how far he walks each day. A brisk 30 minute walk will burn 150 calories; 12 hours of walking will burn a pound of fat. The person should not think in terms of walking 12 hours in one day, but rather an hour or so a day on school days and more on weekends. Walking one hour a day for a year could burn off

25 pounds. Rapid weight loss is not the goal; a lifestyle change is the challenge.

Following is a chart giving estimates for various types of activity and the caloric expenditure involved:

Exercise	Calories Per Hour	Hours To Lose One Pound
Walking	300	12
Bicycling	500	7
Roller Skating	600	6
Ice Skating	375	9
Swimming	600	6
Tennis	500	7
Table Tennis	250	14
Calisthenics	300	12
Jogging	500	7

Keeping a food diary for a two week period may show some eating problems. If one has to think about how much, where, why, and with whom he eats he may become more aware of the subconscious stimuli to eating, thus allowing him to develop alternative lifestyle patterns. If Bobby knows that he always eats when he comes in from school he can plan to play outdoors then, removing himself from the environment associated with eating.

Eating is often due to stimuli other than hunger: boredom, fear, frustration, loneliness, sociability and even habit is responsible for much obesity. Television watching may become a signal to eat. Parents should discuss these facts with the child and help find alternative activities.

Keeping a food diary also helps the child to feel a sense of control and accomplishment. He comes to feel that he is doing something for himself. He will probably be amazed to see how much or how often he eats.

Do not fall into the practice of weighing the child on a daily basis. Every two weeks is a satisfactory timetable for children. Ordinary bathroom scales are often not accurate enough to serve the purpose, but may serve as a rough guideline. If the child can be weighed by the school nurse or in a physician's office the measurements will be more accurate. Remember that two to four pounds a month is quite an acceptable weight loss. Even having no loss of weight, but merely allowing the child to grow to the desired weight by adding height is often satisfactory.

Go through the house today and discard all high calorie and junk foods, especially margarine, oils, and anything made with fats. Read labels. Resolve to never buy them again. You have proven your present diet leads to obesity.

Second helpings may be discouraged by not placing food on the table. Serve the food out on the plate (a small plate makes the portions look more generous) and do not place serving dishes on the table. Place a dish of raw fruit or vegetables on the table for those who feel deprived if they do not have seconds. These foods are low in calories and are quite filling.

Instruct the child to chew each bite until it is a cream. Overweight people often eat as if they were afraid the food was going to be taken from them if not eaten immediately. These people can consume an excess of calories before their satiety level catches up, about twenty minutes after the start of the meal in many people. Putting down the fork or spoon between every bite discourages rapid eating. After the food in the mouth is thoroughly chewed and swallowed pick up the eating utensil and take another bite. This slows the eating process to allow the body to send its satiety signal before the child has time to overeat.

Some parents have tried sending their children to "fat camp" to lose weight. Many obesity specialists feel this is unwise. While the child may lose 20 pounds at camp, when he comes home he will be under the same stimuli that produced the overweight, and will regain the weight. The lifestyle must be corrected, and these changes must be persisted in the rest of the child's life--not just the few months it may take to lose some weight. This may lead the child to believe that he has to be at camp to be able to lose weight; that it is impossible to do so at home.

The caloric restriction for a young person must be carefully planned. Excessive caloric restriction may retard growth. The diet should be plentiful in fruits and vegetables. Most meats contain high levels of fat; hamburger, a teenage favorite, is often 30 to 60 percent fat. Processed meats such as liverwurst, sausage, frankfurters, salami and bologna are all high in fat.

Whole grain breads are more filling than white bread. Use fresh fruit instead of sugary desserts. Drink plain water in place of soda pop.

Do not fry foods. A teflon-coated cooking pan makes oil unnecessary and spares many unnecessary calories.

Vegetables should be eaten with as little preparation as possible. Extensive chopping or cooking destroys vitamins and minerals. Canned vegetables almost always have sugar added to them. Potatoes are not fattening--it is what we put on them that puts on the pounds.

Prepared breakfast cereals should be used with great caution. Many of them are 57 percent sugar. Read the ingredients of any cereal before you put it in your shopping cart. Television advertising is designed to get children to demand these cereals, and parents will have to be prepared to deal with these demands if they allow television. Breakfast is probably the most important meal of the day and should be planned with care.

Many overweight children protest that they should not be fat because they do not eat any more than their slimmer peers. Sometimes it is true that they eat no more than others, but they may be less active, burning fewer calories, and therefore weighing more.

Always keep in view the concept that habits that have been present for years will not be changed overnight. It is a day-by-day effort, but one that will repay both parent and child with the satisfaction and health benefits of normal weight.

OSGOOD-SCHLATTER'S SYNDROME

Osgood-Schlatter's syndrome is a common problem in teenagers. Symptoms include knee pain and stiffness. There may be swelling about the knee and tenderness to pressure. It may occur in both knees at the same time. Pain is often worse with jumping, running, or climbing stairs. It is common in teenagers who participate in sports. It often occurs during or shortly after a growth spurt (516). It is generally a self-limiting process and will subside as the child grows. It is more common in boys, probably because they are more athletically active. It occurs earlier in girls than in boys, most frequently in 8- to 13-year-old girls and 10- to 15-year-old boys. Figure skating and gymnastics may produce symptoms in girls (517). Symptoms typically subside over about a two year period.

The cause is not fully understood, but it is felt that overuse of the joint is a contributing factor. There is overgrowth of bone at the attachment of the patellar tendon. This bone overgrowth may cause a protuberance.

Treatment

Formerly, children with Osgood-Schlatter's syndrome were restricted from physical activity. Now most orthopaedic physicians feel that the child should determine his own level of activity. If the child has pain with a certain activity he should avoid it or at least restrict it. Swimming or bicycling may often be participated in without pain, but activities such as running may need to be limited or eliminated.

Quadriceps-strengthening exercises may be helpful after the acute pain subsides. They will improve muscle strength.

An ice pack placed over the knee is often helpful in reducing pain.

Daily gentle massage will improve blood flow in the area.

An elastic bandage worn during activities may reduce pain.

Quadriceps stretching exercises should be performed during a warm up period prior to exercise.

Steroid injections are sometimes recommended, but some caution that this (or the use of any pain medication) may produce pain relief sufficient to permit the child to unknowingly stress his leg, producing permanent injury. Some have used surgery in the past, but we suggest the above treatments, always remembering that the symptoms generally subside spontaneously.

PICA

Pica (pie kah) is the persistent intake of food or non-food items. Common substances include paint, ice, soil, clay, ice, grass, starch, plaster, paper, coal, chalk, pebbles, hair, insects, buttons, and cigarettes (518). It is estimated that half of all children in the one- to three-year-old group have pica. Most children outgrow it by five years of age. It seems to be more common in areas of low socioeconomic status. Some state that it is more common in blacks. Pica in children is often associated with behavior disorders such as temper tantrums and hyperactivity.

Pica typically begins in early childhood, during the stage when the child puts everything into his mouth in his exploration of the world around him.

The cause is not clearly understood, although a number of reports have appeared in the medical literature of improvement with iron supplementation. Many pica sufferers have anemia and treatment of this anemia leads to resolution of the pica (519). Others cite studies showing low calcium levels in pica. Some have suggested that the pica is actually the body's attempt to get the missing nutrient, but the substances eaten are usually very low in the deficient nutrient. Some attribute pica to stress.

Adverse effects of pica include excessive weight gain, toxins from substances consumed and displacement of wholesome foods. Some substances, such as clay, may reduce nutrient absorption by binding nutrients to them. Lead poisoning may occur if the child eats old lead-based paints which are found in many old houses. Cribs may be painted with lead-based paints which the child swallows after chewing on the crib rails. Intestinal obstruction may occur from balls of grass, hair, fabrics, etc.

Treatment

The child should be carefully watched, and should not be allowed to eat these foreign substances. As the child matures he will distinguish foods from non-foods.

Give one teaspoon of powdered charcoal stirred in a little water drunk through a straw twice daily in midmorning or midafternoon (or two capsules or four tablets). This may reduce the craving and is very helpful to adsorb any toxic substance (except heavy metals like lead) which may have been eaten.

Because many of the substances eaten are crunchy some suggest that the child should be given a diet high in crisp, crunchy finger foods such as whole grain crackers or zwieback, celery, radishes, or carrots (520). These provide chewing experiences for the child.

Pica is twice as common in children who live in homes having pets as in homes without pets (521). Many of these children eat the pet's food. Some think that the children are merely imitating what they see the pet do.

Children who eat non-food substances are often heavy milk drinkers (522). They sometimes refuse solid foods, but consume large amounts of milk. Remove all dairy products from the diet to try to eliminate the craving. Milk is known to produce anemia in children.

Try to avoid problems by recovering or eliminating hazardous or problem materials or objects. Lead paint should be removed down to the original wood. Painted plaster must be removed or covered with new wallboard.

PINKEYE (CONJUNCTIVITIS)

Conjunctivitis is an inflammation of the conjunctiva, the membrane which covers the eye (523). The white portion of the eye may become red. It is sometimes called "pinkeye" and is probably the most common eye problem in children. The eye becomes red, swollen, and produces a discharge which may be watery, yellow, green, or contain pus. While it causes discomfort it generally does not cause pain, although the child may report a sensation of sand in the eye. It may be caused by infection, allergy, chemical or physical irritation. Recovery usually occurs within one to three weeks.

Allergic conjunctivitis may be due to animal danders, pollen, dust, chemical additives, food allergies, medications, swimming pool chemicals, cosmetics, tobacco smoke or air pollution. Children suffering from allergic conjunctivitis typically have redness and itching of the eyes, but no discharge.

Allergic conjunctivitis may be distinguished from other types by the "mag" sign. To check for this gently pull the lower eyelid down while the patient gazes upward. A bulging crescent or half-moon shape is apparent between the sclera and inner edge of the conjunctiva.

Vernal conjunctivitis usually appears in the spring and may continue throughout the summer, clearing in the winter. These children complain of light sensitivity, tearing, itching, and mucous discharge.

Catarrhal conjunctivitis is the most bothersome type. The eyes are red, itchy, burn, and are sensitive to light. The child may have other allergic symptoms such as itchy nose, sneezing, and swollen eyelids. The discharge is thick and may contain pus. The discharge may be so profuse that the child may awaken in the morning unable to open his eyes which are sealed by the discharge. A gentle cleansing with warm water and clean washcloth may open the eyes. This variety is highly contagious and care should be taken to avoid spread. Conjunctivitis-causing bacteria may be carried on towels, clothing, paper, toys or hands. Launder bed and bathroom linens separately from those of other family members. All family members should wash their hands frequently. Keep fingers away from the face.

Conjunctivitis typically occurs in association with the measles.

If the child reports decreased vision or pain, or if you notice that the pupils are irregular, you should consult your health care provider.

Treatment

Cool compresses may prove comforting. Dip four to six thicknesses of gauze or cotton cloth into ice water and wring dry enough to prevent dripping. Place over the inflamed eye, refreshing it as it warms.

The eyes should be gently sponged several times a day with a cotton ball soaked in cool water (523).

Raw grated, blended, or sliced potatoes may be applied to the eyes.

Older children may be more comfortable wearing dark glasses. Do not use eye patches.

Conjunctivitis-carrying bacteria may be carried on towels, clothing, paper, toys, or hands.

The child should not be permitted to rub or touch his eyes, and should wash his hands frequently.

Some children suffering from allergic conjunctivitis are benefitted by a milk-free diet (525).

The child who is prone to conjunctivitis should be protected from chilling, as skin chilling lowers conjunctival temperature and decreases the ability of the conjunctiva to resist bacterial invasion (526).

CONJUNCTIVITIS OF THE NEWBORN (OPHTHALMIA NEONATORUM)

Ophthalmia neonatorum is an inflammation or infection of the conjunctiva of the eye during the first month after birth. There are three common types: chemical, Chlamydial, and gonococcal.

In 1883 gonorrhea was common in pregnant women and many newborns became infected during the passage through the birth canal. This infection often led to blindness. Chlamydial conjunctivitis typically begins five to 12 days after birth, with swelling of the eyelids and the conjunctiva (lining of the eyeball), and redness. There may be a discharge from the eyes.

Gonorrheal conjunctivitis typically appears two to four days following birth, with swelling of the eyelids, inflammation and swelling of the conjunctiva, and profuse discharge from the eyes.

Some bacteria are capable of causing conjunctivitis in the newborn.

These typically begin when the infant is about five days old.

The routine use of antibiotics to prevent neonatal conjunctivitis is cause for concern, as it is known that germs, over time, are able to build up a resistance to antibiotics, making the antibiotic ineffective.

Infants who remain in the hospital for prolonged periods after birth may be exposed to germs in the nursery. Children born at home are at decreased risk of this exposure.

Some feel that the sterile water flushing associated with the silver nitrate administration may have been the factor responsible for the decreased incidence of conjunctivitis of the newborn. If the flushing fluid is saline, heated to 108 degrees and flushing is continued for one full minute, gonococcal germs are very likely to be killed, as they are quite sensitive to even slight heating or chilling. Immediately after the hot saline flush apply an ice water compress, changed every 15 seconds to the infected eyes. Continue the compresses for five minutes. Watch the infant over the next five days for symptoms of conjunctivitis. Get a culture of secretions right away if gonorrhea is suspected.

PINWORMS

Infestation with pinworms (*Enterobius vermicularis*) occurs at one time or another during the lives of most school children. It is said to be most frequent in five to fourteen year olds. The disease is readily spread, and may occur in epidemics. Eggs are capable of infesting another host within about six hours of being laid. Once swallowed they release larvae, which become adult worms, and travel outside the rectum to lay eggs on the skin of the buttocks.

Pinworms are not considered a serious health problem, but they can cause irritation to the hapless sufferer. There is usually intense itching around the anus, and there may be sleep disturbances and irritability due to lack of sleep (527). The slender, quarter-inch long female worm comes out of the anus during the night to lay her eggs, which produces the itching and irritation, and then she crawls back into the anus or dries up. In young girls these pinworms may enter the vagina or urethra (urine tube) producing vaginal and urinary tract infections, and sometimes even bedwetting. A single female pinworm may deposit 10,000 eggs (527), which are designed to survive in even unfavorable conditions. The eggs are too small to be seen by the naked eye and may adhere to door knobs, drapes, and even dust which may float through the air. The child who touches the eggs and then puts his hands into his mouth is readily infected. Thumbsuckers and nail biters are particularly likely to acquire pinworms.

The parent can diagnose pinworms by applying a piece of adhesive tape to a tongue depressor or even the finger, and rubbing or pressing it firmly around the child's anus after a night of sleep while the child is still asleep. This should be done at least two hours after the child falls asleep to be most likely to pick up eggs. The pinworms come out at night while the child is quiet, and this is the only time they may be expected to be found outside the body. The eggs stick to the tape. The tape may be placed under a 10X to 45X magnifying glass or microscope to inspect for eggs. This test should be repeated for six or seven nights in a row, as pinworms may easily be missed on a single examination (527).

Visual inspection may also demonstrate the pinworms. Using a flashlight quickly check the anal area while the child is sleeping (527). This is easier to accomplish if the child is sent to bed without underwear. Inspection must be rapid as the pinworms will quickly retreat back into the anus in response to light. Lights in the room should not be turned on;

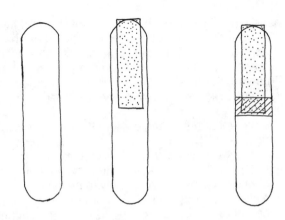

Method of Preparing for Pinworm Exam: Begin with tongue blade and adhesive tape. Wrap tape sticky side out over edge of tongue blade. Wrap a second strip of tape around center of tongue blade to hold tape in place.

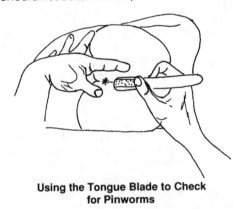

Using the Tongue Blade to Check for Pinworms

the flashlight should be the only light. Pinworms appear as tiny white threadlike creatures, usually less than one-quarter to one half inch in length. This examination should be carried out on six or seven successive nights if worms are not found.

Pinworms are occasionally noticed on the outside of a child's stool. Some recommend that a gloved and well lubricated finger be inserted into the child's rectum, and stool obtained. This may also produce pinworms for examination.

Because pinworms are so highly contagious it is often necessary to treat the entire family to bring about total eradication of the problem.

Treatment

High doses of garlic have been reported effective (589). Use one to four cloves per day for a week depending on the size of the child. Some have reported success with the use of garlic tablets (four to twelve per day) or other forms of dehydrated garlic, but it is likely that fresh garlic is most effective. One physician reported good results with the use of a garlic sandwich made by mixing raw garlic with grated carrots and salad dressing and spread over bread. The garlic should be taken daily for two weeks, stopped for a week, and then taken again for another two weeks.

A garlic rectal suppository is said to be effective in those who do not wish to eat garlic. Use one tablespoon of charcoal four times daily by mouth at the same time a garlic clove is inserted as a suppository. Instead of the clove of garlic, oil of garlic may be combined with cocoa butter, chilled to make firm, and inserted for five nights in a row, with the treatment routine repeated after three weeks.

Likewise, onions are said to be effective in the treatment of pinworms (528). Cut up two onions and allow them to soak in one quart of water for 24 hours. Strain the mixture, and give the child teaspoons of the fluid to drink periodically throughout the day. The solution may be diluted with additional water if the child can be persuaded to accept it more readily in that state. The child should be given an enema before this treatment is started.

A hot or cold water enema using three tablespoons of salt per quart of water may be helpful (529). Use very hot or ice cold to stimulate the reflex to expel the enema. A child under three years of age should be given only one cup of solution, a four to eight year old two cups; three cups may be administered to a nine to twelve year old, and four cups to a teenager or adult. This enema should not be repeated for at least 24 hours. If it is not expelled naturally, insert a finger (well lubricated with petroleum jelly) and massage the lining of the rectum until the salt water is expelled.

Blueberries are reported effective in the elimination of pinworms. The child is given a pint of fresh blueberries four times a day for the first day, then once a day for the following six days (530).

Some say that two raw carrots a day for two days are helpful (531).

All clothing and bedding should be washed frequently in hot water. Care should be taken not to shake the bedding while removing it from the bed as the eggs may be shaken out into the room (532).

All family members should be instructed to wash their hands carefully before meals and after using the toilet. Toilet seats used by infected persons should be wiped with salt water (three tablespoons of salt per quart of water).

The fingernails should be kept short and clean. A brush should be used to clean the nails before bedtime, and nail biting should be discouraged.

Underwear should be changed frequently and laundered promptly in hot water.

The child who has pinworms should not sleep with other people. The child's sleeping room should be cleaned daily. Dust may carry eggs and should be avoided. Dustcloths should be dampened with diluted household ammonia. It is said that closing the house for two days and maintaining a temperature of 97 to 99 degrees will destroy all the eggs. Sunlight is known to kill pinworm eggs, and should be allowed into the house to the greatest extent possible (533).

A hot epsom salt sitz bath may decrease the itching associated with pinworms. Add 1 1/2 cups of epsom salts to one gallon of hot water and have the child sit in it for 20 to 30 minutes. The sitz bath may be given twice a day. Petroleum jelly is also said to soothe itching and may be applied at night to decrease scratching.

It may help prevent reinfestation to dress young children in a one piece sleeping suit, so they are unable to touch the rectal area when they scratch (534).

Children infected with pinworms should shower rather than take tub baths and should use separate washcloths for face and body. The anal area should be washed in cool water morning and evening.

PLEURISY

Pleurisy is the inflammation of the membrane which covers the lungs and lines the walls of the thorax and the diaphragm. These membranes become irritated and rub together with each breath, producing pain. A grating or rasping sound may be heard through the stethoscope or with an ear to the chest as the membrane rubs together. Pain is increased when the patient tries to breathe deeply, cough, or sneeze.

Although most pleurisy nowadays is the result of a relatively benign viral infection, it is important to know that it may be a sign of a much more serious disorder. These include underlying pneumonia, tuberculosis, and even cancer. If there is excessively high fever, prostration, coughing up pinkish sputum, or failure to improve quickly, a physician should be consulted immediately.

Treatment

Fomentations may be applied to the chest continuously until the pain is relieved, and then for ten minutes every two hours (535).

A tight bandage over the chest is often effective in relieving pain.

A hot water bottle may be applied over the painful areas between fomentations if the child is comforted by it. Some children find cold applications, such as ice packs, more effective in providing comfort.

Be careful to keep the child warm, and away from drafts. Sudden, jarring movements often increase pain. Move the child gently and slowly.

PNEUMONIA

Pneumonia is a common childhood disease. It is an infection of the lungs, which may have spread downward from the throat and nose. It may involve only a small section of lung, or both lungs. Involvement of both lungs is sometimes called double pneumonia.

Pneumonia is classified as lobar, bronchopneumonia or interstitial pneumonia, according to the area of the lungs involved. Lobar pneumonia involves the lobes, or large divisions, of the lungs. Bronchopneumonia begins in the tiny bronchioles of the lungs. Interstitial pneumonia is generally confined to the alveolar walls.

Fungi, bacteria or viruses may cause pneumonia. The disease is not highly contagious, and if another person catches the infecting organism from the patient it may produce only mild symptoms such as a sore throat, or no symptoms at all. Viral pneumonia often follows an upper respiratory tract infection such as a cold. The child gradually develops a dry, hacking, nonproductive cough, and increased respiratory rate; his temperature may reach 100 to 104 F. Bacterial pneumonia is generally of sudden onset. The child has respiratory distress sometimes associated with chest pain, and a high fever.

Symptoms include fever, cough, rapid and sometimes difficult breathing, chest pain and sometimes abdominal pain.

Treatment

Fluid intake should be encouraged. This will thin secretions in the lungs, making them easier to cough up.

Children with fever and shortness of breath should be kept quiet, with limited activity. Pneumonia-associated fatigue may persist for several weeks after some types of pneumonia.

Increase air moisture with a cool air vaporizer (536). Change the bed clothing and bed linen as they become damp to prevent chilling.

A hot foot bath (see treatment section) may be used for headache, or to assist in nasal stuffiness. It may also be used to increase body temperature to assist the immune system with mild temperature elevation. The head should be kept cool with washcloths wrung from ice water if the temperature goes above 100-101 degrees F. by mouth, or 101-102 degrees F. by rectum.

Steam inhalations may be given for fifteen minutes every two hours to thin secretions.

Fomentations may be used to the chest every two hours. Keep the heat up for 10-12 minutes, then sponge off vigorously with a cold cloth. Repeat the cycle three times in a series. Dry the chest. Repeat the series as often as every two hours.

A heating compress may be used between other treatments, and at night.

For patients who are not very sick give a hot half bath, followed by a cold water pour and vigorous dry sponging.

Coughing is often helpful in bringing up mucus or sputum, and should not be treated with medications to prevent this function. A heating pad or hot water bottle applied to the chest may ease chest pain, but some receive more relief from an ice bag (524).

The child may be more comfortable in a semierect position. Others prefer to lie on the involved side.

Stuffy nose in infants can be cleared with the use of a bulb syringe as described in the Colds section.

Postural drainage may assist in mucus removal.

Infants with pneumonia should have their position changed every two hours. The head of the mattress may be raised.

Garlic is noted for antibiotic-like, antifungal, and perhaps even antiviral effects; it may be used to good effect in pneumonia. Perhaps one of the easiest ways to administer garlic to a child is to use liquid Kyolic, the Japanese aged garlic preparation. It can be given by a dropper to infants, and up to a teaspoon three times daily in older children.

Recently we have noted that fenugreek tea can be very helpful in relieving the wracking cough associated with bronchitis or pneumonia.

The child should be protected from chilling.

The child's room should be adequately ventilated to allow an abundance of fresh air, but he should not be placed in a draft.

Since pneumonia may vary markedly in severity, from a mild illness not much different from a bad cold, to a rapidly progressive life-threatening condition, the child's progress should be monitored closely. Chills and high fever, rapid shallow respirations, cyanosis (blue color) of lips or skin, or delirium are ominous signs; a physician should be seen immediately.

If treatment of most pneumonias is early, careful, and vigorous, it can usually be controlled.

POISON IVY

About half of Americans are sensitive to poison ivy, which may grow as a vine or upright shrub. The leaves are found in clusters of three, one on the tip of the stalk, and the other two opposite each other. The irritating substance, urushiol, is found in the plant sap and may be carried to unsuspecting victims by animals, tools, or clothing. Even smoke may carry tiny droplets, which may cause symptoms. If a child accidentally gets in poison ivy he should be bathed with soap immediately, and his clothing washed using an alkaline laundry detergent or soap. Waiting more than an hour after exposure makes the bath ineffective. An animal which has been in poison ivy should be washed immediately. Anyone working around poison ivy should wear gloves and long clothing to prevent skin contact.

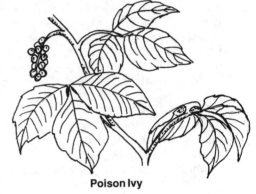

Poison Ivy

Symptoms include severe itching, blisters, and redness and swelling of the skin. Onset of symptoms may begin six hours, or several days after exposure. Symptoms may be expected to subside entirely within two to three weeks.

Treatment

Pain and itching may be relieved in several ways. Ice cubes may be rubbed over the area for twenty minutes at a time, several times a day, allowing the area to air-dry afterward. Compresses dipped in ice water, and applied over the area are also soothing. Some prefer a saline solution made by adding two level teaspoons of salt to a quart of water. Dip clean cloths into the water, wring out enough to prevent dripping, and gently place over the affected area. Change the compress every three or four minutes for an hour, allow the area to dry for an hour, then repeat as needed for symptoms.

Vinegar or lemon juice are reported helpful. Apply liberally to the area. Some prefer to dampen salt and rub it gently into the affected area.

Hot water, as hot as can be tolerated without burning oneself, is often very successful in stopping itch due to any cause within a minute or two (537). The treatment may be repeated as often as necessary.

Goldenseal tea may be used as a rinse or compress. Powdered goldenseal root may be dampened with a bit of water and applied as a paste.

The nearly transparent membrane from between onion sections, or a very thin slice of onion, can be applied to a patch of poison ivy with much relief.

Oatmeal may be ground finely in a blender, dampened with a bit of water to make a paste, and applied (538). Dampened baking soda or epsom salts may be used in the same way (539). An oatmeal or cornstarch bath (a cup of cornstarch or oatmeal) in about 4 inches of lukewarm water in a bathtub is often soothing. Some use about three pounds of epsom salts to a tub of cool water. Pat dry after the bath.

Aloe vera gel is also said to be helpful (540). Banana peel rubbed over the area may be helpful. Others prefer to melt wax, and apply it to the itching area using a small cotton swab (541). Over-the-counter poison ivy medications are often ineffective and may induce allergic reactions.

The child's fingernails should be kept short and clean, and he should be discouraged from scratching, which may contribute to infection.

Sweating aggravates the itching, so the child should be discouraged from strenuous activities that induce perspiration, and should take a shower immediately after swimming.

If the child develops difficulty breathing, severe swelling, or high fever, he should be seen by his medical care provider.

PRICKLY HEAT (MILIARIA RUBRA)

Prickly heat is a common skin condition in children from a few days old upward. It is very common during the first two weeks of life. The immature sweat glands are not functioning properly. It is more common in hot, humid climates, and in overweight children. However, it may occur even during winter months if the child is overdressed. It may also occur with a fever. Some say that ointments applied to the chest to treat colds may contribute to prickly heat.

Children with light complexions seem more inclined to suffer heat rash. Common sites are the diaper area, cheeks, neck, scalp, upper chest, shoulders, back, underarms and skin creases. There may be many tiny pinhead sized pink or red bumps, or even small blisters. They sometimes itch, and the child may scratch them.

The problem may be prevented by keeping the baby or child cool. Avoid overdressing, and use only cotton clothing. Synthetic fabrics such as dacron or nylon should be avoided.

The careful use of a fan or air conditioner is often helpful. Sunbathing should be avoided until the problem clears.

Wet compresses may be used to soothe the itch and also help to cool the child (542). Dip a piece of clean cotton material, such as old bed sheets, in cool water and apply over the affected areas. Freshen the compresses every three to four minutes, as they warm up. Continue for an hour, then allow the skin to air dry. Some like to use a mixture of one part vinegar to three parts of water as the compress solution (543). The treatment may be repeated throughout the waking hours.

Cool baths may also be used, but soap, bubble bath, and oily substances should be avoided. Some like to add one-half cup of baking soda, oatmeal or cornstarch to a small tub of water for bathing. Allow the child to air dry after bathing. Ointments should be avoided as they block sweat glands.

Cornstarch powders are drying and soothing (544), but avoid powders that contain talc.

Encourage fluid intake, and reduce salt intake (545).

Do not use any binding material on the child, such as adhesive tape, plastic, or wet diapers (546).

Symptoms should subside in two to three days (547).

PSORIASIS

Psoriasis is a common childhood disease, although it is rarely seen before the age of three years. The cause is unknown, but there is often a family history. One type of psoriasis frequently follows tonsillitis. Children with chronic psoriasis often continue to have the disease in adulthood.

The outermost layer of skin is produced at a rate six to nine times faster than normal in psoriasis. The scalp, skin behind the ears, arms, legs, hips and back are the most common sites. The scales are often associated with itching.

It has been estimated that two to four percent of Americans suffer psoriasis. It is estimated that 37 percent of psoriasis sufferers have onset before the age of 20. Psoriasis in children is more common in females.

Treatment

The diet should be simple. One man, who had suffered psoriasis for seven years, reported complete clearing of his symptoms when he eliminated meat from his diet (548). Some have successfully used a diet consisting of raw fruits and vegetables, with entire disappearance of the lesions within 12 weeks of beginning the diet (549).

Several patients have reported improvement of symptoms in a diet low in tryptophan. Milk, cheese, and meat all have high levels of tryptophan.

Dairy products, meat, eggs, and poultry are all high in arachidonic acid, a substance broken down by the body into various chemical substances, one of which causes swelling and redness of psoriasis lesions. Persons with psoriasis should use a diet free of these substances (550). The addition of two to four heaping teaspoons of ground flaxseed daily will provide beneficial omega-3 fatty acids which are anti-inflammatory.

A low-fat, sugar-free diet may produce considerable improvement. Psoriasis may be associated with a disorder in fat metabolism (551).

The rice diet (rice and fruit) developed for high blood pressure patients, apparently improves psoriasis in patients who have previously been treated unsuccessfully with various medications (552).

Obesity seems to exacerbate psoriasis. Overweight children should be placed on a weight reduction program.

Some people have improvement with a gluten-free diet. Wheat, rye, barley, and oats contain gluten (553).

Local heat applications have been shown helpful to some. Heat may be applied to the lesions for 30 minutes, two or three times weekly, for a total of six to ten treatments (554).

Alternating hot and cold may help. Apply the heat for two minutes, the cold for two seconds, with alternations continued for 15 to 20 minutes daily (555).

Fever treatments may be used for those who have extensive lesions. Fill a bathtub with water hot enough to raise the body temperature to 102 to 104 degrees. Maintain the fever for 20 to 45 minutes. The head must be kept cool, using ice bags or wash cloths wrung from ice water. Treatments may be given five times a week, if the patient is able to tolerate them. It may require three or four weeks before improvement is noted.

Salt water baths are reported helpful in many psoriasis cases. The program involves four to six hours of sunbathing, interspersed with 20 minutes of sea bathing. Four to six weeks may be required for symptomatic improvement. A cup or two of salt may be added to bath water if you do not live near the sea.

Waterproof tape has been shown to be very effective in the treatment of psoriasis lesions (556). A young lady suffering from psoriasis had a skin biopsy. After the biopsy the physician placed an ordinary Band-Aid over the area. When she returned three weeks later, with the Band-Aid still in place, it was observed that the area covered by the tape had completely cleared, but the area under the pad was unchanged. The doctors were so impressed with this that they covered the remaining areas of psoriasis with adhesive tape and again observed clearing of the lesions. They began studying various types of tapes and dressings on a number of patients, with amazing responses, in which many of them remained clear for as long as a month after application of the tape. Waterproof tape was found to be most effective. Application of the tape continuously for a week or more was more effective than daily tape changes (557). One-third of a group who had adhesive tape placed over their lesions for four weeks had complete clearing. Others in the study showed lesser degrees of improvement.

A daily bath will assist in scale removal. A soft brush may be used to loosen the scales, but care should be taken to avoid irritating the skin, as any trauma worsens lesions. White petrolatum may be applied to the affected areas after the scales are removed. Oatmeal may be added to the bath water.

A starch bath may be soothing to psoriasis patients. Add one cup starch to a small amount of slightly warm water. Stir to dissolve the starch, then add the solution to the bath water. Glycerin may also be added to the bath water (553).

Gentle rubbing with a pumice stone may assist in scale removal. Soak the lesions for 10 to 15 minutes to soften them.

Avoid skin injury. Any type of trauma is likely to increase symptoms. Tight, irritating clothing should be carefully avoided.

Avocado oil or strong burdock root tea may be applied to the lesions several times a day.

Sun exposure is beneficial in many cases of psoriasis. Sunburn should be carefully avoided. Exposure is best done in the morning hours, to decrease the risk of burning. The eyes should be protected during sun exposure (558).

Many report benefit from high air humidity. Dry skin should be guarded against.

Emotional stress should be avoided, as it is known to worsen symptoms in many. Daily out-of-doors exercise aids in stress reduction.

Psoriasis of the scalp may be treated with an olive oil massage, followed by a hot towel compress for 30 minutes, and then a gentle shampoo. Scratching or any form of trauma to the scalp may worsen symptoms.

Topical corticosteroids should be avoided. They merely suppress symptoms, and may lead to adverse effects such as atrophy of the skin.

PUVA (psoralen plus long-wave ultraviolet light) has been used for psoriasis for some years, but recent studies suggest an association between PUVA and skin cancer. Other adverse effects of PUVA include vomiting, nausea, dizziness, dry skin, itching, headaches, skin freckling, and severe skin pain. PUVA has induced cataracts in experimental animals.

A Stanford Psoriasis Day Care Center has been effective in training patients to avoid or cope with many factors that worsen the disease. Knowledge about triggering factors such as burns, cuts, bruises, skin infections, drugs, stress and low humidity assist psoriasis patients to avoid many exacerbations of their disease.

Beta-blockers given for heart problems may produce psoriasis. It is possible that many other drugs have similar effects.

RECTAL ITCHING (PRURITUS ANI)

Rectal itching in children is most frequently due to pinworms. Other causes include antibiotic administration, anal fissures (see section), wet diapers, food allergy, and excessively vigorous cleaning of the rectal area.

The first step in treatment is to check for pinworms (see section), and treat if they are present.

Antibiotics may disturb the natural flora of the bowel, causing rectal itching (559). The flora balance eventually readjusts, but requires time.

Sitz baths (see treatment section) may be given twice a day. Add one-half to one ounce of Purex or Clorox to the water.

Avoid the use of any kind of ointment as they may aggravate the problem. Many of the medicines with "caine" in their name contain allergens which may worsen the problem (560). Ointments also tend to retain moisture which may worsen the condition.

The rectal area should be kept dry and cool (561). Young children may be allowed to go without undergarments to allow maximal air circulation. Place the child on padding in his crib to absorb any urine. Children should not be allowed to remain in wet or dirty diapers for long periods. In older children clothing should be loose-fitting and made of cotton.

After a bowel movement the bottom should be wiped front to back, instead of the commonly used back to front motion. Use wet tissue or cotton to cleanse the area, and pat--don't rub--dry. A hair drier may be also be used. Scratching should be avoided. If itching is intense after a bowel movement a bulb syringe filled with three to four ounces of warm water may be used to irrigate the area, or water may be poured from a cup.

Sun exposure or a heat lamp may be used to dry the area. Be careful to avoid burning.

Soap, dyed or perfumed toilet tissue, and deodorants may produce an allergic reaction which leads to rectal itching. Soap is highly alkaline, and may change the normal acidity of the skin.

Milk, cola drinks, tea, citrus fruits and juices, chocolate, nuts, popcorn, highly seasoned and spicy foods, cinnamon, cloves, and other spices, and tomatoes are all known to be capable of causing rectal itching in people sensitive to them (560,562).

Two teaspoons of charcoal powder may be stirred into a glass of water and taken four times a day. Mineral oil or other laxatives may irritate the colon, inducing itching.

A warm goldenseal tea bag may be applied to the rectum for about half an hour to relieve itching. A witch hazel compress may also be used, or a cotton ball dipped in witch hazel may be placed inside the rectum. Aloe vera gel can be applied at bedtime.

RECTAL PROLAPSE

Rectal prolapse, protrusion of the rectal mucosa out of the anus, is most common in children under five years of age. The tendency for it to occur in young children is felt to be because of their lack of a sacral curve in the spine, which provides support for the rectal tissue. This curve develops as the child matures. Prolonged straining and poor nutrition are felt to be common causes. Constipation, chronic diarrhea, cystic fibrosis, and neurological or anatomic abnormalities were the most common causes in one study, but in almost ten percent of cases in the study no cause was determined (563).

The mother may see bright red to dark tissue protruding from the anus after a bowel movement. The child may have a sensation of distention of the anus. There may be mucous or bloody discharge. The child typically appears entirely well between episodes of protrusion. Early in the course of the process the prolapse may subside spontaneously, but each bowel movement loosens the rectal tissue from the supporting wall a little more, and eventually the point is reached that the prolapse must be manually replaced (564). The parent may reduce this prolapse by placing the child face down on the mother's lap. Older children may be placed in the knee-chest position. Cover the finger with a piece of toilet paper. Gently press the mass back into the anus and hold it in place for a few moments. When the rectal tissue is back in the anus withdraw the

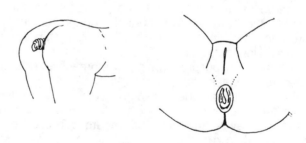

Rectal Prolapse

finger, leaving the tissue in place. It will be expelled with the next bowel movement. The tissue is used to permit withdrawal of the finger without pulling the mass out again. A well-lubricated finger may be equally effective. After the finger is withdrawn a cotton wad should be applied to the anus and the hips taped together to provide compression to the area (565). Some suggest having the child lie face-down in bed, elevating the foot of the bed to provide a gentle upward pressure. This may produce spontaneous replacement.

Constipation should be carefully guarded against. Straining at the stool increases pressure in the rectum and causes further tearing of the tissue from its supporting wall. Placing the feet up on a stool during bowel movements produces a more anatomically correct position for the passage of the stool in older children.

Attempts to toilet train that demand straining in an attempt to pass a bowel movement should be avoided.

Some have reported good success in the treatment of rectal prolapse by the insertion of a cone-shaped piece of ice into the rectum after the bowel movement (566).

REGURGITATION

Regurgitation, the return of food from the stomach, is different than vomiting, and is fairly common during early infancy (567). Typically, regurgitation involves only small amounts of returned food. Regurgitation is felt to be due to immaturity of the upper end of the stomach, and disappears as the child matures. It is almost always gone by the time the child has been walking for three months, but clears up by eight months of age in most children. If the child is growing normally it is generally not cause for concern.

There are a number of measures which the parent can take to decrease regurgitation. Many newborns regurgitate for several hours after birth, emptying the stomach of blood, amniotic fluid and other substances which have been swallowed during the delivery.

Treatment

Avoid overfeeding the child, as this distends the stomach. A full stomach makes regurgitation more likely (568). Feeding times should be kept to 20 minutes or less, and should be at least two-and-one-half hours apart, and preferably four to five, with longer intervals at night.

Burp the baby when he pauses during feedings, but do not interrupt sucking. This interferes with his feeding rhythm, and may cause him to cry, and swallow more air.

Tight diapers put pressure on the stomach and should be avoided. Double diapers may also cause problems (568).

Breast feeding alone, with nothing else added, not even water, is the ideal food for at least the first six months. But for the older child, thickened feedings may be helpful to curb regurgitation. Cereal may be added to the child's feeding to thicken it. Breast milk may be expressed and cereal added.

Keeping the child upright for 30 to 45 minutes after feedings is often helpful (569). Place him in his infant seat after each feeding.

RHEUMATOID ARTHRITIS, JUVENILE

It is estimated that there are 250,000 juvenile rheumatoid arthritis patients in the United States (570). Onset is before 16 years of age, with symptoms of limitation of motion, pain or tenderness on movement, swelling and redness of the joint. Symptoms persist more than six weeks, and other causes of joint pain such as infection, cancer, rheumatic fever, and connective tissue disorders must be ruled out. There is no specific test for juvenile rheumatoid arthritis; diagnosis is often made by ruling out other possible causes.

Peak onset is one to three years of age, with another in the eight to twelve year old group. Juvenile rheumatoid arthritis may occur in infants only six months of age.

Juvenile rheumatoid arthritis was first described by George Still in 1897.

The cause is not understood, but it is felt that something causes the immune system to begin manufacturing antibodies which attack the linings of the joints. Arthritis sometimes appears after an infection. There are three main subgroups of this disease: systemic, polyarticular (many joints), and pauci-articular (few joints).

In systemic onset disease symptoms include fever, lace-like rash, joint pain and stiffness and irritability. Wrists, feet, ankles, knee and elbow joints are most frequently involved. The joints become swollen and may be tender to touch or motion. Joint pain is often worse when fever is present, and pain and tenderness varies throughout the day, and from one day to the next (570).

Eighty percent of children with this type of juvenile rheumatoid arthritis will go into remission, with little or no disability. Symptoms often decrease during the first year after onset. The remaining twenty percent may progress to disabling disease. These children often are retarded in their growth and short in adult height.

The fever spikes may reach 103 to 105 degrees F., and often appear in the late afternoon, although some children have two fever spikes a day. After several hours the fever typically returns to normal. There are sometimes chills with the fever. The rash usually occurs on the trunk and proximal extremities, but in some cases even the soles and palms of the hands may be affected. The rash often appears with fever increase, disappearing as the temperature returns to normal. It is light colored initially, with variation in intensity during the course of its presence. The rash appears and disappears rapidly and is not associated with any skin peeling or residual symptoms. A few patients report itching with the rash, but this is not always present. Stress, heat exposure, and skin trauma may worsen the rash.

This type of juvenile rheumatoid arthritis is slightly more common in boys. Onset of symptoms may be at any age.

Children with polyarticular rheumatoid arthritis have symptoms in many joints, typically the hand joints, but the knees, ankles, elbows, neck, toes, feet, temporomandibular joint, shoulders and hips may be involved. Joint involvement is often bilateral. The joints feel warm to the touch, swell, and become red and tender. Fatigue is common. Some develop skin nodules, particularly on such pressure spots as the elbows, hands, knees, heels, scapulae, sacrum and hips. Fever and rash are usually not present. Children with this type of rheumatoid arthritis typically have more than five joints involved, and symptoms often persist for long periods. This type seems to be more common in females.

Polyarticular juvenile rheumatoid arthritis is the most common type, with this group making up one-third to three-quarters of the total cases of juvenile rheumatoid arthritis. The prognosis in this type is also the best of the three types.

Pauciarticular juvenile rheumatoid arthritis usually involves fewer than five joints. The large joints, such as the elbows, knees and ankles may be bilaterally involved. This type of rheumatoid arthritis is more common in females, and symptoms usually appear before the child reaches five years of age. Symptoms may progress to become a polyarticular type disease.

Many of these children also suffer chronic inflammation of the iris and ciliary body of the eyes. They may become light sensitive and have eye pain. Serious loss of vision may occur if this is not promptly and properly treated.

Treatment

A double-blind study of allergies in rheumatoid arthritis suggests that environmental and nutritional factors play a role in connective tissue disorders. Of 30 patients with rheumatic symptoms, 86 percent showed rheumatic symptoms in response to allergy tests. A single patient sometimes had a musculoskeletal allergic reaction to as many as ten tested extracts. Many of these patients also demonstrated nervous, respiratory, gastrointestinal and vascular system reactions. Soy, coffee, egg, milk, sugar, alcohol, beef, lettuce, orange, pork, potato, tobacco and yeast were common offenders.

Diet may play a major role in the treatment of rheumatoid arthritis. As early as 1935 references to food-induced rheumatoid arthritis began appearing in the literature. The frequency of these reports has increased down through the years.

Two Wayne State University physicians have reported marked improvement in arthritis sufferers placed on a fat-free diet. They had placed overweight patients on a fat-free diet to reduce their weight, and observed improvement in their joint symptoms within a few days. When fatty foods were returned to their diet the symptoms returned within 72 hours (571).

Another group of patients placed on an animal-product free diet showed improvement in their symptoms. Twelve of a group of twenty patients were fasted, then begun on a strict vegan diet, without strong spices, tea, coffee, alcoholic beverages, or refined sugars. They demonstrated less pain and improved joint function (572).

About one-third of a group of patients studied at Vanderbilt University and the University of Florida stated that certain foods worsened their disease. Preservatives, pork, beef, sugars, alcohol, chocolate and caffeine were the most commonly listed troublemakers (573).

A study from Israel reports an association between milk allergy and juvenile rheumatoid arthritis. A 14-year-old girl who had a six year history of juvenile rheumatoid arthritis showed recovery after milk proteins were carefully eliminated from her diet (574). When milk was intentionally or accidentally reintroduced into the diet the symptoms again appeared. Dr. W. G. Crook has reported joint swelling as an allergic reaction to milk, and other researchers have demonstrated that multiple systems may be involved in the manifestations of milk allergy. A three-week trial of milk protein elimination may be of great benefit. Another study has shown rheumatoid-like lesions in laboratory animals given cow's milk for 12 weeks (575).

A 38-year-old woman with an eleven year history of progressive rheumatoid arthritis was placed on a diet eliminating milk, butter, and cheese. She began to feel better three weeks after starting the diet, and eventually her morning stiffness completely disappeared and inflammation almost completely subsided. This patient had previously been tested for milk allergy with negative results (576).

Several years ago Dr. Norman Childers reported an association between nightshades (potatoes, tomatoes, eggplant, peppers and tobacco) and arthritis. His latest studies from the University of Florida reveal that milk may worsen symptoms of rheumatoid arthritis (577).

Dr. Bernard M. Zussman, of the University of Tennessee Allergy Clinics reported rapid relief of rheumatoid arthritis symptoms in a group of patients when eggs, wheat, cereal, milk and some fruits were eliminated from the diet. He reported that skin tests for food allergens were ineffective; a trial of a diet eliminating the suspected foods was the most effective method of determining the allergens. (See Food Allergies Made Simple for further information on food allergens.)

Wheat is a frequent cause of rheumatoid arthritis symptoms. Of a group of 87 patients studied, 41 were shown to be allergic to wheat (578). This grain should be totally eliminated (including wheat bran and wheat starch) for a three month trial for persons with rheumatoid arthritis.

Heat is one of the standard treatments for any type of arthritis. As a treatment for arthritis, heat comes down from ancient history, and may be applied in several ways: fomentations, hot baths, whirlpool, heat lamps, and melted paraffin among others. See the treatment section for instructions. Because sensation and circulation in the skin may be reduced heat treatments must be used with care to avoid burning the patient. Diabetics and people with impaired sensation are unable to recognize that they are being burned, and unfortunately, are more likely than others to burn quickly.

Heat treatments should be continued for 20 to 30 minutes and may be carried out one to four times a day. Hot baths are helpful in the relief of morning stiffness, and can make exercise easier by reducing pain and muscle spasm. Alternating hot and cold baths, called "contrast baths" also have a place in the treatment of juvenile rheumatoid arthritis.

A hot bath is a simple treatment which can readily be carried out in the home. The tub is filled with water at about 100 degrees F. The child gets into the tub and the water temperature is raised to about 104 degrees F. by the addition of hot water. Use a water thermometer to maintain the temperature at 104 degrees for 30 to 45 minutes if the child is 12 years of age or older. Under the age of 12, use the following schedule: 3 minutes in the hot bath for age 3 or under; after age 3, add 1 minute per year until age 12. Smaller children can be treated 2 or 3 times a day if necessary. The water level should be up to the neck and a cold towel or compress may be applied to the head to cool it. At the conclusion of the bath the child should be sponged with cold water and put in bed until perspiration subsides. As some people become nauseated with heat treatments this treatment is best carried out on an empty stomach, although the child may be given fluids freely during the bath. Some adults have shown what was termed "striking" improvement with fever treatments raising the body temperature to 104 degrees F. for two or more hours. Even a hot shower, although not as effective as a tub bath, may produce muscle relaxation with pain relief.

Some report improvement with cold applications rather than heat. Cold applications may be more effective in acute phases, while chronic phases are usually best helped by heat. Dr. Peter Utsinger, of the Philadelphia Germantown Medical Center, reported that 24 rheumatoid arthritis patients had significant pain relief, improvement of range of movement, and greater muscle strength after four weeks of what he calls "Baggie-therapy." The treatment consists of putting six ice cubes and a quart of cold tap water in a Baggie, placing it on top of the affected joint with another under the joint. The Baggies were wrapped in a towel and kept in place for 20 minutes. Treatment was carried out four times a day. Initial discomfort disappears after about three to five minutes (579,580). Paraffin baths often bring great benefit, but some children are afraid to put their hands in the hot paraffin. Paraffin may be applied to the skin at a temperature higher than water temperatures without burning. A paintbrush may be used to apply the paraffin to the affected joints. Paraffin does not dry the skin as does water, and leaves it feeling soft. It is particularly helpful in treatment of small joints.

Exercise, both passive and active, is essential in juvenile rheumatoid arthritis to ease pain, relief stiffness, and prevent freezing of the joint. (In passive exercise the joints are gently moved by another person; in active motion the joint is moved by the patient himself.) Exercise assists in maintaining normal joint position and function, thus reducing the possibility of muscle contractures (permanent muscle shortening), improves circulation in the joint and encourages movement of fluid collected in the joint.

Joints should be moved through their range of motion to the point that discomfort begins, held in that position for 5 to 10 seconds, and released. Each movement should be repeated three to ten times in each of two daily exercise sessions. Exercise periods should be carried out only after stiffness has subsided. Heat or cold treatments may be given before exercise sessions to increase mobility and comfort of the joints.

Those who have access to a swimming pool may benefit from pool exercise periods. The water supports the joints, reducing stress. Exercises may be carried out in a whirlpool or even a home bathtub.

Swimming and bike or tricycle riding are often good exercise for juvenile rheumatoid arthritics, but competitive sports should be avoided (581). Extensive walking, kicking, jumping, or running should be avoided if the hips or legs are involved. Exercise should be out-of-doors with sunlight exposure.

If symptoms are worse after exercise or post-exercise pain continues for more than two hours, the program should be reduced slightly, with fewer repetitions and a reduction in extremes of motion range. Excessive exercise may cause an increase in inflammation.

Exercise should be balanced with rest. Regular sleeping hours at night and rest periods during the day are recommended. Proper position in bed is essential. If the child is lying on his back he may have a small pillow under his head or in the curve of the neck to stabilize the head. Arms raised over the head increase vital breathing capacity. The child lying on the abdomen should have a pillow in a comfortable position under the chest and abdomen. The mattress should be firm. A plywood board one-half to three-quarters of an inch thick may be placed under the mattress to provide firm support. While lying on the abdomen the feet should hang off the end of the mattress in a neutral position.

Dr. Jack Soltanoff of West Hurley, New York, reports that garlic is very helpful in arthritic pain relief. He states that one clove daily may be chewed and swallowed. We have chopped it finely and stirred it into a salad or sprinkled it on top of other foods (582). Those who object to the odor may use the odor-free garlic capsules or tablets. Parsley is said to counteract the odor.

A garlic poultice may be used on painful joints. Peel two large heads of garlic, chop and soak in one-half cup of warm olive oil for five minutes. Dip a thick sock in hot water and wring out the excess water. Fill the toe with the garlic-olive oil mixture, and rub it over the painful joint for three to five minutes (582).

A Rusk Institute of New York physical therapist, Barry Ostrow, suggests wrapping diced garlic in a hot damp washcloth and rubbing the painful area for 15 to 20 minutes. For those who prefer cold to hot applications the garlic may be placed in a damp washcloth and frozen. Joint pain of new onset may be treated with the application of the cold garlic pack for ten minutes every two hours for the first 36 hours. Chronic pain may be treated with ten to twenty minute hot applications two or three times a day.

In adults, fish oils are being enthusiastically recommended for inflammatory arthritis patients. Anti-inflammatory prostaglandins are produced by the omega-3 fatty acids in fish oils. We do not recommend fish oils because of their cholesterol content, often excessive amounts of vitamin D, their aggravation of diabetes and possibility of contamination with viruses and heavy metals. Flaxseed oil has the beneficial Omega-3 fatty acids, and may be used in a dosage of one to two teaspoons a day mixed into cereal. English walnuts and flaxseed are also high in omega-3 fatty acids. Take six walnuts or two tablespoons of ground flaxseed once daily.

The herb feverfew has anti-inflammatory properties. Smaller children can use one-third to one-half cup of the tea three times a day, with up to a cup three times a day for older children. One caution is that feverfew has been reported to cause allergic symptoms in those who are allergic to ragweed or the chrysanthemum family.

Massage, properly carried out, is helpful in stimulating blood flow and relaxing muscles. Heat should be applied before massage, and long, gentle, smooth massage strokes toward the heart should be used. Massage which causes severe pain should be stopped immediately.

Aspirin has anti-inflammatory properties and large doses are often given in the treatment of juvenile rheumatoid arthritis. Reye's syndrome, changes in liver function, stomach irritation, blood clotting problems, kidney irritation, ringing in the ears and tooth erosion are some of the adverse effects of aspirin use.

The child should be encouraged to lead as normal a life as possible. School activities and other social events help the child feel "normal," and not unlike other children. Fatigue is common and some children will need a shortened school day to allow rest periods.

Some children will need splinting of the affected joints to prevent contracture. At rest, joints assume a flexed, more comfortable position and if permitted to remain in this position for long periods may produce permanent shortening of muscles.

RINGWORM

Ringworm is a term applied to fungus infections which may invade the body, hair, or nails. There are four main types of ringworm--ringworm of the scalp (*Tinea capitis*), the body (*Tinea corporis*), the nails, and the feet (Tinea pedis). Ringworm of the feet is also called athlete's foot. (See section on Athlete's Foot.)

Ringworm of the body begins as small, red flat or slightly elevated ring- or oval-shaped sores, which may be moist, crusted, dry or scaly. The centers heal as the sores enlarge, spreading outward in a circular fashion. This manner of spread is responsible for the name of "ringworm." Worms are actually not responsible for the disease.

Ringworm of the body may be spread by direct contact with infected individuals, or by contaminated clothing. Animals may also transmit the disease. It may be acquired when walking barefoot at swimming pools, in showers, or other areas where infected people may be barefooted.

Ringworm of the scalp is most common in school children, and is highly contagious. The child may lose hair in infected patches. The key to preventing ringworm is keeping the skin clean and dry. Briskly rub the skin and nails with a coarse towel after bathing, to remove the outer layer of dead skin, where the fungus often gains entrance.

Treatment

Avoid scratching the lesions. The fingernails should be cut short, and the hands washed frequently.

Children who have ringworm should not sleep with others; their bedding should be washed separately from that of other family members.

Crusts and scales may be removed by applying saline compresses for 10 to 15 minutes three times a day.

Freshly cut garlic is reported very effective in curing ringworm. A report from the Medical Journal of Australia (590) told of a girl who treated one arm with traditional medicine and the other arm with freshly cut garlic three times a day. The garlic-treated arm healed in 10 days, while the arm treated with prescription medication required three to four weeks to heal. The garlic may be blended with a little water, and applied as a poultice, compress or soak. CAUTION: Some people are allergic to garlic and should not use it. Raw, weepy or ulcerated skin may be irritated by the garlic.

Castor oil, apple cider vinegar, thymol oil, aloe vera gel, and goldenseal tea applied several times a day have all been reported to be very effective. Plain vinegar one to four times daily for 30 days will usually cure even stubborn cases on the feet or body. Wash the area thoroughly and dry by brisk and prolonged rubbing before applying any of the substances. One report in the medical literature indicated that ordinary table salt dampened with a little petroleum jelly to make it stick, may be applied twice a day to the lesions. The area should be shaved if in a hairy place, and the ointment rubbed in until the area becomes tender.

If there is extensive disease the child may be placed in a tub of warm water to which one-half cup of apple cider vinegar has been added. Allow the child to soak for 30 minutes two or three times a day (583).

As heat and moisture encourage fungus growth it is best for the child to avoid getting hot and sweaty during periods of infection (584).

Underwear should be cotton, and changed twice daily. Tight clothing should not be used as it will prevent aeration.

If swelling is present a compress solution may be made by adding one teaspoon of salt to one pint of water. Apply the compresses four times a day (584).

Ringworm of the Scalp (Tinea Capitis)

Ringworm of the scalp is generally found only in children. It is especially common in socio-economically deprived, uncared for children. There are occasional outbreaks in schools.

It may be transmitted from hair brushes, barbers' tools, hats, or even theater seats. If the skin has been bruised or broken it is easier for the fungi to enter the body.

The hair should be shampooed daily. The hair should be kept short, but it is not necessary to shave the head. Short hair makes it easier to apply the medications to the involved areas of the scalp. If the hair is cut at home the hair clippings should be carefully collected and burned. Scissors, combs, and other instruments used in the hair cutting should be boiled after use. Clothing worn by child and parent should be sterilized.

ROSEOLA INFANTUM

Roseola infantum, also called exanthema subitum (585), is a disease of very young children. Symptoms include a fever, often 104 to 106 degrees F., which may last for three to five days, and suddenly disappear as a rash occurs (586). The fine, pink rash is largely confined to the trunk, but there may be some on the neck, arms, and legs. Some children have red throats, swelling of the lymph glands, runny nose, or swelling of the eyelids. One physician reported that almost all children developed droopy eyelids immediately prior to the onset of roseola infantum. During the illness the child may be irritable; a few have diarrhea or vomiting, but there are few other signs of illness. They may eat and play normally. It is most common in children between six months and two years of age, but it has been known to occur up to 14 years of age. The incubation period is about nine days. One episode of the disease produces permanent immunity. Convulsions may occur, but are generally self-limited and do not recur. They generally do not require therapy. Antibiotics are not helpful. Complete recovery is the general course of the disease.

This disease may rarely cause a serious problem. It has been known to cause bone marrow arrest at times; usually the bone marrow, which recovers in two to four days, can "catch up" so quickly that nothing is noticed. But in children who have a hemolytic anemia, such as sickle cell disease, the bone marrow is already working at full steam. If it stops production for even a short time, the hemoglobin may drop precipitously, requiring hospitalization and perhaps transfusions. If a child has a hemolytic anemia, special precautions should be taken to avoid roseola.

Treatment

Sponging baths or hot half baths may be used for fever (587). Warm baths (see treatment section) will often shorten the period of fever, and bring on the rash sooner.

Fluid intake should be encouraged. This will help control the fever and make the child more comfortable.

The room temperature should be kept cool, and fresh air should be provided day and night.

SCABIES

Scabies is an infestation of the skin by *Sarcoptes scabiei*. These small eight-legged mites mature in 10 to 14 days, and live for about 30 days. After mating the female may lay 10 to 25 eggs before she dies. Children infested with mites usually have about 20 of them. If they become dislodged from the body they remain alive and able to infest another host for at least 36 hours, and perhaps up to eight days.

Scabies is also called "the itch" or the "seven year itch." It is common in the United States and peak incidence is late summer and early autumn. There are itching wheals, vesicles, papules or threadlike burrows in the skin with an overlying eczematous dermatitis. Itching is worse at night and with heat. Scabies is found in all social and economic groups. Contact is the sole requirement for infestation; even a handshake is sufficient. Clothing and bed linen may also be involved in transmission of the disease. Outbreaks often occur in areas where persons live in close proximity, and often entire families develop infestations simultaneously.

The female mite burrows into the skin, forming tunnels in which to deposit eggs. For several weeks she will continue to burrow, depositing a few eggs a day. The eggs hatch in four to five days. Warmth, as from a warm shower or bed clothing, stimulates mite activity.

Onset of symptoms begin 2 to 6 weeks after infestation, with severe itching. It may be so intense that the child is unable to sleep. Gray or skin-colored ridges appear in the skin.

The most frequent sites of involvement are the finger webs, hands, wrists, elbows, underarms, waist, and feet. Skin above the neck is rarely involved, except in infants.

Mites are most active at night, and itching is most intense then. Scratching may induce secondary infection, and inoculate mites in new areas. A rash due to an allergic response may appear about a month after the primary infestation.

The disease is more common in girls than in boys, and older children and young adults are most often the victims of this affliction. Several reports have appeared in the medical literature of people who developed scabies after contact with infested dogs.

Treatment

Cool soaks, starch baths, or calamine lotion may be used for itching.

Garlic applications may be helpful. Blend a garlic clove in one cup of cold water. Wet a strip of cloth in the garlic water, apply to the affected area, cover with a piece of kitchen plastic, and hold the poultice in place with any kind of bandage for two to eight hours.

A salve made from anise seeds is reported effective against scabies.

Lindane or Kwell (gamma benzene hexachloride) has been widely used, but it has been shown that this pharmacologic agent can be absorbed from the skin into the blood. Convulsions and even death have occurred in animals absorbing large amounts of Kwell through the skin. Convulsions have been reported in children after its use (591). If this product is used the child should not take a warm bath before the application as skin hydration may increase systemic absorption of the medication.

A preparation of flowers of sulfur in a petrolatum base is a safer method of treatment. However, it has a faintly unpleasant odor and will stain clothing (588). A five percent mixture may be used for children. Sulfur ointment P.P. is 97 to 100 percent effective. The child should take a warm, soaking bath before application of the sulfur ointment. Apply ointment from the neck to the toes each night for three to five nights. He should not bathe during the treatment period.

Bed linens and clothing should be laundered frequently in hot water (140 degrees F). Dry cleaning or ironing will also kill the parasite. Scabies will not survive temperatures greater than 120 degrees F. for longer than five minutes.

Fingernails should be kept short and scratching discouraged.

It may be necessary to treat all members of the household at the same time as the mite is easily spread.

SICKLE CELL DISEASE

There are several types of sickle cell disease (592). Our discussion will focus on sickle cell anemia, the most common.

The disease is due to abnormalities in the blood hemoglobin. It is more common in blacks, with an estimated incidence of 1 case per every 600 births in the United States. It is generally not apparent until after the child is six months of age, as he retains large amounts of fetal hemoglobin for several months after birth.

The blood cells take on an elongated shape, and become stuck in tiny blood vessels, obstructing blood flow in the area. The resulting lack of oxygen in the area leads to the severe pain which these patients often experience.

Highest rates of sickle cell disease occur in countries where malaria is common.

Sickle cell disease runs a course of exacerbations, called "crises," and remissions. Some children have a weekly crisis, others go several months between them. Some children have mild symptoms during these crises; others have severe symptoms. Crises may be brought on by dehydration, infection, stress, trauma, exposure, lack of oxygen, and strenuous physical activity. Symptoms may be present for one day or several weeks. General measures to improve overall health are particularly important in these children.

Symptoms during crises may include anemia, pain, enlargement of the spleen, lack of appetite, paleness of the skin, weakness, yellowing of the skin, and fever. Symptoms often increase as the child matures. The spleen is gradually scarred over the course of years, the liver often becomes firm, tender, and enlarged. If sickling occurs in the brain blood vessels the sickle cell patient may suffer seizures or a cerebrovascular accident (stroke). These appear most frequently in children under ten years of age. Some feel that hyperventilation may predispose to cerebrovascular accidents. The heart often becomes enlarged, and a murmur may be heard. A lung infection causes fluid collection in the lungs, and these children are very susceptible to pneumonia. The kidneys are often damaged over the course of years, with associated hematuria (blood in the urine) and inability to concentrate the urine. Urinary tract infections and renal failure are common, and the child may have to get up during the night to urinate. There may be infarcts or infections in bones, leading to severe pain. The small bones of the hands and feet are particularly susceptible in young children. Leg ulcers, eye changes, and priapism (painful, persistent erection of the penis) are all common.

These children mature more slowly than normal (593). Physical and mental development are often slower than that in unaffected children. Adults are often shorter than would be expected. Sickle cell patients have reduced life spans. Women who become pregnant are at increased risk of complications such as miscarriage, eclampsia, and pulmonary disease. The greatest risk of death is before five years of age (594).

Treatment

Water is the treatment of choice for sickle cell anemia. It should be drunk in generous amounts, and applied externally in the treatment of fever, pain, and leg ulcers.

Dehydration is a common problem, and must be guarded against (594). These children require more fluids than the normal child, as their kidneys are often unable to concentrate urine. Some of these children with kidney impairment need six to eight quarts of water per day (594). The child should be trained to take water on a regular basis throughout the waking hours. Water intake should be increased during hot weather, or during heating treatments. The urine should be kept pale in color at all times.

Tea, coffee, and cola drinks should not be given as they stimulate fluid loss. Tea also interferes with iron absorption. Cranberry juice may increase acidosis, which may worsen symptoms. These children should be given a simple diet free from added salt (no salt added at the factory, stove, or table), and free of sugars and free fats (margarine, mayonnaise, fried foods, cooking fats and salad oils). Low levels of sodium (salt) in the blood have been shown to decrease sickling. See Appendix 2 for a low salt diet.

They should use iron rich foods frequently, as they tend to have anemia, due to excessive breakdown of blood cells. Iron supplements, however, are probably best avoided, as iron deficiency has been shown to reduce sickling.

Fever should be treated with adequate fluids or hot half baths. The cause of the fever should be determined and treated.

Hot and cold fomentations are often effective in relieving pain. Warm baths, showers, or whirlpool, if available, are also helpful.

Prolonged breath holding and underwater swimming may decrease oxygen levels in the body, precipitating problems (595).

Because irritation and trauma may lead to problems clothing should not be restrictive or tight (593). The child should not remain in positions which hinder free blood flow. Any skin breaks should be cleansed promptly and steps taken to prevent the development of infection.

The child should be protected from chilling or excessive heat. Dress him appropriately for the weather conditions.

Warm baths are often effective in relieving priapism. Treatment should begin as quickly as possible after the onset of the erection. The longer the priapism has been present the more difficult it is to relieve (594).

Exercise should be done to the child's tolerance, but he should not overdo. These children often lack stamina, which will limit their activity (594). Parents should be careful to avoid over-protectiveness. These children may be restricted to bed because of acute pain during crises. Passive range-of-motion exercises should be carried out, and as symptoms resolve the child should be started on a progressive walking program. Any exercise program should allow rest periods between activities.

Hot and cold applications over leg ulcers may hasten their resolution. Packing them with common table sugar mixed with betadine to a peanut butter consistency twice daily will greatly encourage healing. Keeping the leg elevated is also helpful. Wet-to-dry dressing changes every two hours during the day assist in healing. These are carried out by dipping some sterile material, such as gauze in normal saline (1 teaspoon salt to 2 cups water) and applying the wet dressing over the ulcer. As the bandage dries it adheres to the wound. At the time of dressing change the dead tissue adheres to the gauze and is pulled off the wound.

Some children develop lesions over the shins. These seem to respond best to elevation of the leg and hot compresses.

The child should have adequate rest and sleep on a daily basis. A regular schedule of rising time, meal times, and bed times will enable the body to best synchronize its circadian rhythms.

SINUSITIS

Sinusitis is an infection or inflammation of the lining of one or more nasal sinuses. These sinuses are bony air cavities in the head. There are eight of them in the adult, but infants and young children have only four.

Symptoms of sinusitis include runny nose, pain over the sinuses, "toothache," or pain behind the eyes, cough, swelling, circles around the eyes, fatigue, irritability, lack of appetite, sore throat, bad breath, headache, and low grade fever. They typically have a cough which is often worse during the night or while lying down, and in the early morning. Onset often follows a cold, but allergy is a common cause of sinusitis. Chilling, fatigue, weather changes, or swimming may also cause symptoms of sinusitis.

Treatment

Helping the child keep the nasal passages open so he can breathe is impor-

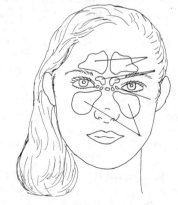

Location of Sinuses

tant. Very young children are unable to blow their nose, nor can they breathe through their mouth. The parent will need to suction the nasal passages using a rubber syringe. Administer saline drops (see cold section for preparation instructions) after syringing, allow the child to lie quietly for ten minutes, and suction again.

Saline nose drops may be helpful also for the older child. Have the child blow his nose to clear secretions, then lie down on a flat surface. Drop the nosedrops into one nostril at a time, allowing the child to remain quiet for about ten minutes to allow the drops to drain downward. If the nose is still stuffy, the child may blow his nose again, and the drops applied the second time (596).

A vaporizer may make breathing easier (596). Some feel that adequate humidification of the home and a low temperature will help prevent sinusitis attacks. Steam inhalations may be given for 20 to 30 minutes three times a day (597). See treatment section for procedure.

The child should be encouraged to take lots of fluids. Water is the beverage of choice, although clear herb teas may be used. Peppermint tea is helpful (598). Garlic tea, made by boiling four cups of water, removing from the heat and adding crushed garlic cloves, is reported helpful in the relief of nasal stuffiness.

Heat from a heat lamp, heating pad, or warm compress may be applied over the sinuses (596). A towel may be wrung from hot water and applied over the sinuses for five minutes. Sponge the area with a towel wrung from cold water, and reapply the hot towel. Repeat three times, finishing off with the cold. Some like to use a peppermint leaf compress over the affected sinuses. Others recommend breathing through a hot towel (600). A small child may be frightened by this procedure.

Some prefer cold applications to warm. For these people crushed ice may be placed in a plastic bag, and the bag wrapped in a slightly moistened towel and applied over the involved sinuses (599).

A hot foot bath (see treatment section for procedure) will often help clear nasal stuffiness. The hot water draws the blood from the head into the feet. Keep the feet in hot water for 20 to 30 minutes and conclude the treatment by a brief cold water pour to the feet. The patient should then be placed in bed until sweating stops. The hot foot bath may be carried out several times a day.

Cigarette smoke should be avoided as it worsens sinusitis.

The child should not swim during sinusitis attacks. Swimming and diving may wash nasal infections into the sinuses, and chlorine is irritating to nasal passages.

Antihistamines are ineffective and may even be harmful. They may thicken the mucous lining the sinuses hindering its ability to move secretions. Decongestants may decrease blood flow in the nasal membranes, providing an environment favorable for the growth of unwanted organisms (601).

Sniffing warm salt water up into the nose may help clear excess mucus. Use one-half teaspoon of salt in eight ounces of water.

Over-the-counter or prescription nose drops should not be used as they produce a "rebound phenomenon" with worsening of symptoms.

Allergies are the most common cause of chronic or recurrent sinusitis. Milk, wheat, corn, and yeast are the most frequent offending foods; but coffee, chocolate, all soft drinks, food additives, artificial colorings, sugar, preservatives and sweeteners are also causes.

Chilling should be avoided, as it induces vasoconstriction, lowers leukocyte response and impairs phagocytic capabilities (603). Room temperatures should be kept constant, as sinusitis is often aggravated by temperature changes (604). Air conditioning may worsen symptoms.

The child should be instructed to blow his nose gently, rather than forcefully.

Elevating the head while the child is resting is often helpful in easing breathing, and decreasing swelling of the face. The head of the bed may be elevated two to four inches by placing blocks under the bed legs, or the child may be propped up on several pillows. If one nostril is more obstructed than the other, placing the child in a position with that side elevated may assist in opening the nostril. The child should be encouraged to rest on his side rather than his back (602).

The child should be encouraged to participate in physical exercise out of doors if he is not very ill. Exercise helps open nasal passages, and both infrared and ultraviolet light are helpful in the treatment of sinusitis.

Splashing the face with cold water followed by vigorous drying will shrink the inferior turbinates. After this procedure the child should sit leaning forward slightly and gently blow his nose until it is clear, then sit upright, close his mouth tightly, and breathe slowly through the nose.

Mechanical vibrators are helpful in some cases of sinusitis. Seventy percent of a group reported pain relief after a vibrator was placed in the midline of the forehead or over the most tender site. The vibrator was used for 45 minutes twice a day for 30 days. Patients often reported improvement within five minutes of beginning treatment, although some required up to 25 minutes to obtain maximum benefit (605).

Warm moist compresses may be applied to swollen eyes.

SLEEP WALKING (SOMNAMBULISM)

Sleepwalking is common in normal children, with most children probably sleepwalking at least once during their childhood. The exact incidence of sleepwalking is difficult to determine, as it is often not reported to the health care provider. The child who has night terrors may develop sleepwalking as the night terrors disappear. Sleepwalking is felt to be a manifestation of immaturity of the nervous system rather than a sign of mental problem. Sleepwalking is more common in boys, who mature more slowly than girls, and tends to run in families (606). These children are also often bedwetters (696) and may suffer migraine headaches. Many of them also talk in their sleep. These children may be light sleepers who are easily awakened (608). Sleepwalking does not seem to occur in very young children but may appear by the age of four or five. It often disappears as the child matures. Sleepwalking may occur once a year or several times during a week. Incidence of episodes is felt to be highest in the 11 to 12 year old group. Children who begin sleepwalking at a young age seem to be more likely to outgrow it quickly; one study reported that children who began sleepwalking before ten years of age were likely to stop by fifteen years of age (609).

Onset is usually within three hours of going to bed (610). The episode starts as the child suddenly sits up in bed. His eyes are open but he seems indifferent to his environment. He may return to sleep without getting out of bed but may get up and walk about the house or even go outdoors. The parents should see that he does not hurt himself but they should not attempt to awaken him or to get him to return to bed. If returned to bed before he is ready he is likely to get up again.

Although the cause of sleepwalking is not clearly understood it has been observed that children who are put to bed shortly after a heavy meal, children who are overly fatigued, or who have missed previous sleep are more likely to sleepwalk (606). Children who have food sensitivities are more likely to sleepwalk. Food sensitivities should be sought for by the "elimination and challenge" diet. While stress does not seem to be the factor responsible for sleep walking it has been observed that it may increase the incidence. Several reports have appeared indicating that sleepwalking episodes may start during, or shortly after an illness in which the child had a fever (607).

A single episode may last just a few minutes or an hour. The child engages in what appears to be purposeful activity including such activities as dressing, going to the bathroom, or talking in mumbled form which makes no sense (606). When the activity is completed he returns to bed, resumes sleep, and the next morning feels rested, generally without any recall of the event (610).

SORE THROAT (PHARYNGITIS)

Sore throat is caused by an infection or inflammation. It may be due to allergy or associated with another illness such as a cold, the measles, a bacterium or a virus. The child may have swollen lymph glands, headache, lack of appetite, and fever with the sore throat. Infants who are too young to complain of sore throat may cry during feedings or refuse to eat.

Children who have persistent postnasal drip may have sore throat due to repeated throat-clearing.

Sore throat due to Streptococcus is often called "strep" throat. This type of sore throat is uncommon in infants but Streptococci may be cultured from about 10 percent of sore throats in the five to sixteen year old group. Certain of these cases are actually viral sore throats with streptococci being in the throat as a chronic state, even when no sore throat is present. With a true streptococcal sore throat onset of the illness is rapid with fever up to 104 degrees F., extremely severe sore throat, headache, enlargement of lymph nodes in the neck, conjunctivitis, and sometimes associated abdominal pain. There may be a glistening or white discharge on the tonsils which are very red and swollen. Swallowing may be difficult. There may be hoarseness, cough, and diarrhea. Dr. Frank Oski, a prominent professor of pediatrics, reports a direct relationship between strep throat and milk drinking.

Viral sore throat accounts for more than 90% of all sore throats in children, according to *Emergency Decisions*, January, 1986. This type is slower in onset, with symptoms of a common upper respiratory infection. There may be fever, headache, cough, and muscle aches. Occasionally there is associated nausea and diarrhea.

Parents who have recurrent episodes of streptococcal sore throat should have throat cultures done on their family pets according to Dr. Stewart M. Copperman of New York. He reports that in 40 of 100 cases of recurrent streptococcal pharyngitis household dogs or cats were found to have positive cultures for Group A beta-hemolytic streptococcus. After the animal was treated the family had no more recurrent, persistent streptococcal sore throats (611,612). This report underscores the desirability of limiting exposure to pets, and all pets except aquarium or terrarium animals must have separate quarters at some distance from the family. After touching pets children must wash hands and nails thoroughly.

Treatment

Warm or cold compresses, depending on the child's preference, may be applied to the throat (613). If warmth is preferred a heating pad, hot water bottle, or warm towel may be used. A cold compress squeezed from ice water and continually refreshed or an ice bag may be used in children who prefer cool compresses.

The child often has a poor appetite and he should not be forced to eat. Adequate hydration is essential. An abundance of fluids should be provided and encouraged. Citrus fruits should be avoided as they are often irritating to the sore throat (614). Cool liquids are usually preferred and ice chips may be acceptable (613).

Fever may be treated with warm baths or hot mitten friction. Ice water may cause chilling with constriction of skin blood vessels which forces the blood to the interior of the body preventing cooling of the skin surface. Alcohol should not be used for sponging as the fumes may be toxic, and it may chill the skin (615). With a warm bath the white blood cells and the immune proteins become more active, the skin blood vessels are dilated and the infection comes under the control of the body's immune system. Increased air humidity is helpful (616), particularly for very young children who cannot gargle. Pans of water placed on heaters, humidifiers, or steam from running hot water in the bathroom may all be used. A pan of water placed on the kitchen stove will provide escaping steam which the child can be encouraged to inhale.

Children over three years of age can often gargle after being shown the procedure (617). Warm saline water made by adding 1 teaspoon of salt to one glass of water makes a satisfactory gargle (615).

A heating compress to the throat is an excellent treatment for sore throat (617). Pharmaceutical nose drops may produce a rebound worsening of symptoms if used for more than a day or two (616). Saline nose drops are very helpful for all ages, and very young infants may obtain quick relief if the parent suctions the nasal passages with a bulb syringe (see section on colds).

Petrolatum applied under the nose will help prevent skin irritation from a runny nose (616).

The parent should wash the hands carefully after caring for the child, to prevent spread of the infection (616).

STUTTERING

Stuttering, or speech difficulties, are common in young children who are just learning to speak. Boys stutter more often than girls, probably due to their slower physical development. It has been estimated that 25 percent of all children stutter at some time during their development, but others think the percentage is even higher than that. It has been said that 90 percent of all children have some type of speech abnormality during the process of learning to speak, but only one percent of children truly stutter (618). Speech problems often are merely due to the fact that the child's speaking ability does not develop as rapidly as his thought processes (619). The body seems to concentrate on the development of one part of the body at a time and other parts temporarily fall behind in development (619). A child may have increased speech difficulties during periods when his ability to walk is developing rapidly. Speech problems generally resolve by the time the child is six or seven years of age. Most cases of speech abnormality disappear over two or three months if the problem is properly handled. Researchers feel that proper handling on the part of parents may prevent what is really a temporary state from becoming a permanent problem.

Stuttering does seem to run in families to a mild degree, but it is felt that environmental factors are probably more important than genetic. However, current research suggests that a child does not begin stuttering because he hears someone else doing it (619). The child's personality may also play a role.

Treatment

Parents should avoid calling attention to the child's speech difficulties. They should remember that it is just as normal as falling off a bicycle while learning to ride. No parent tells his child to "slow down" so he won't fall off his bike! Siblings, relatives, and teachers should be instructed to make no comment about the child's problem. Calling the child's attention to it increases the risk he will become concerned about it, and increase the rate at which it occurs, and prolong its presence (619).

If the child expresses concern over the problem to his parents the parent should tell him that everyone makes mistakes while they are learning to speak, and even after they have practiced speaking for many years they may sometimes have difficulty getting their words out. These children are often relieved to be told that many children have the same problem; they are not the only one.

The parents should guard their speech to the child. It should be slow, but not so deliberately slow that the child feels that the parent is "speaking down" to him. The parent should pause for two or three seconds between the time the child ends his speech until the parent begins to speak in response. This will demonstrate to the child that there is no need to hurry with speech (619).

The parent should spend time alone with the child on a daily basis. Pleasant, enjoyable conversation should be engaged in. Such activities as reading to the child and asking him to tell you what he thinks is occurring in pictures, or asking him questions about the story encourage speech. Verbal games such as asking the child to name all the red objects in a room may also be used. Ask the child to tell you his favorite story or of some experience he has recently had (619).

Do not attempt to correct a child's grammar during times of speech difficulty. He can learn proper grammar later; it is important not to call attention to the child's speech in any way during times of speech difficulty (618).

Basil Jones, a pediatrician, reports curing a number of cases of stuttering by removing milk from the child's diet. His observations suggest that food allergies may cause stuttering in some children (697).

When the child speaks the parent should provide eye-to-eye contact if at all possible. A study reported by Dr. Edward Conture, professor of communication sciences and disorders at Syracuse University, revealed that the mother's interaction with the child had a very definite impact on the child's speech problems. Mothers who turned from their child when he stuttered, who avoided eye-to-eye contact or expressed displeasure with their child's performance had children with greater incidences and prolonged duration of stuttering (698).

When the parent cannot stop what she is doing to provide eye-to-eye contact she may still respond to the child's conversation by head nods, questions, or "uh-huhs." The parent should talk "with" the child, not "to" the child.

The parent should not supply a word which the child is stumbling over. He should wait quietly and patiently for the child to say the word. He should not tell the child to "hurry up" and say a word, or to "slow down."

Stress often increases stuttering in young children (619). Parents should protect the child from unnecessary stress. Violent television programs or movies, frightening stories, family conflicts and change in the home environment may stress the child beyond his ability to cope. A regular schedule provides a comforting factor for stressed children (619). They should have a simple diet, plenty of out-of-doors exercise, and should be protected from excessive fatigue.

STYE (HORDEOLUM)

A stye is a "boil" on the eyelid around an eyelash follicle, oil or sweat gland. Styes are common in children and adolescents. A painful red lump may appear, then over two to three days the lump comes to a head and drains pus. It is generally caused by one of the staphylococcus bacteria and may be contagious. Failure to drink enough water to keep the eyelid secretions thin can contribute to the cause, as can inadequate hand washing.

Treatment should be begun at the first sign. Use warm, wet compresses three to six times a day for 15 to 30 minutes at a time (620). Saline solution for an eyewash made by adding one-half teaspoon of salt to eight ounces of water (621) may be used if the eye itself becomes inflamed. After the stye drains compresses should be continued until all drainage ceases.

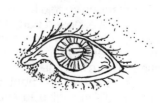

Stye

The stye may just gradually disappear or may form a head and drain. The hands should be washed carefully with soap and water before and after touching the child's eye or face for the treatments.

The child should have his own towel and washcloth, and not touch those of other family members (621). These must be laundered daily. Discourage the child from rubbing his eye, as the bacteria may be spread.

Styes are particularly common in adolescent girls because of incomplete removal of eye make-up at night (622). Any eye makeup used prior to the onset of the stye should be discarded as it may be contaminated. Mascara should not be kept longer than three months as bacterial growth may occur (623).

Refined, fried and highly processed foods should be eliminated from the diet (624). Avoid meats, dairy products, white flour, salt, oils, tobacco and alcohol. A good diet will increase the body's ability to resist bacterial invasion.

SUNBURN

Sunburn is common in both children and adults, and results from overexposure to ultraviolet rays. Sunlight contains both visible and invisible light rays. Ultraviolet B rays are the more harmful of the rays.

Sunburn has been shown to produce premature wrinkling of the skin and has been associated with skin cancers. The darker the skin the more protection the person naturally possesses against sun-related skin problems. Sunburn during childhood may have lifelong consequences.

With sunburn the skin becomes red, hot and tender. There may be associated fever, chills, headache, nausea, and abdominal cramping (625). Symptoms may begin 2 to 4 hours after sun exposure with maximum symptom intensity in about 24 hours. In severe cases there may be blistering and peeling of the skin.

Prevention

Prevention of sunburn is the goal. Maximum ultraviolet B ray exposure occurs from 11 A.M. to 3 P.M. (625). Outdoor activities should be well before or after these hours when possible, especially for fair skinned, blue-eyed persons. Length of exposure should be gradually increased, beginning with about ten minutes and increasing five to ten minutes per day so long as no sunburn occurs. Redheads and children with freckles have more sensitive skin and are more likely to burn with sun exposure. With the sunburn very fair people may develop a feeling of faintness or may actually faint and develop a fever up to 102 degrees F.

Sunscreens should be used when prolonged sun exposure is necessary. Apply to all exposed parts of the child's body, with special attention to the hands, ears, neck and head. Reapply the sunscreen if the child has perspired enough to wash it off. Be certain to use sunscreen, not suntan lotion. There is some question as to whether or not sunscreens are safe for infants less than six months of age. Some children even older than six months are sensitive to substances in sunscreens and may develop an allergic reaction. Sunscreens have also been shown capable of preventing sun-induced vitamin D production, which may lead to rickets.

Children are more susceptible to sunburn than adults and should wear long sleeves, long pants and a hat when out of doors for long periods.

An overcast day will not prevent sunburn. Sun glare off water, sand, sidewalks or snow may contribute to sunburn (626).

Treatment

Cool tap water soaks or a tepid bath will rehydrate the skin and decrease the inflammatory process. Two or three tablespoons of baking soda may be added to a tub of water (626). Avoid the use of soap during bathing.

Cool compresses of baking soda and water, vinegar, aloe vera or colloidal oatmeal may be soothing to the sunburned child.

Water intake should be encouraged (626).

Over-the-counter sunburn medications often contain substances such as lidocaine or benzocaine to which many people are intensely sensitive. Furthermore, they give no more relief than very simple, less-expensive home remedies.

SWIMMER'S EAR (OTITIS EXTERNA)

Swimmer's ear is a condition in which the outer ear canal becomes inflamed, swollen and red because of infection following water in the ear. Water in the ear canal washes away the protective waxes normally found in the ear canal, allowing the infection to gain a foothold.

Tenderness and pain, discharge from the ear canal, difficulty hearing, and itching are common symptoms. Touching the ear often causes pain. There may be a feeling of fullness in the ear.

Children who go swimming are more likely to develop swimmer's ear, although hot, humid climates may be sufficient to cause the problem. Shampooing the hair, or water which enters the ear canal during bathing may also contribute. Chlorinated water is more likely to cause swimmer's ear than salt water (627). Injury, as with the use of a hair pin or cotton swab to clean the ears, may also predispose to swimmer's ear.

Treatment

The key element of treatment is keeping the ear clean and dry. During periods of active disease the child should not be allowed to swim. After symptoms clear and he resumes swimming he should shake his head on coming out of the water to remove as much water from the ears as possible. A hair dryer set on low may be used to dry the ears several times a day. Pull the ear up and out to straighten the ear canal and allow free flow of air (628). Soft ear plugs should be used during swimming but the firm ear plugs may damage the ear lining, decreasing the ability of the skin to protect against invasion. Ear plugs should also be worn by susceptible persons while bathing and shampooing the hair.

Heat from a hot water bottle, heating lamp or heating pad may be effective in pain relief (629). Heat should not be applied for longer than 15 minutes at a time.

Commercially available drops are sold in drugstores to prevent or treat swimmer's ear but these may be easily made up at home. Several formulas have been suggested:

(1) One ounce of plain rubbing alcohol

One ounce of white vinegar (5% acetic acid) (630)
(2) One ounce of white vinegar
     One ounce of 70% ethyl alcohol

Use either of the two formulas, whichever is easier for you to make up. Place several drops in each ear before and after swimming, and at bedtime in the following manner. Wash your hands, warm the eardrops in hot water if they have been kept in the refrigerator and have the child lie down. Pull the ear down and back in a child under three years of age to straighten the ear canal, allowing the drops to flow easily into the ear. In children over three years of age the ear should be pulled up and back to straighten the canal. Allow the drops to run into the ear until the ear canal is completely filled. Turn the child on the other side which will allow the drops to run out of the ear. Then dry the ear with a facial tissue as well as possible. Repeat with the other ear. If the child complains of severe pain from the drops, the drops should be discontinued and the ear drained and dried.

Water may be substituted for the alcohol in the ear drop formulas if the child is sensitive to alcohol, although the resulting solution will not dry so easily or completely.

TEAR DUCT BLOCKAGE (DACRYOSTENOSIS)

Dacryostenosis is blocking of the tear duct which carries tears from the eye to the back of the nose. In about six percent of normal, full-term infants this duct is not open at the time of birth. Symptoms appear shortly after birth. The parents will notice excessive tearing or continuous watering in one or both eyes (631). Tears may run down the face even though the child is not crying. There is no redness of the eyelid or eye. The eyelashes may be crusted with discharge from the affected eye. There may be a small lump in the inner canthus of the eye, which is merely the full duct (632).

In the past some pediatricians have elected to surgically open the tear duct but recent studies have demonstrated that simple massage is usually effective in opening the duct. Most cases clear by 12-16 months of age without any surgical procedure.

Signs of dacryocystitis (infection of the lacrimal sac) include redness of the skin, swelling of the duct, fever and purulent discharge. Dacryocystitis can be treated with hot saltwater compresses. Use a clean cloth dipped in a salt water solution made by adding one-half teaspoon of

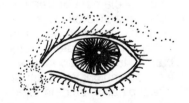

Full Tear Duct in Dacryostenosis

salt to eight ounces of hot water. Allow the solution to cool enough to avoid burning the child. Wring the cloth out until it ceases dripping and place it over the eye. As the cloth dries out dip it into the saline solution again and reapply. Leave the compress on for an hour, remove it for an hour and repeat the treatment (633).

Some infants have mucocele, which appears as a bluish mass. If the white of the eye becomes red, redness and swelling appears along side the nose, or yellowish or white discharge appears in the corner of the eye, the child should probably be evaluated by your health care provider. Massage should be stopped at the first sign of infection to avoid risk of spread.

Mucus collected in the corner of the eye can be removed with clean, damp cotton ball or cloth.

Although a large percentage of ducts open spontaneously, some prefer to assist the natural process. Using clean hands, with short fingernails, the parent should place the tip of the finger over the corner of the eye and gently, slowly, push the finger downward in an effort to force the lacrimal sac fluid through the closed off drainage tract. This should be carried out repeatedly for about one minute, three to four times a day (634). Some parents prefer to use a cotton-tipped swab for the pressure and massage. Some-times a pop is felt as the duct opens and the problem immediately resolves.

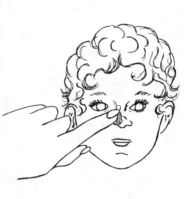

Massage Technique for Dacryostenosis

This treatment may need to be carried out for six or eight months in some children.

THRUSH (ORAL CANDIDIASIS)

Thrush is an infection of the mucosa of the mouth by Candida albicans (635). It occurs in approximately four percent of all infants, with onset often within eight to nine days after birth. Infants of mothers who have vaginal yeast infection may be exposed during birth, but infants of non-infected mothers may be exposed in the newborn nursery.   Infants of diabetic mothers are unusually susceptible, as are infants born with cleft palate or cleft lip (636).

Symptoms include white patches in the mouth which may look like milk curds. Milk curds are easily rubbed off but thrush sticks to the oral tissues, and when removed leaves a red, raw appearing area (635). In severe cases discomfort may hinder food intake. Infection is more common in bottle-fed infants (637); it is felt that breast milk contains substances which assist the infant's immune system to resist the infection (638).

Infants who have been given antibiotics often have thrush invasion due to the elimination of the normal oral bacteria.

Treatment

Bottle nipples and pacifiers should be soaked in 130 degree F. water for fifteen minutes between each use (639). Mothers who are breast-feeding should wash their nipples well with plain water after each feeding.

Cleanse the infant's mouth with plain water after every feeding. Inspect carefully for indications of thrush and begin treatment at the first indication of it.

Antibiotics and steroids destroy competing bacteria, making the child more susceptible. Some recommend swabbing the infant's mouth with the mother's saliva to establish a flora which will provide an environment unfavorable for the growth of Candida (640).

Use a cotton-tipped applicator to swab the infected areas with a saturated solution of baking soda three or four times a day. You may wish to try to carefully remove all lesions adherent to the oral tissues which are within easy reach.

Candida is sensitive to garlic and the mouth may be swabbed out with a garlic solution several times a day. Make the solution by blending one peanut size clove in one cup of water until smooth.

Five bay leaves may be simmered in 2 cups of water for twenty minutes, the leaves strained out, and the solution used as a mouthwash for thrush. Be certain the solution is cool enough to avoid burning the infant. The tea may be kept in the refrigerator for a day but should be made up fresh every two days. Use a sterile dropper to place the tea in the baby's mouth twice a day.

TICK BITES

Ticks drill into the skin but it takes several minutes for them to accomplish this. They may readily be removed before they accomplish this. Grasp the tick with tweezers or the fingers and pull gently but firmly with an unscrewing motion. If the tick has accomplished his drilling do not attempt to just yank him out. Part of his body may be left behind, causing an infection.

If tick body parts are inadvertently left in the skin during the removal use a clean needle to remove them, just as you would pull out a splinter.

The tick may be covered with fingernail polish, petrolatum, alcohol or kerosene and gently removed after a few minutes using tweezers. Wash the area with soap and water. Because tick bites may be associated with several diseases the area should be observed for a few days for any signs of infection, redness, tenderness or pus. Lyme disease is one of the most rapidly spreading tick-borne diseases, the deer-tick being the vector. In areas where Lyme disease is endemic children may need to wear long sleeves and trousers and use approved insect repellents when playing outside. Parents should inspect children carefully when they come into the house. Family pets, especially cats, have been found to harbor the deer-tick and have been responsible for a number of cases of Lyme Disease. Any generalized, unexplained rash should be seen by a physician in areas endemic for Lyme Disease and Rocky Mountain Spotted Fever.

TICS

Tics are sudden, purposeless, involuntary, repetitive body movements (641) such as head movements, face jerks, eye twitches or blinks, shoulder movements or arm movements. They may persist for a few weeks and spontaneously disappear, but in other children persist for several months. They appear irregularly and are worse at some times than at others. The head is most often the area affected, with the shoulder, trunk and lower extremities involved less frequently. The child may attempt to disguise them by performing some associated movement to make the tic appear part of a purposeful movement. Incidence of the movements increases when the child is under stress, and cease during sleep. Sometimes the child may voluntarily suppress them, but there is often a rebound effect after cessation of voluntary control, with a higher incidence of movements (642). Boys are affected more often than girls (643) and a family history is reported in about half of all cases. However, it is likely that the family history is much higher than the reported incidence, as tics are transient, and unless severe and unremitting are not likely to be reported to the family physician or even a topic of common knowledge among family members. One study reported that the average tic duration was four-and-a-half years (644).

Average age of onset is reported to be 7 to 12 years of age, although cases have been reported in 2 year olds and may develop in adolescence. Up to 35% of children have tics at some point in childhood and most of these disappear spontaneously over a few months. The child may begin with one tic, such as jerking the head, and this tic may disappear only to be replaced by another such as wiggling the nose or blinking the eyes (695). Children with tics often have associated behavior disorders such as nightmares, attention deficit (hyperactivity), bedwetting or sleepwalking. Sometimes the tics first appear after the child is given a medication to treat another behavior disorder (645).

Some tics are vocal and may involve repeated sounds such as throat clearing, coughing, sniffling, grunting, barking, repeating the words of others or in severe cases, obscene language. Vocal tics are less common in children than in teenagers or adults. Tics may be associated with the use of a number of medications, or illness such as sinusitis or any type of infection. The child may begin the movements in response to local irritation such as hair in the eyes, clothing that is too tight, or other annoyance and the motion may persist even after the condition is corrected. Such factors should be looked for and removed immediately, as the tic will not improve so long as they are present. Children may also imitate tics they observe in other people.

Tics are classified in one of two groups. Simple tics generally involve only one movement, which may disappear only to be replaced by another tic. Up to one-quarter of all tics in children are of this type. This type of tic is the most likely to resolve spontaneously, often within six months.

Complex tic disorders may involve numerous movements and are more likely to include vocal tics. The tic is chronic, with variation in severity of symptoms from day to day. This group also includes Tourette syndrome, which manifests as motor incoordination with echolalia (the involuntary repetition of words just spoken by other persons) and coprolalia (the involuntary use of obscene or vulgar words). Children with complex tic disorders may manifest more complex tic movement including retracing steps, twirling, squatting, touching or hitting himself or others, jumping, kicking, or stamping the feet.

Treatment

The family should ignore the movement as much as possible. Scolding the child only places more stress upon the child. He is often ridiculed by his classmates and friends, and may try to avoid them. Instead, the parent should direct his attention toward the general improvement of the child's well-being.

The child's program should be evaluated to see if too much is expected of the child. Schooling should be delayed in these sensitive children as both the curriculum and the other students will have an adverse effect on the nervous system. If he runs from one activity to another all day long he may have a program beyond his tolerance. He should have ample time for vigorous out-of-doors exercise in useful, purposeful activities such as yard work or gardening, with a parent if possible. Competitive sports should be carefully avoided. Television, radios, comics, funny papers, and other stimulating factors including movies should be carefully eliminated (647). However, in restricting these activities the child should not be made to feel that he is being punished.

The diet should be simple and non-stimulating (648). Coffee, tea, soft drinks, sugar, honey, molasses, syrup, spices, vinegar and other irritating foods should be eliminated.

The child should have a regular schedule seven days a week and 365 days a year. He should arise at the same time every morning, have meals at the same time and go to bed at the same time every evening. He should have adequate sleep every night (648).

The child may discuss with the parent his inability to control the movements and the embarrassment this problem causes him. In these cases the parent may wish to guide him in some exercises which may be helpful. It must be remembered that every child is different, and what will help one child with a tic will not help another. In most cases "benign neglect" will resolve the problem.

A deep breathing exercise may be helpful. The child should take a slow, deep breath as he raises his arms up above his head, then breathe out slowly as he lowers them (648). Repeat the steps for ten minutes at a time three or four times a day. The child's attention should be focused on the exercise, which will divert his attention from the tic.

The child may be instructed to stand in front of a mirror to observe his tic, then voluntarily reproduce the tic five times. Interestingly, these children may have a very difficult time reproducing the tic, and often must make great effort to accurately reproduce it. It is felt by some that this brings the tic under his voluntary control as he learns which muscles are involved.

A third exercise consists of having the child remain motionless for as long as possible. The period of time should be very short at the beginning of the exercise, and slowly, gradually increased in duration, until he can remain motionless for at least five minutes (649).

Medications such a haloperidol are often recommended in the treatment of tics, particularly in Tourette syndrome and others of long duration, but the parent should be aware of the severe adverse effects that may be associated with this medication (650). It may cause sleepiness, memory and concentration difficulties, Parkinson-like symptoms, tremors, muscle rigidity, drooling, shuffling gait, fatigue and muscle weakness. The child may become depressed or apathetic, irritable, unwilling to go to school and overly dependent on others.

TOEWALKING

Many children begin learning to walk by appearing to be walking on their toes. The child actually walks on the balls of his feet rather than the toes. This is normal for the first few months of walking. An infant held upright will attempt to stand on his toes. If toewalking persists after the child reaches the age of four or five years it may need evaluation by your health care provider. Some normal children continue toe walking until they are seven or eight years of age. Toewalking may run in families (651), and is more common in boys. Activity is not limited nor does the child complain of pain. Many of these children are clumsy and they are often hyperactive.

Toe walking may be due to a number of factors but probably the most common physical cause is tight heel cords.

Children who have "normal" toewalking are able to put their heels on the ground and may even be able to walk flatfooted for short distances. They are merely more comfortable in the toewalking position. If your child spends part of his time walking flatfooted you may be fairly certain he will eventually do so consistently (652).

There has been a recent increase in the incidence of toewalking. This is felt by some to be due to the hours that young children spend in walkers requiring them to walk on their toes in order to move about. It becomes a habit for the child and is outgrown when the child is no longer in the walker (653).

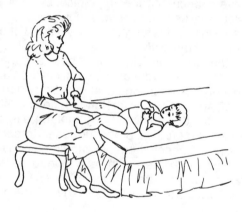

Stretching Exercise for Toewalking Done by Parent

Children with tight heel cords may often be helped by gentle stretching exercises carried out by the parent. The foot should be flexed up toward the knee, held for ten seconds, and released, repeating the stretch twenty to thirty times several times a day. The parent should be careful to keep the toes straight up and not turned toward either side (654).

Children three or four years of age may stretch their heel cords by standing with their toes on a book at least two inches thick.

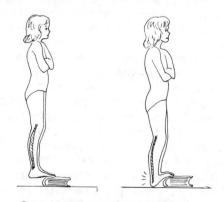

Stretching Exercise for Toewalking Done by Child

They should lower the heels to the ground, hold for ten seconds, then lift the heels off the floor and repeat for twenty or thirty times at each session. The child should not bounce up and down during the exercise as this will cause contraction of the muscle rather than stretching. If these exercises are unsuccessful and the child persists in toe walking casting may be carried out. Recent studies suggest that surgery to lengthen the heel cord has often been carried out unnecessarily. Some children with persistent toe walking have physical abnormalities such as autism, short tendo calcaneus, spastic diplegia, Charcot-Marie-Tooth disease, cerebral palsy, muscular dystrophy or other neuromuscular disease.

TONGUE TIE (ANKYLOGLOSSIA)

Tongue tie is a very rare problem (655) but unfortunately many children have been subjected to an unnecessary surgical procedure to correct it.

Tongue tie is abnormal shortness of the frenulum linguae, the tissue which attaches the tongue to the bottom of the mouth. Children with true tongue tie have speech and feeding difficulties. They may have abnormal dental development because of poor tongue function. With true tongue tie the child is unable to stick his tongue out or to lift it off the bottom of the mouth to touch the roof of the mouth.

The tongue is normally short at birth, and the band tight (655). It stretches in use, and by one year of age most children are able to stick the tongue out of the mouth. Never should surgery be performed until after the child is one year of age. Even with tongue tie the child may not suffer speech impediment, or if he does have one, there is no guarantee that clipping the frenulum, the surgical procedure used to correct tongue tie, will solve the problem. A speech therapist should be consulted.

Parents of children with true tongue tie should evaluate whether the associated risks (bleeding, infection, scar tissue formation and injury to the openings of the salivary ducts) are worth the advantages to be gained (656).

TONSILLITIS

Tonsillitis is an inflammation of the tonsils which is caused by bacterial or viral infection (657). It is a common problem between the ages of two and seven years of age. It is particularly common in children who attend school and are exposed to the infection there. Some children have four or five acute infections during the course of a year. Symptoms include sore throat, fever, swollen tonsils, palpable lymph nodes and difficulty swallowing. The tonsils may be swollen and red, and have yellow or white patches on them. Children less than six or seven years of age may not complain of sore throat even with tonsillitis (658), but may appear lethargic or sleepy. Symptoms may resolve over seven

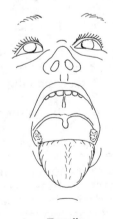

Tonsils

to ten days. In the past repeated episodes of tonsillitis were considered indication for tonsillectomy but we have recently begun to understand that by the time the child is eight or nine years of age he begins to outgrow the problem (657). There are no known permanent adverse effects even from repeated episodes of tonsillitis. Deaths from tonsillitis are almost unknown but deaths from tonsillectomy are not.

Enlarged tonsils and palpable cervical glands appear in almost all children two to eight years of age. It is during this time that the child develops his own immunity. Lymph gland enlargement is common during this time. Enlarged tonsils are not necessarily a sign of infection; they may be large only because they are performing a large task of boosting the immunity. Chronically infected tonsils may be small and tonsils which are large may be small when examined two weeks later. Sore throat may be due to factors other than tonsillitis and some studies have shown that removing the tonsils does not decrease the incidence of sore throat.

Tonsillectomy should not be entered into lightly. Several studies indicate that children who have had tonsillectomy are at increased risk of pneumonia, bronchitis, common colds, pleurisy, acute cervical lymphadenitis, multiple sclerosis, Hodgkin's disease and poliomyelitis. The increased incidence of respiratory tract infection following tonsillectomy is often greater than the tonsillitis associated illness. Some feel that tonsillectomy predisposes to the later development of leukemia (659). It may also contribute to the development of such diseases as AIDS by reducing the body's ability to resist opportunistic infections (660). The tonsils play a role in the body's natural defense system and their removal forces other areas of the body to attempt to take over their function. These organs were designed by the Creator to defend against infection--they were not placed there in error. Their location allows them to capture germs which enter through the mouth and throat (661). They also produce antibodies, which assist in fighting infection (662). Removing the tonsils and adenoids is removing the disease fighting equipment--not removing the cause of the disease.

Tonsillectomy is often recommended in the treatment of ear infections or reduced hearing. One must question the validity of this as a justification for surgery, as many childhood ear infections are untreated or inadequately treated. If these ear infections were very likely to produce hearing loss we would have many more deaf people walking around the country. Ear infections are often undetected and although children may show temporary hearing loss, repeat testing several years later shows normal hearing.

Adenoids are often removed at the time of tonsillectomy. The adenoids are often prominent in young children; by adulthood they usually disappear entirely. Everything said for keeping the tonsils can be said to be advantages for keeping the adenoids as well.

Studies which show an improvement in symptoms after tonsillectomy show significant changes only for the first year after surgery. After then there appears to be no significant benefit from tonsillectomy but the complications mentioned begin about that time. Asthma onset after tonsillectomy is not uncommon.

Treatment

The finest treatment we have for tonsillitis is sucking on charcoal tablets as lozenges, or even better, nibbling all day on a paste made from charcoal powder mixed with water. Add a few drops of water to two tablespoons of charcoal powder. The charcoal is soothing to the throat and it removes substantial quantities of germs from the throat surfaces.

Sucking on crushed ice may be helpful in pain relief (657). An ice bag may be applied to the throat. An ice collar or flannel wrung from ice water and changed frequently may be used. Cool bland liquids may be given frequently.

The tonsils may be swabbed with lemon juice for pain relief (663).

Fluid intake should be encouraged, as it will assist the body in eliminating toxic substances.

Constipation should be avoided, and treated if present. Drinking hot water first thing in the morning may produce a bowel movement in some; others may require an enema.

Hot or cold compresses may be applied to the throat, depending on the child's preference.

Gargling with hot salt water is often soothing (664). Add one teaspoon of salt to an eight ounce glass of water. Gargling may be repeated every 15 minutes. Goldenseal tea may also be used as a gargle (665).

A heating compress may be applied to the throat between other treatments. See the treatment section for technique.

A cool-mist humidifier may assist in relieving throat irritation (666).

Steam inhalations may be used several times a day (663).

Fever may be treated with a hot half bath followed by cold mitten friction.

Symptoms of allergy may be mistaken for tonsillitis (677). These children often have worsening of their symptoms after tonsil removal. Elimination of the most common food allergens may be very helpful, even curative, in these children.

Tonsillitis is more common in children who are exposed to their parent's cigarette smoke (668).

People who own dogs who have streptococcal infections of the eyes may acquire the infection and develop tonsillitis (669).

Hot foot baths are helpful in symptom relief. A hot foot bath, combined with alternating hot and cold applications to the throat may be carried out two or three times a day. Apply heat for five minutes, then cold for five minutes, with three changes of each. Finish off the treatment with a cold mitten friction.

Garlic is a natural antibiotic and may be given in any form the child will accept it.

General measures to improve the health should be undertaken. Children should have a regular schedule with adequate rest every day. The diet should be low in sugar and fats, and contain fresh fruits and vegetables daily. Out-of-doors exercise should be taken every day. Refined foods, such as white bread and white rice should not be used.

ULCERATIVE COLITIS

Ulcerative colitis is an inflammation of the colon. It is most common in the 10 to 19-year-old age group (670). There are often other family members with a history of allergic disease such as hay fever, asthma and eczema. It is more frequent in Caucasians and among those of Jewish descent.

The inflammatory process may involve the entire colon or only intermittent patches. Symptoms include abdominal pain and cramping, diarrhea, mucous or blood in the stool, and rectal discomfort. The diarrhea is often worse during the night and early morning hours, but may persist around the clock in severe cases (671). There are intermittent recurrences and resolution of symptoms. Onset of symptoms may be sudden or slow, and symptoms vary from mild to severe in intensity (670). In severe cases growth may be retarded. There may be associated anemia, joint pains, edema, and clubbing of the fingers.

Treatment

Food allergy may be the most common cause of ulcerative colitis. Milk and gluten are the most commonly incriminated foods, but eggs, wheat, tomatoes, beef, condiments, citrus fruit, beans, apples and strawberries may induce symptoms. Milk allergy tests are ineffective and a trial period of strict elimination of all milk and milk products should be tried in all cases of ulcerative colitis. Gluten is found in wheat, rye, barley and oats. Millet and rice are generally well tolerated.

Very hot or very cold foods may irritate the gastrointestinal tract and stimulate peristalsis leading to evacuation of the bowel. Such stimulants as coffee, tea, chocolate, colas and carbonated beverages should be avoided, even in small quantities.

All foods should be eaten slowly, and thoroughly chewed. Overeating, which leads to distention of the colon, should be avoided. The meals should be taken on a regular schedule.

Babies should be breast-fed rather than bottle fed (672). Most ulcerative colitis patients were fed cow's milk during infancy rather than breast-fed.

Activity should be encouraged to the limits of the child's tolerance. These children may require encouragement to do what they can to help themselves and to live as normal a life as possible within the limitations of their disease.

The child may have 15 or more episodes of diarrhea during a day. Care must be taken to provide good perineal care during episodes of diarrhea. Sitz baths may be soothing. Cooked carrots, charcoal powder, or carob may assist in the control of diarrhea and some report benefit from the pectin found in bananas and apples. Cooked brown rice or rice water is also reported helpful. If charcoal is used, take a heaping teaspoonful with each loose stool. It is a very effective remedy for diarrhea.

Heat applications to the abdomen may be used for pain relief (673). Use fomentations to the abdomen for twenty minutes once a day.

In the past patients with ulcerative colitis have been given a low-fiber diet, but recent studies suggest that high-fiber diets are often well tolerated and actually improve the condition.

A number of drugs are felt to induce or exacerbate symptoms of ulcerative colitis (674). General measures should be taken to improve the overall health. Daily out-of-doors exercise decreases stress which is felt to play a role in exacerbations of the disease. Competitive sports are stressful and should be eliminated.

Some people are sensitive to chemicals found in city water. These people show improvement when placed on distilled water.

A cold sitz bath for 15 to 30 minutes with a simultaneous hot foot bath may decrease diarrhea. Use a wash tub from the hardware store for the cold water, which should be at about 92 to 94 degrees F., and a foot tub for the foot bath with water at 108 to 112 degrees F., depending on the child's heat tolerance. Be careful to avoid burning the child.

Some are benefitted from the use of eight ounces of freshly prepared cabbage juice immediately before each meal.

Fever treatments have been helpful in some cases of ulcerative colitis. The patients in the study group were given 2 1/2 hours of heat treatment, with rectal temperatures maintained at about 104 degrees F. They were given three treatments a week, with a total of about 12 treatments (675).

Some herbal teas may be helpful: peppermint, catnip, slippery elm bark and goldenseal are all recommended. Aloe vera gel may be soothing. A small goldenseal and pectin retention enema has been useful for some. Use one teaspoon of goldenseal powder and two teaspoons of pectin powder. Pectin may also be taken by mouth. Goldenseal capsules may be taken three times a day.

Abdominal pain may be treated with hot compresses over the abdomen, with a simultaneous hot foot bath.

UMBILICAL HERNIA

An umbilical hernia is a weak place in the umbilicus (navel) allowing the protrusion of abdominal organs into it (676). It is a common condition and rarely requires surgical treatment, even when they are as large as an egg. There are seldom any complications. It is most common in premature infants, in black infants, and in infants of high birth weight. It tends to run in families. It may be present at birth, or appear only when the child coughs, strains or cries (676).

Treatment

Time is the best treatment for umbilical hernia. A study reported in 1962 showed that most cases of umbilical hernia healed by the time the child was six to twelve months of age. Umbilical hernias which persist to the age of six or seven years may heal spontaneously, without surgery, as the muscles of the abdomen strengthen.

For many years parents have taped the hernia, sometimes using a coin to hold the hernia in place. Recently physicians have come to understand that the main benefit of this treatment is the psychological treatment of the parent (677). The child often develops a reaction to the tape, and some feel that taping the hernia actually hinders its cure, as it weakens the muscles whose function is to close over the hole which allows the protrusion. The muscles are exercised and strengthened as the child crawls and walks (678).

URINARY TRACT INFECTION

Urinary tract infections may cause symptoms of painful urination, cloudy or foul-smelling urine, frequency and urgency of urination, backache and fever. Young children may have associated nausea and vomiting, diarrhea, loss of appetite, bed wetting, fever, abdominal pain, irritability, fatigue and urinary retention. Symptoms may be very mild in infants and young children.

Before the age of two the child may be unable to explain his discomfort. The parent should watch for fever, foul-smelling urine, crying on urination, blood in the urine, loss of appetite, and irritability. Older children, who have been potty trained, may begin wetting their pants or wetting the bed at night.

One of the principle underlying causes of recurring urinary tract infection is a food sensitivity. The food or the reaction to the food causes the bladder surface to become irritated. These irritated surfaces are unable to resist infection by common germs in the same way the nasal membranes are more susceptible to infection in a person with hay fever.

Urinary tract infections are most frequently caused by germs which are normally found in bowel movements. Infections limited to the kidneys are called pyelonephritis, those involving the bladder are called cystitis, and those involving the urethra are called urethritis.

Urinary tract infections are common in children, especially in infant boys and older girls. It is felt that respiratory tract infections are the only infections which occur more frequently in children. Children from two to six years of age seem to have the highest incidence of urinary tract infections (679).

Children with urinary tract infection often have pain when voiding, and frequency of urination. However, local irritation of the vagina or urethra may produce these symptoms and the parent should carefully inspect this area for any signs of irritation if a girl complains of burning on urination. Irritation may be due to dyes in clothing, laundry detergents, soaps or poor hygiene. Yeast infections, masturbation, pinworms or trauma may also cause burning on urination.

Older girls are felt to have urinary tract infections more frequently than boys because their urethras are short and straight, allowing bacteria ready entrance to the bladder. If they use the toilet tissue wiping from front to back, the bacteria are not so readily carried to the mouth of the urethra.

Soaking in a bathtub filled with soap or bubblebath may make it easier for contaminated water to enter the urethra and bladder of girls (680). One study showed that dye placed in soapy bath water could be recovered from the bladders in a large percentage of females.

A tendency to urinary tract infection seems to run in families, especially those having allergies.

Treatment

Recurring urinary tract infection should be investigated with an elimination and challenge diet (Appendix 1) to discover any irritating foods the bladder may be sensitive to, causing it to be unable to resist infection.

Fluid intake should be encouraged. Urinary stasis is felt to be an important factor in urinary tract infection. Urine which remains in the bladder provides opportunity for chemical irritation and bacterial growth. Cranberry juice is said to decrease the ability of bacteria to stick to the urinary tract cells, allowing them to be more readily flushed out of the body (681). Frequent urination, which flushes out the germs, and dilution of strong and irritating urine are the goals of increased fluid intake. Avoid the use of carbonated beverages, tea, coffee or alcohol (682).

Bubble bath has been shown capable of causing irritation of the urinary tract in children. A number of cases of urinary frequency, urgency and pain on urination have been reported in children using bubble bath. Within a week after stopping the use of bubble bath the symptoms disappeared. Shampoo in the bath water may have a similar effect (685, 686).

The use of soap to wash the genital area may produce irritation (687). Plain water should be used to cleanse the genital area in those who are sensitive to soaps. Many feminine hygiene products may produce allergic reactions. Scented or colored toilet tissue may be irritating.

Sitz baths (see treatment section) may be useful, 20 to 30 minutes several times a day (679).

The toilet tissue should be used to wipe from front to back and discarded after one wipe (679). Parents cleansing the child at the time of diaper change should follow the same procedure. The hands should be carefully washed after each toilet use.

Boys should be trained to rinse under the foreskin regularly if it is retractable.

Cotton underwear, without dyes or colorings, should be used. Clothing should be loose enough to allow air circulation.

Urinary tract infection in some children may be due to constipation. Apparently fecal retention can produce bladder neck obstruction. The full rectum displaces the bladder, probably preventing the passage of urine. In one study, cure of constipation led to urinary tract symptom improvement in 36 of 45 children. There was recurrence of urinary tract symptoms in those children whose constipation was not corrected (688).

Protein intake should be reduced in children who have strong smelling urine. Milk contains very heavy protein (689). It is also a very common food causing allergy or food sensitivity.

Many children try to retain their urine to avoid the pain associated with urination. Having the child urinate while sitting in a tub of warm water may be helpful.

Children should be taught to avoid holding their urine for prolonged periods.

Children who have urinary tract infections should take only short tub baths (showers are probably better), and should not be allowed to sit in wading pools for long periods.

If urinary symptoms persist in spite of vigorous preventive and treatment measures, a urologist may need to be consulted to rule out congenital or acquired obstructions or defects in the genitourinary tract. Persistent symptoms in girls are being increasingly reported in cases of molestation, often by family members.

VAGINITIS AND VULVOVAGINITIS

Vaginitis is an inflammation of the vagina (690). When the inflammation involves both the vulva and vagina it is called vulvovaginitis. These are common problems in children. They may be caused by germs, yeast infections, parasites such as pinworms, masturbation or irritation from chemicals.

Symptoms include itching, frequent painful urination, and vaginal discharge which may be foul-smelling and profuse. A small amount of vaginal discharge is normal. There may be swelling of the perineal area. The child may have severe discomfort on urination, walking or sitting. She may become irritable, and restless, and scratch the genital area with her hands or rub against furniture in an effort to relieve the itch.

Treatment

Sitz baths are often soothing but gauze compresses may be applied to the area if sitz baths are not available. Use a solution of 1 teaspoon of salt to one quart of warm water for the compress solution. Sitz baths may be given two or three times a day using plain water, colloidal oatmeal, baking soda or starch. Local irrigations with a saline solution may also be used. Corn starch powder may be applied to the perineum to assist in keeping the area dry.

Bubble baths and soaps should be avoided. Vaginitis may be caused by common antibacterial tub cleansers, antibacterial soaps, female deodorant sprays or antibacterial agents in swimming pools or whirlpools. Scented toilet tissue causes vaginal irritation in some (691).

Plain white cotton panties should be used, and changed frequently. Synthetic fabrics tend to retain moisture, encouraging growth of germs. Girls should not be permitted to sit in wet clothing, such as a bathing suit, for long periods. Clothing should be loose, allowing air circulation in the area. Tights, jeans, sleepers, wool clothing and leotards should not be used while the girl has vaginitis. Clothing should be thoroughly rinsed to eliminate all detergents which may produce irritation.

Girls should be trained to wipe from front to back after using the toilet (690) and to wash their hands carefully before and after using the toilet. The perineum should be cleansed gently after every use of the toilet. While she has an infection, while she is sitting on the commode, after each toilet use pour one quart of very warm water or very cold water over the area and pat dry afterward. In severe cases the hair dryer may be used to hasten drying (692).

Many young children insert foreign bodies into the vaginas as a part of the exploration of their bodies. It gets trapped behind the hymen and causes irritation, pain or chronic discharge. Use an otoscope, the instrument used to look into the ears, to find a foreign object. A blood-tinged discharge suggests a foreign body. Examination should be carried out for foreign bodies in every child with vaginitis. Parents should be reassured that this self-exploration is normal and does not mean that their child is "bad." (693)

Vaginitis due to Candida is associated with a thick, white, sometimes cottage cheese-like discharge (694). There is often intense itching. This type of vaginitis is common in diabetic children, those who have received antibiotic or steroid therapy for other conditions, or those who have been taking oral contraceptives. A diet low in free carbohydrates is often helpful to these children. Sitz baths with vinegar water (one cup to a gallon of water) are suggested.

Trichomoniasis vaginitis is associated with a thin, yellowish-green, foamy discharge. There may be itching and/or burning in the vulvar area. Nonspecific vaginitis cannot be traced to a specific cause. There may be a clear or gray discharge, often with a fish-like odor. Gonorrhea, although not as common today as formerly, may also produce vaginitis.

If the perineal area is red and inflamed, vegetable oil, such as olive oil, may be used as a cleansing agent in the place of soap, or the area simply rinsed multiple times with clear water.

Pinworm-induced vaginitis will generally resolve with treatment of the pinworms.

VOMITING

Vomiting is the return of the stomach contents through the mouth. The stomach contracts and forces its contents up through the throat and out through the mouth. Vomiting is a symptom, rather than a disease. It may be due to about sixty different abnormal conditions, but fortunately, most cases of vomiting are not indicative of severe illness (700). The child who gains weight and grows normally, and who appears alert and happy but vomits occasionally most likely does not have any serious abnormality (699). Half of all infants experience occasional vomiting, which may be due to poor feeding techniques, immaturity of the gastrointestinal tract, or a multitude of other factors. Young children often spit up which is to be distinguished from vomiting. Small amounts are often spit up whereas vomiting may produce larger amounts. Other children regurgitate their food. See discussion of this elsewhere in this book.

Cyclic Vomiting

Some children develop a pattern of repeated vomiting which is called cyclic vomiting. These children usually have allergic diseases such as rhinitis, eczema, asthma, allergic conjunctivitis or hives. Many of these children later develop migraine headaches and there is often a family history of migraines. Onset of symptoms begin in late infancy and typically disappear at about nine or ten years of age. These episodes may occur every few weeks, on a somewhat regular basis. The attack often begins with a mild headache, fatigue, restlessness and pale skin. Vomiting begins and may continue for several hours. The child vomits everything he is given and may retch with even an empty stomach. There may be fever, irritability and abdominal pain. Some children have associated diarrhea or constipation. They generally have no appetite and prefer to be left alone and allowed to lie quietly. Symptoms may persist for about four days, then suddenly subside, and the child returns to normal until the next attack. Unless these attacks are very frequent the child continues to grow normally. The frequency of the attacks gradually decreases over time until they entirely disappear. It has been noted that fatty or fried foods cause attacks in many of these children but a number also react to other foods, including oranges (701). Low-protein, low oxalate diets have recently been shown helpful to these children. Oxalates are found in large amounts in oranges, cocoa, chocolate, rhubarb and tea.

Treatment

Withhold all food and fluid for two hours after a vomiting episode. Begin with a teaspoon or two, depending on the age of the child, of clear fluid such as water or herbal tea, given every 20 minutes. Older children may be given ice chips, with instruction to melt them entirely in the mouth before swallowing. If vomiting recurs do not give anything for another hour. If the child does not vomit again the fluid intake may be slowly increased. After six to eight hours bland foods such as mashed potato, applesauce, rice, toast or banana may be given. If this is well tolerated for about 24 hours the child may be started on his regular diet, but fatty or greasy foods, milk, and spices should be omitted for several days.

Breast or bottle fed infants should be burped frequently during feeding. They should not be encouraged to finish a bottle of milk they do not want. Overfeeding is a common cause of vomiting in very young children. If the child is being breast-fed limit his feeding to one breast, to prevent overfeeding. Place him on the other breast at the next feeding. As the vomiting subsides he may again be given both breasts but his nursing time should be limited. After 24 hours without vomiting normal feeding may begin. Some children benefit from being burped before feeding but some children protest that they are hungry and want to eat right now (702). Crying increases swallowed air, which fills up the stomach, overdistending it, and may lead to vomiting. Eating too rapidly causes more air to be swallowed. Using a nipple with a smaller hole will slow down the rate at which the child can obtain the milk, and allow more time for the stomach to empty (703). Too small a hole in the nipple, however, leads to air swallowing, so a bit of experimentation may be required to determine the proper size nipple hole for your child. Bottle propping may also cause vomiting. The child should be fed in an nearly upright position.

Clearing the nasal passages before eating (see colds section) may be very helpful in children who have a cold. The mucus in the back of the throat may cause them to vomit.

Young children should be handled gently for several hours after feedings (700).

If you notice that a particular food causes the child to vomit it should be eliminated from the diet. Many infants are allergic to milk, and vomit or have diarrhea after taking it. A trial of a milk free diet in children who repeatedly vomit may be very helpful. Eggs are another food which often cause vomiting (701). Gluten allergy may also cause vomiting. Gluten is found in wheat, oats, rye, and barley.

Young children may be placed on the right side for an hour or so after a meal to permit the food to leave the stomach more readily. Use a rolled up towel behind the child's back to prop him up (704). Older infants may be placed on the stomach, with their heads turned to one side. Do not place a young child on his back after feeding, as he may inhale the vomitus and choke. Some children do best if they are placed semi-upright in an infant seat for several hours after eating.

Bad dietary practices are probably the most common cause of vomiting in children. Overeating, new foods, any spices and all highly seasoned foods, "junk foods," poorly chewed food, and irregular eating habits are sufficient to induce stomach emptying. Feedings should be given on a regular schedule.

The child who vomits repeatedly should be given a low-fat diet. Fat slows stomach emptying, encouraging fermentation, which in turn leads to irritation (703).

Care should be taken to prevent dehydration in these children. If your child cries without tears or has not passed any urine for more than eight hours he may be dehydrated. See the section on diarrhea for instructions for home-made rehydration solutions for children who are vomiting repeatedly. Carob powder is helpful in vomiting. Mix it in water and give through a baby bottle for young children; older children may eat it with a spoon. Catnip tea is often soothing and quiets the upset stomach.

If the child has an associated fever, cool cloths may be applied to the forehead.

One of the finest remedies for cyclic vomiting is charcoal. Stir one heaping tablespoon in a quarter cup of water or juice and serve with a straw. If the powder is not available use eight tablets or four capsules. May be repeated each time the child vomits.

Peppermint tea is sometimes soothing, as is barley water (for those not allergic to gluten). Rinse one-half cup of barley well, add to two cups of water and bring to a boil. Simmer for ten minutes, strain and serve.

The child's clothing should be loose enough that it does not constrict the abdomen. The compressed stomach will be able to hold less food (705).

Vomiting is often associated with intestinal infections such as "stomach-flu," or with diseases such as ear ache, colds, croup, motion sickness, or urinary tract infections. Other symptoms presenting at the time of onset of vomiting may provide clues to the cause.

Food poisoning may cause vomiting in children, as it does in adults. If others who have eaten the same food are also showing signs of illness you may suspect food poisoning.

Many medications may cause vomiting (700). Aspirin, aspirin substitutes, many antibiotics, and some asthma medications, are known to cause vomiting in some children. Any drug the child is taking should be considered suspect.

Blockage of the intestine may cause vomiting. If the child vomits green or yellow fluid, and has a swollen, hard stomach, and seems generally ill, his vomiting may be due to intestinal obstruction.

Vomiting is often associated with meningitis (infection of the spinal cord and coverings of the brain) or encephalitis (infection of the brain). These children usually have fever, headache, stiff neck, irritability, and do not want to move. Young children may have bulging of the fontanel (soft spot) on top of the head. These children require immediate professional attention.

A child with severe infection may vomit. The child with infection may have a high fever, have poor skin color, seem to be dazed or not know what is going on about him, and generally look and act ill. These children need professional attention.

Vomiting is a sign of Reye syndrome. This syndrome often occurs following a viral illness, particularly if the child has been given aspirin to control fever or pain. Associated symptoms include behavior changes, lethargy or sleepiness, and irritability. Take your child to the emergency room immediately if these symptoms develop following an illness.

A blow to the head which causes a concussion may induce vomiting.

If your child vomits blood and has not had a recent nosebleed he may have severe stomach irritation. Aspirin may cause bleeding, or he may be suffering from a viral disease which damages the lining of the stomach. Blood which has been in the stomach for a while looks like coffee grounds when it is vomited.

If vomiting is associated with blood, or green or yellow material, the child has severe pain in the abdomen, the abdomen is hard to the touch or swollen, there is severe diarrhea with the vomiting, the child shows signs of dehydration (see section on diarrhea), the child has had an injury to the head or abdomen recently, or the child's behavior changes suddenly he should be evaluated by his health care provider.

WART (VERRUCAE)

Warts are round, raised, rough skin growths. Physicians sometimes call them verrucae, a term coming from the word "verruca," which means "a steep place" because they thought warts looked like "small hills" on the skin. They are probably the most common skin abnormality in children. Peak incidence is in the ten to nineteen year old group, and 70% of all wart patients are between the ages of 10 and 39. Warts are more common in girls than in boys. It is felt that ten to sixteen percent of the population have warts. They are caused by a virus (not handling frogs or toads), and are considered mildly contagious, although the method of spread is not completely understood. Up to half of wart sufferers have other family members who also have them. New warts occur in infected people more often than in those who have no warts. The incubation period is felt to be from one to eighteen months. It is felt that the skin surface must be broken to allow the virus to enter the body. Picking at warts and scratching may spread the virus.

Some researchers feel that the frequency of warts has increased in the past twenty years. They have observed that warts are less common in tropical regions of the world.

Warts most often occur on the extremities, but may occur on any skin surface. There are several different types of warts. A study carried out on children under 16 years of age revealed that 70% of warts were the common wart, 24% were plantar warts, 3.5% were flat warts, 2% filiform and 0.5% acuminata. United States studies have shown a plantar wart frequency of 2.8 to 6.8 percent (706).

The common wart (verruca vulgaris) also called infectious or viral wart, occurs often in adolescents, and is less commonly seen in prepubertal children. They rarely occur before the age of five years, with peak incidence in the 14-15 year old group. They may be one-eighth to one inch in size, and tan, brown, black or flesh-colored. They may be smooth or rough in texture. They occur anywhere on the skin but are most common on the hands and fingers and about the knees and nails. They are often found around the nail folds of nail biters. There may be a single wart, or a cluster. They enlarge over time. They are generally not painful unless they appear under the fingernails or in areas where they are subject to pressure. About two-thirds of these warts will resolve within two years and 90 percent within five years. Over a two-year period about two thirds of the warts in a control population resolved, but approximately half of these patients developed new warts during this period.

Children with allergies seem to have warts more commonly than nonallergic children, and warts in these children are often resistant to treatment.

Children who suffer atopic dermatitis (dermatitis due to allergic reactions) are more likely to have warts. One woman developed common warts in locations where she was exposed to cobalt and nickel, metals she was allergic to.

No form of treatment is known to be 100 percent effective, and treatment is often more effectual in young children than in adolescents or adults. Warts resolve spontaneously in children more often than in adults.

Flat or plane warts (verruca plana) are most common in prepubertal and adolescent girls. They may be brown or tan and are usually less than 2 mm. in size. They may be flat rather than raised. They often occur in groups, sometimes of 50-100 warts. They may become itchy and red as they begin to regress. They are often found on the face, neck, arms, hands, and legs, where they may be spread by shaving. A scratch in the skin may lead to a line of warts.

Plantar warts (verruca plantaris) occur on the sole of the foot, or occasionally on the palm of the hand, and may be painful. They are very common in school-age children, but are rarely found before the age of 5 or 6. Peak incidence appears to be from 12 to 14 years of age. They are rare after the age of 25, and occur with about equal frequency in both boys and girls. There may be only one wart, or a cluster of them. Clusters of 40 to 50 individual warts sometimes grow together into a large area called a "mosaic wart." They are felt to be spread by walking barefoot. Some feel that flat feet, orthopaedic defects, athletic injuries or improper footwear predispose to plantar warts. Girls who wear poorly fitted shoes may develop plantar warts in pressure areas. Plantar warts appear most often under the forefoot and toes of older girls and women, perhaps because of high-heeled shoes. These warts occur more often in people who have a chronic problem with damp feet. Keeping the feet dry is felt to be helpful in both preventing and treating this type of wart. Cotton socks which will absorb perspiration and soaking the feet in diluted tea may be helpful in the prevention of damp feet. Before puberty, 30-50 percent of plantar warts resolve spontaneously within six months. They may persist for longer periods in older people.

Digitate or filiform warts are most common on the face, often around the mouth, nose, and eyes. They may be mistaken for skin tags. Shaving may cause the spread of these warts.

Condyloma acuminata are also called fig warts, genital warts, moist warts, pointed warts or venereal warts. They are found on the genitals and are felt to be transmitted by sexual contact. They are typically white to pink in color.

Many authorities feel that treatment of most warts is both unnecessary and unwarranted. They point out that about 67 percent of warts disappear spontaneously within two years. They have been observed to resolve more rapidly in boys. The number of warts present is not felt to influence the course of resolution. Regardless of the method of treatment there is a high recurrence rate. No wart treatment in current traditional medical use is satisfactory, and no method has been demonstrated to be superior to others. Before embarking on a professional treatment program that could result in permanent scarring the parent should consider the importance of treatment. Children who are teased because of their warts may wish to have them treated, but often warts are no problem to children; the parents are the ones who demand treatment. Treatment of warts around the nail bed may cause damage to the nail plate, resulting in temporary changes in the appearance of the nail. Children who persist in chewing, picking at, or biting on their cuticles or nails may be very difficult to treat. They may also acquire warts on their face or mouth from these activities. If the child persists in picking at or chewing on a wart the parent should cover it with a bandage.

It is interesting that meat handlers have more warts than do non-meat handlers (23.1% vs. 9.9%). It may be that the meat carries the wart-inducing virus (707).

Treatment

If one decides to treat a wart he should remember that the first rule is to do no harm with the treatment. There are many toxic chemicals currently used in wart treatment. We feel that these substances are best avoided. Spontaneously resolving warts heal without scarring, but unwise treatment may leave lifelong skin changes.

Redness and itching of the wart may suggest that the wart is responding to the treatment program.

Livia Warszawer-Schuarcz, M.D. of the University of Plastic Surgery at Rebecca Sieff Government Hospital, in Safad, Israel, reports the successful treatment of warts, including plantar warts, with a very simple procedure. She places the inner side of fresh piece of banana skin over the wart and holds it in place with tape. Fresh banana skin is applied daily after the area is washed. She reports that pain decreases and the wart softens within one week. Once a week she scrapes off the thickened, hard, outer layer of skin. The maximum time required for complete disappearance of the warts in this study was six weeks, and Dr. Warszawer-Schuarcz reported no recurrences in a two-year follow-up study (708).

Adhesive tape has proven very effective in treatment of some warts. Waterproof tape is applied snugly (but not so tight as to hinder blood circulation) over the wart and allowed to remain for 6 1/2 days. The tape is removed, the wart exposed to the air for 12 hours, and the tape reapplied for another 6 1/2 days (709). The wart may be gently scraped every two weeks during the treatment program. The warts generally disappear within four to six weeks of treatment. Surprisingly, the physician who reported this method of treatment has observed that treating one wart may be sufficient to induce regression of other warts on the body.

Castor oil or any sweet oil may be rubbed on warts several times daily. Use an emery board or pumice stone periodically to remove the dead skin.

A tiny wad of cotton may be soaked in freshly squeezed pineapple or lemon juice, castor oil or wheat germ oil, and taped over the wart. A piece of fresh crushed pineapple pulp may be taped over the wart. It is said that the wart will be dissolved with persistent treatment.

A saturated table salt solution is said to cure warts in three to four weeks. Soak a cotton ball or the gauze portion of adhesive bandage in the solution and apply it to the wart nightly (710). The wart may also be soaked for twenty minutes three times daily in a solution made by dissolving 1 1/2 teaspoon of ordinary table salt in one-half cup of water.

Comfrey poultices are said to be helpful (711). Puree a handful of fresh comfrey leaves in a blender, place a small amount of the paste into a small gauze pad, and apply to the wart nightly.

Aloe vera pulp, a slice of raw potato, or a thin slice of garlic may be applied to the wart twice daily until the wart disappears.

Juice from white cabbage (712), sour apples, figs or milkweed are said to be effective wart treatments. Apply one drop daily as long as necessary.

Simple soaking of the wart for 30 to 90 minutes twice a week in hot water kept at 113 to 118 degrees F. cured more than half of the patients in one study (713).

Sunlight exposure sufficient to cause a slight redness of the skin has been reported useful (714).

Two patients have been reported to have developed multiple flat warts while receiving tetracycline (715). It is possible that other medications may have a similar effect.

WASP STINGS

Wasp stings are painful, and are often frightening to young children. Wash the sting, then gently remove the stinger without squeezing. Cold applications, wet table salt, baking soda, meat tenderizer, or a charcoal poultice may be applied for pain relief. After six hours heat is the preferred treatment.

WHOOPING COUGH (PERTUSSIS)

Whooping cough is an infection of the respiratory tract. The name comes from the severe spasms of coughing, which cause the child to make a "whooping" sound as he attempts to draw air through the narrow glottis. "Pertussis" means "intensive cough" (716).

Whooping cough is not so common in the United States as it was previously. Despite this, during 1984, cases of pertussis were reported in almost every state in the country.

Pertussis is spread by airborne droplets. Symptoms begin an average of seven to ten days after exposure. It is highly contagious. Peak incidence is in late summer (716). For some unknown reason it is more common in females than in males. About 90% of cases occur in children less than nine years of age, with ten percent occurring before the child is one year old (717).

The disease is described in three categories. The first is called the "catarrhal stage," which manifests with cold-like symptoms of runny nose, stuffy nose, and sneezing. There may be mild cough. The disease, at this point, is often considered to be merely a cold. The child may lose his appetite, and complain of headache. This stage lasts for seven to ten days. As the disease process continues the cough becomes more vigorous and more frequent, particularly at night. Secretions develop which are thick, sticky, and profuse.

During the second stage, the "paroxysmal stage," there are violent episodes of coughing, which may last for several minutes. They may occur once or twice a day, or fifty times. As the child gasps for air he makes the whooping sound which gives the disease its name. The child may drool, and become quite anxious. There may be associated vomiting during the coughing. The child's face may turn red, or his skin may become blue due to lack of air. The coughing episode is often followed by vomiting. He may become exhausted by the coughing. The eyes may bulge and the tongue protrude. Nosebleeds, conjunctival hemorrhages, and rectal prolapse may be associated with this stage. This stage may last a couple of days, or four weeks, but in most cases continues for about two weeks. The coughing episodes gradually decrease in severity and frequency.

The third stage is the "convalescent stage." This stage continues for three or four weeks, and is manifest by a chronic cough, of less intensity than previously.

Treatment

Cough medications, sedatives, expectorants, and antispasmodics are ineffective in the treatment of whooping cough (716). Young children may require suctioning of the nose and throat (see cold section for procedure).

Fluid intake should be encouraged between coughing episodes. Water may well be the best available cough syrup. Seeds of fenugreek steeped in boiling water and sipped at intervals have been very helpful in soothing the paroxysmal cough. Adequate water intake will assist in thinning the secretions, making them easier for the body to eliminate. Small amounts, given frequently, are generally better tolerated than large amounts (718). The diet should be light, and free of oils and sugars. If the child vomits up food or fluid he may be fed again immediately after vomiting, as there is often a refractory period then during which he will be able to retain food.

A tepid bath in water at about 99 degrees F. for 10 to 15 minutes, with the head or face kept cool with an ice pack or wet washcloth is said to be very helpful in whooping cough. The child receives great relief and often sleeps afterward. Coughing episodes seem less frequent. The bath brings the blood from deep in the body to the surface, decreasing congestion.

Sudden temperature changes, chilling, dust, smoke, physical activity, and excitement may all promote coughing episodes. These should be guarded against. The parent should talk quietly to the child, calming him during coughing episodes.

Some children benefit from a humidifier or steam kettle in the room (719).

The bedroom should be well ventilated day and night, but drafts should be avoided.

Petroleum jelly may be applied under the nose and around the lips to prevent skin irritation from the nasal discharges and the vomiting. Always rinse the mouth after vomiting if the child has permanent teeth, to prevent etching the enamel.

Garlic is said to be helpful in whooping cough (720). Use one-half teaspoon of garlic powder for each 20 pounds of the child's weight. Sun bathing is also said to be helpful. Expose both sides of the body but avoid drafts, chilling, or sunburn.

TESTS YOU CAN DO

A number of simple tests can readily be carried out by the parent. A number of these are described in the section on the physical examination.

Blood Pressure

The words "blood pressure" refer to the pressure in the arteries, rather than in the veins. One is actually measuring the pressure of the blood against the artery walls. The heart contraction is called systole, the resting phase is called diastole. Blood pressure is therefore recorded as systolic over diastolic (e.g. 120/80). The difference between the systolic and diastolic pressure is called the pulse pressure. This should normally be between 30 and 40.

Blood pressure is determined by measuring how high the pressure pushes a column of mercury up a glass tube, and is recorded in millimeters of mercury (mmHg).

When blood pressure is measured the person should have been sitting quietly for at least five minutes before the pressure is taken. The legs should not be crossed. The person should not talk during the blood pressure readings, as talking causes elevation of the blood pressure. Inhaling tobacco smoke (your own or someone else's) will raise the blood pressure, as will caffeine, heavy exercise, chilling, drinking hot or cold beverages, a full bladder, pain, or a heavy meal just prior to the reading. If you are taking your own blood pressure do not squeeze the bulb with the hand the pressure is being measured in.

To measure blood pressure one generally uses a blood pressure cuff called a sphygmomanometer, and a stethoscope. These items are readily available at drug or department stores, or mail order companies. Aneroid sphygmomanometers have a pressure gauge attached to a dial and should be checked against a mercury sphygmomanometer annually, to insure accuracy.

Cuff size should be taken into consideration when measuring children's blood pressure. If too large a cuff is used readings will be low; too small a cuff will give high readings. A cuff with a bladder width of 5 cm. and a length of 8 cm. is recommended for infants with a midpoint arm circumference of from 7.5 to 13 cm.; children with

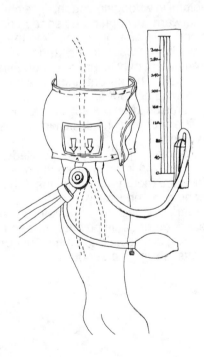

Checking the Blood Pressure

an arm circumference of from 13 to 20 cm. should use a cuff with a bladder width of 8 cm., and length of 13 cm. As a general rule, the cuff should cover two-thirds of the upper arm.

To measure blood pressure the person should be seated comfortably, with the relaxed arm supported and at heart level. The person should extend his arm, palm up, and open and shut his fist about ten times to ensure relaxation. Find the brachial artery on the inside of the elbow. Wrap the cuff snugly around the arm, placing the bladder over the brachial artery. The bottom edge of the cuff should be about an inch above the elbow bend. Place the stethoscope over the brachial artery and inflate the cuff to about 140 mmHg as quickly as possible. If sounds are heard pump the cuff up another 20 mmHg. Continue until no sounds are heard. Begin deflating the cuff at the rate of about 5 mmHg a second until the first sounds are heard. Systolic pressure may be read to the nearest 2 mmHg. Continue deflating the cuff until sounds disappear. Read diastolic pressure to the nearest 5 mmHg.

If you have difficulty hearing the sounds deflate the cuff entirely and ask the child to raise his arm above his head, and open and close the fist several times to stimulate circulation. Reinflate the cuff after the arm is returned to the resting position. If extremely difficult to hear, pump the cuff up to 200 mmHg while the arm is being held above the head, lower the arm, and take the blood pressure.

Pressing too firmly on the artery with the stethoscope will cause elevated blood pressure readings. Use as light a pressure as possible.

Blood Sugar

Blood sugar (or glucose) is often measured in the home. These tests require that the finger be pricked to obtain a sample of blood. There are plastic strips with small pads onto which the blood sample is dropped, and then the pad color is compared with the chart provided with the kit. Glucose meters are also available. The drop of blood is dropped on one of the strips, and the strip placed into a meter, which reads the glucose level. To be accurate the instructions must be followed carefully.

Small lancets are available which make obtaining the blood sample fairly easy. These lancets may be cleansed and reused, but if used too many times they become dull. The finger should be cleansed with soap and water, and thoroughly dried. Any water on the skin will influence the final results. The fingerstick should be done along the side of the finger, rather than in the middle where most of the nerves are located. The center of the finger is also more likely to be calloused which may make it more difficult to get the lancet through the skin. After the skin has been pricked the finger should be turned downward, and the blood "milked" with gentle massage until the blood drop falls on the pad.

If using the visually read strip wait the specified time before comparing the pad with the chart. Anyone with a color vision problem should use another type of system for blood sugar measurement.

The strips can be cut in half and still provide accurate readings, but decrease the cost of each test.

Dental

Plaque disclosing tablets are available in many drugstores. These contain a dye which adheres to any plaque on the teeth. To determine if the child's toothbrushing methods are adequate he should be given one tablet to chew for about one minute after he has brushed his teeth. The remaining material should be spit out. Inspection of the mouth will reveal red areas where the plaque still remains. The child needs to pay special attention to these areas when he brushes his teeth. This procedure may be carried out for several days in a row, until the child has developed a technique which leaves little or no plaque on his teeth. The dye gradually disappears over a few hours, and will be gone in the morning.

The parent may do a preliminary search for cavities. He will need a penlight and a dental mirror for this procedure. Place the mirror behind the area you wish to inspect and shine the light onto the mirror. Look for holes or blackish colored areas. Give special attention to the areas between the teeth, the crevices on the top of the teeth, and the gum line.

Hemoglobin

Hemoglobin tests are used to evaluate anemia. Levels of 10 to 13 grams are normal for children. A dipstick test is available, or a hemoglobinometer may be used. Follow instructions carefully for whichever method you are using.

Temperature

Many mothers use the back of their hand as a thermometer gauge, but for a more accurate measurement a thermometer is needed. There are plastic strip thermometers available, which are just stuck to the child's forehead, but many question the accuracy of these. Electronic thermometers are fast and easy to use, but are more expensive than the common glass thermometer.

The child's temperature should not be measured orally for 20-30 minutes after he has consumed either hot or cold food or fluids. Temperature measurements, regardless of where taken, will be abnormally high after a hot bath or vigorous exercise.

To measure the child's temperature with a glass thermometer clean it thoroughly with rubbing alcohol or soapy water. Do not use hot water as it may break the thermometer. Shake the thermometer mercury down to below 95 degrees F. For oral readings the thermometer should remain under the child's tongue with his mouth tightly closed for at least three minutes. Rectal temperature readings require that the thermometer be left in place for three minutes, but armpit measurements take five minutes to be accurate.

To read the thermometer hold it by the end opposite the bulb. Your fingers over the bulb may raise the temperature. Hold the thermometer in good light, but not close enough to a light bulb that it will be affected by the heat given off by the bulb. Slowly roll the thermometer back and forth until the column is clearly visible. On most thermometers the long lines indicate full degrees, and each small line indicates two-tenths of a degree. Most thermometers are marked in Fahrenheit (F.) degrees, but a few are centigrade (C).

See the discussion of vital signs in the section on the physical examination for further discussion of this procedure.

Transit Time

If your child is bothered by constipation you may wish to measure how long it takes for food to pass through his body. This is called the "bowel transit time." Africans on a high-fiber, unrefined diet have demonstrated a transit time of between 33 and 34 hours, but transit times longer than 80 hours have been shown in children on refined diets. A test substance such as charcoal, which will make the stool black may be given to the child, and the stool watched for the last signs of it. When it has disappeared you know how long it takes for food to pass through the body. A child on a diet with adequate fiber should be expected to pass the charcoal within 36 to 48 hours.

Urine

Strips of plastic with patches attached may be use to check for sugar, blood, acidity, ketones, and albumin in the urine. These are available in many drugstores. The sticks are simply dipped in the child's urine and the resulting colors compared to a test pattern provided with the sticks. Some tests check only one item, such as sugar.

It is important to follow carefully any instructions given with the particular kit you are using. The urine container must be clean and dry, and should be carefully washed to remove even the slightest trace of detergent or soap. If distilled water is available use it for rinsing the container. The container should be somewhat tall and slim, to make the urine rise high enough that the dipstick may be entirely covered. Do not use the test after the expiration date. All strips should be stored in a cool, dry, dark place, with the lid tightly closed.

The first urine of the morning is most likely to reveal any abnormalities, as it is the most concentrated. Testing should be carried out as soon as possible after the urine has been collected. Examine the urine for color, and cloudiness. Red, pink, or red-orange urine may be due to foods such as rhubarb, blackberries or beets, various food colorings, or some drugs. Yellow-orange or bright yellow urine may be due to dehydration, anemia, poor kidney function, foods such as carrots, some drugs, or thyroid disease. If the urine is blue-green or green it may indicate gallbladder or liver disease, or it may be due to some drugs.

Remove one of the strips from the bottle and close the container carefully. Do not touch the pads with your fingers. Dip the strip into the urine for one or two seconds, gently tap it against the edge of the container to remove excess urine, and place it against the chart provided with the kit. Some test kits should be read within a specific time after removing the strip from the urine. Check the instructions with your kit, and follow them carefully.

High sugar levels may suggest diabetes. The urine may contain sugar if the child has been eating a lot of sweets lately.

Ketones are also found in diabetics or during times the child is not eating. Ketones are produced when the body begins burning fat for energy, and lack of food intake, or increased metabolism due to fever may cause elevated levels. Most dipstick tests measure ketone levels as negative, trace, small, moderate or large amounts.

Albumin (or protein) levels often become high in association with a kidney problem. High intakes of protein foods, mustard and other irritants, and some poisons may cause high levels of protein in the urine. Protein levels are often temporarily increased in response to body chilling, acute anxiety, or vigorous physical exercise. A simple test for urinary protein is to slowly add about one teaspoon of white vinegar to the urine. The urine will become cloudy if protein is present.

The pH is a measure of acidity. Seven is considered neutral. As levels increase they become more alkaline, and as they decrease they become more acid. Alkaline levels may suggest a urinary tract infection, but may occur merely because the child is eating a diet high in alkaline foods. A high intake of citrus fruits may produce alkaline urine, while a diet high in such foods as fish, meat, cranberries or prunes will cause the urine to be acid. Milk is said to be able to prevent urinary acidity.

Blood in the urine may indicate injury to the kidney, or urinary tract disease. If much blood is present you will be able to see it. Vigorous physical exercise may jar the kidneys, causing blood in the urine, but this disappears within a day or two. Sickle cell anemia may also cause blood in the urine.

Tests to measure specific gravity of urine indicate how well the kidneys maintain fluid output. They measure the amount of solid material in the urine. The more solid material the higher the specific gravity reading. An inexpensive tool called a urinometer or hydrometer may be used, or one of the dipstick tests you purchase at the drugstore may be used to measure specific gravity. Normal readings range between 1.005 and 1.025, with higher readings indicating more concentrated urine. The urine tends to be most concentrated in the morning, so highest readings should be expected at that time. Urinometers should be checked for accuracy by filling it with distilled water, and checking to see that the reading is 1.000. Some dipstick tests measure bilirubin. Liver or bile duct disease may cause bilirubin excretion in the urine. This will often cause the urine to be dark red-orange in color. Bilirubin, a result of breakdown of hemoglobin, is normally excreted from the body in the stool, and its presence in urine is always abnormal.

There are several tests on the market to evaluate for urinary tract infection. Some of these involve the use of cultures, but simpler ones using nitrite dipsticks or leukocyte dipsticks are also available.

Nitrite dipsticks measure nitrites which are produced by gram-negative bacteria. High levels of bacteria from an infection may lead to high levels of nitrite in the urine. Because bacteria require several hours in the urine to produce nitrites the urine tested should have been in the bladder at least four hours. The first urine of the day is the best for this particular test.

Leukocyte dipsticks measure the number of white blood cells. These cells are the body's disease fighting mechanism, and their presence in large numbers indicates that the body is attempting to fight off an infection.

All urine tests should be done on what doctors call a "midstream" sample. The area should be cleansed with soap and water, and thoroughly rinsed. A small amount of urine should be voided, then one or two ounces of urine caught in a clean, well-rinsed container, and the remainder of the urine voided into the toilet.

TREATMENTS

BAKING SODA BATHS

These are helpful for itching. Add four to twelve ounces of baking soda (sodium bicarbonate) to a tub of tepid water.

CHARCOAL POULTICE

Use for pain (joints, abdomen, ear, throat, chest, etc.), painful or swollen lesions, boils, poison ivy, or over the back or front of the trunk to remove toxins from the body.

A charcoal poultice may be made by pouring a small amount of water into powdered charcoal to make an easily spreadable paste, then spreading it on a paper towel or cotton cloth. Fold the edges of the towel in to hold the charcoal in place. Charcoal powder can be messy--handle it gently. Place the compress over the area to be treated, being generous around all sides, cover with plastic, then with an old towel. The poultice may be held in place with safety pins, an ace bandage or adhesive tape. Be certain the charcoal does not leak out, as it is sometimes difficult to remove from fabric.

CHEST PACK (HEATING COMPRESS)

Uses: chest diseases such as colds, pleurisy, bronchitis, influenza, pneumonia, and cough.

Equipment: Bath towel, large safety pins, plastic garbage bag, and cotton cloth 8 to 10 inches square.

Procedure: Thoroughly warm the patient with a very warm tub bath. Dip the cotton cloth in cold water and smooth over the chest. Cut a slit in the garbage bag bottom for the head and a slit in both sides for the arms. Slip over the head as a shirt. Cut off the excess around the waist. The plastic will prevent any evaporation. Wrap the bath towel snugly around the chest, high up under the arms. Pin with safety pins, being certain that the edges fit snugly against the body to prevent any chilling from fanning.

This pack may be left on overnight for cough, but in acute toxic illnesses it may be changed every hour. This is usually more effective than cough syrup, especially when copious water-drinking is also promoted and the extremities are kept warm.

COLD COMPRESS

Uses: Fever, nausea and vomiting, headache, abdominal pain, arthritis, eye afflictions, sprains, any pain.

Equipment: A folded washcloth or towel, ice water or crushed ice.

Procedure: Wring the washcloth or towel from ice water, and apply to the area to be treated. Refresh the cloth as it begins to warm up from body heat. Crushed ice may be enclosed in a folded washcloth or towel and applied to the area.

Vomiting may sometimes be controlled by the application of a cold wet cloth over the stomach and another to the throat. In severe vomiting the compress may be held snugly against the skin with another cloth or thin towel. In fevers when mouth temperatures go above 100 degrees a cold cloth on the forehead may prevent some of the sensation of weakness, and assist in recovery.

COLD MITTEN FRICTION

Uses: Any infection, cough, fever, or reduced immunity, fatigue, convalescent stage of most illnesses, stimulation of circulatory or nervous system, multiple sclerosis, or to finish a heating treatment.

Equipment: Cold water, terry cloth mittens

Procedure: Dip the mitts into the cold water, squeeze until no longer dripping, slip onto your hands, and rub briskly. Begin with the arms, rubbing in a vigorous alternating back and forth motion from the hand upward toward the shoulder in brisk strokes, adjusting the pressure according to the sensitiveness of the patient. Repeat two or three times, then dry briskly with a rough towel. Proceed to the chest, abdomen, legs, and back.

This treatment is often more effective when it is preceded by a hot fomentation or hot bath which warms the patient.

EAR IRRIGATION

Uses: to rinse wax, foreign bodies, or insects out of the ear, for earache.

Equipment: Ear syringe, warm water, ear basin.

Pull the ear up and back to straighten the ear canal. Look into the ear canal to be certain the eardrum is not ruptured. If you are unsure, have it checked by your health care provider.

Direct the water into the ear with the stream against the wall of the ear canal, not straight down toward the eardrum. Continue washing until the water is clear. If the purpose of the irrigation is to clean out ear wax, drop warm water, olive oil or hydrogen peroxide in the ear at least half an hour beforehand, and preferably the night before, to soften the wax.

ENEMA

Uses: Constipation, cleansing, clearing toxicity, pain anywhere; at the onset of a cold or flu.

Equipment: Hot water or other enema solution, enema bag from pharmacy

Less pressure and less fluid are given in a pediatric enema than an adult enema. Even plain water enemas should not be repeated many times as they may induce water intoxication. Never should a child under age 15 be given more than one enema in 24 hours. Young children may suffer electrolyte and fluid imbalances from the commercial hypertonic phosophate solution enemas. Soap suds enemas may cause rectal irritation and inflammation of the colon, and should not be used.

Saline enema fluid may be prepared by adding two teaspoons of salt to one quart of water. The fluid should be lukewarm at the time of administration. Infants may be given the solution with a enema bulb syringe available at most drugstores.

An infant less than one year of age should receive about four ounces of fluid; a one to three year old child may be given six ounces. Eight ounces may be given to the three to six year old, and twelve ounces to a child from six to twelve years of age. Older children and adults may be given 16 to 32 ounces. Infants will be unable to retain the enema fluid, and should be positioned over a bed pan or receptacle to minimize cleanup. If your bathtub has a removable drain plug, the bathtub may be used to good advantage as it is easily cleaned after the enema. Allow the child to lie down in the tub and expel the enema and bowel movement into the tub. A small tip is thoroughly lubricated and gently inserted two or four inches into the rectum. The enema bag should not be hung higher than 18 inches above the child's hips, and the fluid should flow gently and slowly into the colon.

An older child may be turned on his left side, with a towel under his hips. He should be instructed to retain the fluid, and should be helped to the bathroom for expulsion at the proper time. Pinching the buttocks together may assist the child to retain the fluid. The child and area should be thoroughly cleansed at the conclusion of the procedure.

Have the child lie on his back or left side. Pour water into the bag, expel air from the tube by running some water out, and clamp the tube. Apply petroleum jelly to the nozzle and insert gently into the rectum. Only a small amount of water is necessary for a young child, one to two cups for every 25 pounds of weight. The enema bag should not be more than two feet higher than the hips. Allow the water to flow slowly, encouraging the child to retain the fluid for several minutes. If cramping or a strong urge to expel the fluid occurs, having the child pant like a dog will often relieve it. Never give a child more than one enema at a time, and never repeat on the same day. If the water is not expelled it can be absorbed to cause serious dilution of blood minerals. Sometimes water return can be encouraged by putting petroleum jelly on your small finger, and inserting it into the rectum to massage the rectum with broad strokes.

FOMENTATIONS

Uses: pain relief, chest congestion, warming chilled patient

Water, properly applied, can have a dynamic effect on the body. Care in treatment is necessary to avoid adverse effects.

Fomentations are readily applied to any part of the body and are very effective in pain relief, or promoting healing of infection in tissues or organs beneath the fomentation.

Equipment: 4 large bath towels or fomentation pads, 4 medium bath towels or fomentation covers, aluminum foil, hot oven, ice water, wash cloth

Procedure: Moisten one of the large bath towels, fold, and wrap in aluminum foil. Place in a hot oven at about 375 degrees for about 15 minutes or long enough to become quite hot. Fold a dry towel and spread over the part to be treated. Unwrap the moist towel from the foil and place it over the dry towel. Cover with two folded dry towels to retain the heat.

A canning kettle with rack may also be used to heat the fomentation pads. Put a few inches of water in the pot, roll the fomentations loosely and place on the rack in the kettle. As the water boils steam will rise, heating the pads.

Dampening the pads slightly before placing them in the kettle will help them heat faster, but they should not drip water when taken from the kettle. Use tongs or mitts to remove the hot pads and spread them out on a fomentation cover. Wrap them quickly to retain heat, and apply to the body part to be treated. Several layers of bathtowels may be needed between the skin and fomentation to prevent burning, but these towels should be removed as the fomentation cools, to provide as much heat as possible without burning the patient.

Young children, diabetics, and the elderly are at increased risk of burning, and must be watched carefully. Slipping a hand under it or lifting the fomentation off the body part for a few seconds will provide some cooling, but if the pad is very hot more towels should be placed between the skin and fomentation pad.

A fresh, hot fomentation pad should be applied as soon as the current one begins to cool (about three to five minutes). Wring a washcloth out of ice water, remove the cooling pad, and quickly wipe the treated area with the cold washcloth for 15 to 30 seconds before applying a new hot pack. The cycle should be continued for at least 20 minutes, but cases of severe pain may require 30 to 60 minutes. End with the cold friction.

The patient should be covered with a sheet or blanket, depending on the room temperature to help keep the towels warm and prevent chilling. This treatment, properly given, may induce profuse perspiration.

HEATING COMPRESS

Uses: sore throat, cough, constipation, pain, infection, sedation, hepatitis, backache, ulcerative colitis, cold.

A heating compress may be applied to any part of the body. It is applied cold, and gradually warms up, increasing blood circulation in the area being treated.

Equipment: One or two strips of cotton or linen cut to fit the area to be treated, a piece of cotton cloth large enough to cover the first layer, a plastic strip large enough to cover the two inner layers, a strip of synthetic material or wool flannel cut to fit the area being treated and large enough to cover the plastic covering, safety pins, cold water.

Procedure: Dip the cotton or linen strip into cold water, wring to prevent dripping, and mold snugly over the body part to be treated. Cover this strip with the plastic. Be sure none of the damp cloth sticks out from under the plastic. Wrap snugly, but not so tight that it is uncomfortable. Cover the plastic with the wool flannel or synthetic material strip and pin in place. Leave the compress on for half an hour to overnight. When the compress is removed rub the skin with cold water or alcohol.

HOT FOOT BATH

Uses: headache, stomachache, pelvic infections, chest congestion, fevers, and sprains.

Equipment: Foot tub, large pail, trash container, or bath tub, hot water, thermometer, sheet, two towels, blanket, ice water.

Procedure: Fill the foot tub with water as hot as the child can tolerate without burning him. For children who do not like hot water you may start the treatment with cooler water and gradually add hot water to increase the temperature. Those who tolerate hot water well may be started with 110 degree water. Spread the blanket over a chair, and the sheet over the blanket. Have the child sit in the chair, place his feet in the hot water, and wrap the sheet and blanket around him. Wrap one towel around the neck to catch sweat and trap heat. Add more hot water as tolerated, continuing the treatment for 20 to 30 minutes. At the conclusion of the treatment pour ice water over the feet, rub briskly to dry and put the child in bed for 30 minutes, or until perspiration ceases. Redress in dry clothing.

HOT HALF BATH

Uses: A hot half bath may be used in a number of diseases. It is effective in raising body temperature, enabling the body to more effectively fight disease.

Equipment: Bath tub, two washcloths, bath thermometer, pan of ice water, two to four towels.

Procedure: Fill the tub with water 100-110 degrees F., depending on the age and initial body temperature. The child should be placed in the tub in a manner to cover as much of the body as possible with the water. When sweating begins wring one of the washcloths out of the ice water and apply it to the head, applying a freshened cloth every time the washcloth warms up. It is important to keep the head cool at all times.

A child one to three years of age may be left in the water for three minutes; and thereafter one minute for each year of age. When the time is up, stand the child in the tub, pour cold water from the shoulders down, covering all of the skin, lifting the child up to get to the feet, the cold pour lasting about 10 to 20 seconds. Rub briskly to dry, dress, and put to bed for 30 minutes or more.

HOT BATHS FOR FEVERS

Keep the face and head cool. Follow all baths with 30-60 minutes reaction in bed.

Age of Patient	0-3 years	4-7 years	8-12 years	13-19 years	20 up
Initial Oral Temperature	99°-103°	99°-103°	99°-103°	99°-103°	99°-103°
Initial Water Temperature	106°	106°	106°	106°	106°
Water Temperature					
After 30 Seconds	110°	110°	110°	111°	112°
Length of Bath	3 min.	7 min.	12 min.	13-19 min.	20 min.

Age of Patient	0-3 years	4-7 years	8-12 years	13-19 years	20 up
Initial Oral Temperature	103° & over	103° & over	103° & over	103° & over	103° & over
Initial Water Temperature	104°	104°	104°	104°	104°
Water Temperature					
After 30 Seconds	104°	105°	106°	110°	111°
Length of Bath	3 min.	5 min.	5 min.	7-10 min.	10-12 min.

HOT WATER BOTTLE

Uses: bruises, sprains, pains, warmth, earache.

Equipment: Hot water, water bottle, towel or large knit cap to fit over the water bottle.

Procedure: Fill the bag about one-third to one-half full of hot water from 115 to 125 degrees, and remove excess air by placing the bag on a flat surface, and pressing with your hand, holding the mouth up to prevent the water escaping. Screw the top on before lifting the bag off the table. The hot water bottle may be covered with a towel or the cap. Be careful not to burn the child with it. For an adult, boiling water is used in the bag, and it is filled half full or entirely full, depending on its use.

HYDROGEN PEROXIDE MOUTHWASH

Uses: mouth ulcers, pyorrhea, bad breath, stained teeth, gum boils.

Add one-half cup of 3% hydrogen peroxide to half cup of water. Rinse the mouth three times a day.

NEUTRAL BATH

Uses: to reduce fever, calm a nervous or mentally ill person, induce sleep in insomnia, treat rashes, and reduce blood pressure.

Procedure: Use water from 92 to 98 degrees F. The room should be reasonably warm, but not hot. Continue the bath from 15 to 60 minutes. It is often useful when sleep is slow in coming. It may be soothing to the child who is suffering from hives. At the conclusion of the bath, dry the child with as little motion as possible, and put him in bed. Avoid chilling.

OATMEAL BATH

One pound of old-fashioned oatmeal may be placed in a cotton bag and put in a tub of water. After it has been thoroughly wet the closed bag may be squeezed repeatedly to extract the mucilaginous material which is the soothing principle.

ONION CHEST POULTICE

Steam two large onions until quite soft. Mash one onion in a cloth bag or pillowcase over an area large enough to cover the chest. Apply to the front of the chest. Repeat with second onion and apply to back of chest. Cover with kitchen plastic to prevent drying of the compress and wetting of the sleep clothing. Hold in place with snug fitting sweat shirt or roller bandage pinned snugly, but not bindingly, around the chest. Leave on overnight. Often works wonders for whooping cough and croup syndrome.

PEPPERMINT TEA

Uses: sedation, sleep (and paradoxically for stimulation), cystitis, stomachache.

Add one cup boiling water to one teaspoon of peppermint leaves, allow to steep for five minutes, strain and drink.

POSTURAL DRAINAGE

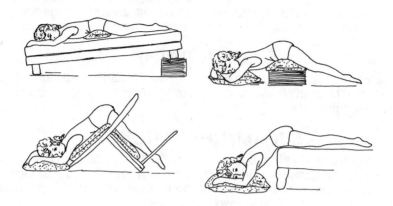

Positions for Postural Drainage
Each position should be maintained for 20 minutes two or three times a day.

SALT BATH

A cup of table salt (sodium chloride) may be added to a tub of tepid water to treat simple dry skin. The bath should be continued for 15 to 20 minutes.

SALT GLOW

Equipment: Salt, water, foot tub filled with warm water
Procedure: Place the foot tub in the bathtub or shower. Have the child stand in the foot tub filled with warm water. Wet the child's skin and your hands. Pick up about one teaspoon of salt, and rub it between your hands. Then rub it on the skin, starting with the chest, then the back. Give this treatment gently the first time, but repeated treatments may be given with more vigor. The objective is to make the skin glow pink. At the conclusion of the treatment have the child shower, or pour a bucket of 80 to 90 degree water over him.

HOT SITZ BATH

To administer a hot sitz bath in the home the patient may be seated in an ordinary bathtub with knees flexed to keep the feet in the water. Water temperature should range from 105 to 110 degrees, and the child should remain in the bath for about 15 minutes. At the conclusion of the bath pour cold water over the treated area or rub with a cold, wet towel, then dry.

SPONGE BATH

Uses: To reduce fever, or to cleanse the skin.
Equipment: Small basin or pan of water 60-120 degrees, two or three

small towels, sponge or small towel, large towel, sheet or blanket.

Procedure: Dip the sponge or small towel into the water in the basin. Begin by bathing the arm. Uncover the arm, bathe it, return it under the covers, and proceed with the other arm. Proceed to the chest, abdomen, legs and then the back. The patient should be covered other than the part being bathed.

STARCH BATHS

Dissolve one cup of starch in a quart of water and add the solution to tepid bath water. The bath should be continued for 15 to 30 minutes. Complete the bath by patting dry.

STEAM INHALATIONS

Place a pan or tea kettle to boil on the stove. Form a cone from newspaper with one end of the cone over the child's face and the other end over the pan. This may be used for ten minutes every hour. Be careful that the child does not burn himself or catch the newpaper on fire.

WET ABDOMINAL GIRDLE

Uses: Constipation, sedation, sleep, skin rashes

Equipment: Linen strips or two layers of cheesecloth 8 to 10 inches wide and long enough to wrap around the body two times,
flannel cover long and wide enough to cover the linen strip, safety pins

Procedure: Dip the linen in water at about 65 degrees F., wring dry, and wrap quickly around the abdomen. Smooth snugly to the skin. Cover with a flannel strip and pin in place. Be certain that none of the damp cloth is uncovered. The girdle should be left on overnight. It sometimes produces local skin irritation. If this occurs omit the treatment for a few nights, then resume.

WET COMPRESSES OR DRESSINGS

Uses: Inflamed, oozing, and itching skin, to remove scales and crusts. Plain tap water is adequate for many of these problems.

Procedure: Cotton material, such as muslin, clean bedding, handkerchiefs, old diapers, or flour-sack dish towels are most suitable for wet compresses. Cut the material in strips and fold two to four layers thick over the area to be treated. Water should be at room temperature. Dip the material into the water, wring out until damp, but not dripping, and apply snugly to the skin. The dressings will begin to dry by evaporation in five to ten minutes and should be removed, dipped in the water again, wrung out and reapplied. Compresses may be applied for 20 to 30 minutes as often as every two hours during the day or even continuously in severe disease. Less severe problems may be treated with compresses two to three times a day. Gently pat the skin dry at the conclusion of the treatment.

Dressings need not be sterilized, but should be laundered every 24 hours.

After 48-72 hours the acute phase should have subsided and compresses should be discontinued to avoid excessive dryness. If large portions of the body must be treated, baths may be more efficient.

Compresses should not be covered with plastic to decrease evaporation as this increases local heat, and may worsen symptoms.

WET SHEET PACK

Uses: To treat fever, psoriasis, pemphigus, eczema and many other dermatological problems, sedation.

Equipment: Blankets, sheets, container of cold water 60-70 degrees F.

Procedure: Lay the blanket out on a flat surface. Dip the sheet into the water, wring dry and place over the blanket. Have the child lie on top of the sheet and wrap it snugly around the child's body, making sure the sheet comes in contact with the body as much as possible. Wrap the blanket up over the sheet and pin in place.

Hot fomentations given before this treatment may produce a better reaction. The feet should be warm at the beginning of the treatment.

For small children, large cotton bath towels may be used in place of the sheet. You may want to use several to cover the entire body.

To treat fever the sheet should be covered with a snugly wrapped wool or synthetic blanket to prevent evaporation. If the patient becomes chilly rub his limbs to warm him or put hot water bottles in several places over the body. Leave it in place for two to three hours, or until the mouth temperature goes up one to two degrees. At that time remove the pack, give a cold mitten friction, and allow the patient to sleep. Upon awakening, the temperature is usually down.

Some patients enjoy having an electric fan blowing gently on the head during the treatment.

APPENDIX 1: COMMON FOOD ALLERGENS

1. Milk is the most common food allergen in the United States. Common sources of milk include whole, dried, skim, 2%, and buttermilk, custards, cheese, cottage cheese, cream and creamed foods, yogurt, sherbet, iced milk, and ice cream. Traces of milk are found in butter, breads, and many commercially prepared foods. Examine all foods for milk products such as lactose, milk solids, sodium caseinate, sodium lactate, milk fats, and whey. Dr. Frederick Speer, of the Speer Allergy Clinic, says that all patients allergic to cow's milk are also allergic to goat's milk.

2. The kola nut family includes cola and chocolate. Both of these foods contain caffeine, as do coffee, tea, mate, cocoa, and many soft drinks.

3. Corn is found in corn syrup, and is used in the manufacture of nearly all chewing gum, candy, prepared meats (luncheon meats, sausages, wieners, bologna), many baked goods, canned fruits and fruit juices, jams, jellies, sweetened syrups, pancake syrups and ice cream. Hominy, grits, tortillas, Fritos, burritos, tamales, and enchiladas contain corn. Cornstarch is often used as a thickener in soups and pies. Corn flour may be found in baked goods. Most American beer, bourbon, Canadian whiskey, and corn whiskey contain corn. Corn oil should be avoided. Cornmeal is used in mush, scrapple, fish sticks, pancake and waffle mixes.

4. Egg is capable of being such a potent allergen that even the odor of egg may produce symptoms. Many vaccines are egg-based. Baked goods, French toast, icings, meringue, candies, mayonnaise, salad dressings, meat loaves, breaded foods and noodles contain egg.

5. Legumes (the pea family) include peanut, soybean, and licorice. Mature ("dry") peas and beans are more likely to induce reactions than are green or string beans, or green peas. Many people sensitive to the legumes are also allergic to honey, probably because in the United States honey is gathered primarily from plants in the legume family. Soybean concentrates are common in baked goods, meats, and many manufactured foods. Soybean oil is the most commonly used oil in margarines, shortenings, salad oils, etc. Peanuts are able to produce severe reactions, including shock.

6. Citrus fruits including oranges, lemon, grapefruit, tangerine and lime are common allergens.

7. Tomato and apples are common in prepared foods. Apple is found in apple vinegar, pickles, salad dressings, etc. Tomato is found in meat loaf, soups, stews, pizza, catsup, chili, salads, tomato paste and juice, and many other prepared foods. Potato, eggplant, tobacco, red and bell pepper, cayenne, paprika, pimento, and chili pepper are all in the same family as tomato.

8. Wheat and small grains such as rice, barley, oats, rye, millet and wild rice may induce allergic reactions. This group also includes cane sugar, molasses, bamboo shoots, and sorghum. Wheat is the most allergenic, rye the least. Rye bread contains more wheat flour than rye

flour. Buckwheat (not a grain) is a useful substitute for wheat. Wheat is found in many dietary products including all baked goods, gravies, cream sauces, macaroni, noodles, spaghetti, pie crusts, cereals, pretzels, chili and breaded foods.

9.   Spices and food additives often induce allergic reactions. Cinnamon is found in catsup, candies, chewing gums, cookies, cakes, chili, prepared meats, apple dishes and pies. People who react to cinnamon usually react also to bay leaf. Pepper (black and white), cumin, basil, balm, horehound, marjoram, savory, rosemary, bergamot, coriander, sage, thyme, spearmint, peppermint, and oregano often cause reactions. Amaranth and tartrazine are probably the artificial food colors most likely to produce symptoms. They are common in carbonated beverages, breakfast drinks such as Tang and Hi-C, bubble gum, popsicles, Kool-aid, Jello, and many medications.

10.   Pork is the most common meat allergen, but oyster, clam, abalone, shrimp, crab, lobster, all true fish (such as tuna, salmon, catfish and perch), chicken, turkey, duck, goose, pheasant, quail, beef, veal, lamb, rabbit, squirrel, and venison may all produce symptoms.

APPENDIX 2: LOW SALT DIET GUIDELINES

A low salt diet can be very difficult for an adult to accept. However, children who have never been trained to like the taste of salt will readily adjust to it. A vegetarian diet is most healthful and easy for persons needing a low salt diet.

Salt is found in many prepared foods, and food labels must be read carefully to avoid it. Avoid any sodium compound. Baking powder, sodium bicarbonate, sodium benzoate, sodium carbonate, sodium caseinate, sodium hydroxide, sodium pectinate, sodium stearoyl-2-lactylate, sodium hexametaphosphate, and monosodium glutamate, are all salt or contain large amounts of salt and should be avoided.

Fresh fruits and vegetables are low in sodium. They should be cooked simply, without the addition of salt during cooking or at the table. Frozen vegetables may have monosodium glutamate added during the processing. Frozen lima beans and peas are often placed in a brine solution during the freezing process. Vegetables frozen in cream sauces must be avoided. Canned vegetables often have salt added during the processing.

Cereal grains contain only small amounts of sodium, but salt may be added during the processing. Instant oatmeal or Cream of Wheat have disodium phosphate added during the processing. Most commercial dry cereals are high in salt. Instant mashed potatoes and quick-cooking rice have salt added during the processing.

All dairy products, meat, fish, all sea food, poultry, and eggs are high in salt, and are best eliminated from the diet. One ounce of cheddar cheese contains about 210 mg. of sodium.

Cured meats and fish should not be used. Bacon, ham, kippers, smoked fish or tongue, sardines, and canned meats should be avoided, as should all luncheon meats such as sausage and frankfurters. Kosher meats are often high in salt, as salt is used to remove the blood from the meat. The salt penetrates into the meat and cannot be entirely removed by rinsing. Fresh fish is sometimes frozen with salt before it arrives at the market.

Crackers, potato chips, salted popcorn, pretzels, and many commercially available snack foods are high in salt.

Bread must be made without salt, milk, or baking powder. Most commercially available breads, rolls, biscuits, and muffins contain salt. Saltines, soda crackers, graham crackers, and any product made with self-rising flour contain salt. Puddings, Jell-O, rennet tablets, all commercially produced pies, cookies and cakes should be avoided. Any food made with baking powder or soda should be avoided. Any dessert containing nuts is very likely to have large amounts of sodium. There are salt substitutes available, but many of these contain ammonium or potassium, which should be avoided in patients with renal or liver disease, both of which are common in sickle cell patients.

Many seasonings may be used in place of salt. Acceptable ones include almond extract, anise seed, basil, bay leaf, coconut, dill, fennel, garlic, lemon juice, marjoram, mint, onion, garlic, cumin, oregano, parsley, peppermint, vanilla and other flavorings, sage, sesame seeds and thyme. Seasonings such as Accent, garlic salt or onion salt, bouillon cubes, catsup, celery salt, celery seeds, celery flakes, celery leaves, horseradish, meat extracts and sauces, meat tenderizers, mustard, olives, parsley flakes, pickles, relishes, saccharin, soy sauce, tomato sauce and Worcestershire sauce are high in sodium.

Drinking water may contain large amounts of salt. The sodium content of city water varies from location to location. It may be necessary to use bottled water. Check with your local health department.

Soft drinks bottled in areas of the country with a high sodium content in their water may be high in sodium. Many soft drinks contain sodium saccharin, an artificial sweetener. Ginger ale is high in sodium.

Some water softeners add considerable amounts of sodium to the water.

Sucaryl, saccharine containing foods, chocolate syrups and other commercially prepared syrups should not be used.

Dried fruits must be selected carefully. Sodium benzoate or sodium flavoring may be added to fruits during the drying process. You can readily dry your own at home, without the use of preservatives.

Many medications, both prescription and over-the-counter, contain high levels of sodium. Baking soda (sodium bicarbonate) is a common home remedy for "heart burn," but is high in sodium. Many antacids, headache medications, cathartics, sleeping medications, and alkalizers contain large amounts of sodium or other salts.

There are several cookbooks on the market which assist in the preparation of a low-salt diet. Such products as mayonnaise, catsup, and salad dressings may be prepared in the home kitchen using a blender. Tomato paste may be prepared in the home kitchen without the addition of salts or high-sodium spices.

APPENDIX 3: SALICYLATE-CONTAINING FOODS

Almonds
Apples
Apricots
Aspirin
Blackberries
Boysenberries
Cherries
Cider
Cider vinegar
Cloves
Cucumbers
Currants
Dewberries
Gooseberries
Grapefruit
Grapes
Lemons
Melons
Mint
Nectarines
Oranges
Peaches
Peppers
Pickles
Plums
Potatoes
Prunes
Raisins
Raspberries
Root beer
Strawberries
Tomatoes
Wintergreen, oil of
Yellow Number 5 Tartrazine

BIBLIOGRAPHY

1. Pediatric Annals 16(10)834-843, October 1987
2. British Medical Journal 283:311, July 25, 1981
3. Behrman, Richard E. M.D. and Vaughan, Victor C. III, M.D., Nelson Textbook of Pediatrics, 12th Edition, Philadelphia: W. B. Saunders, 1983, p. 940-941
4. Journal of the American Medical Association 168:2333, 1958
5. Fulton, James E. Jr., M.D. and Black, Elizabeth. Dr. Fulton's Step-by-Step Program for Clearing Acne. New York: Harper and Row, 1983
6. British Medical Journal 292:1167, May 3, 1986
7. Behrman, op. cit., p. 944-945
8. Rudolph, Abraham. Pediatrics. 18th Edition. Norwalk, CT: Appleton & Lange, 1987
9. Blood 68(4)803-9, October 1986
10. Hayman, Laura Lucia, R.N., Ph.D., FAAN, and Sporing, Eileen, R.N., MSN. Handbook of Pediatric Nursing. New York: John Wiley, 1985, p. 247
11. Klinische Paediatrie 197(4)355-9, July-August 1985
12. Hayman, op. cit., p. 253
13. Rudolph, op. cit., p. 1018
14. Paediatria Danubiana 6(2)97-105, 1949
15. Annals of Nutrition and Metabolism 30:324-330, 1986
16. Rudolph, op. cit., p. 1018
17. Postgraduate Medicine 82(2)62, August, 1987
18. GP 20:85, 1959
19. Clinical Allergy 11(6)549-553, 1981
20. Annals of Allergy 42:160-165, March 1979
21. Journal of Allergy 27:382-3, 1956
22. Weinstein, Allan M., M.D. Asthma: The Complete Guide to Self-Management of Asthma and Allergies for Patients and Their Families. New York: McGraw-Hill, 1987
23. Brunner, Lillian, R. N. and Suddarth, Doris, R.N. The Lippincott Manual of Nursing Practice. Philadelphia: Lippincott, 1982, p. 622
24. American Journal of Public Health 72:574-579, 1982
25. Medical Tribune, January 22, 1975
26. Journal of the American Medical Association 169:1158, March 14, 1959
27. British Medical Journal 1:669, March 18, 1978
28. Medical Journal of Australia 2:614-617, November 28, 1981
29. Journal of Allergy 45:310-319, May 1970
30. Helvetica Medica Acta 20:433-434, November 1953
31. Allergy 38:211-212, 1983
32. Journal of Asthma 22(1)45-55, 1985
33. Emergency Medicine, July 15, 1985, p. 51-53
34. Journal of the American Medical Association 231:1017-1018, 1975
35. Pediatrics 45:150-151, January 1970
36. Science News Letter 85:374, June 13, 1964

37.   Homola, Samuel, D. C. Doctor Homola's Natural Health Remedies.
      West Nyack, NY: Parker Publishing Company, 1973, p. 43
38.   Medical Journal of Australia 1:612, April 24, 1976
39.   Medical Self-Care, Summer, 1981, p. 44-47
40.   Pediatric Clinics of North America 16(1)31-42, February 1969
41.   Munchener Medizinische Wochenschrift, October 5, 1909
42.   University Hospital Bulletin, June 1935, p. 19
43.   American Practitioner, July 1948, p. 708
44.   Arzneimittel-Forsch 6:445-450, 1956
45.   Phipps, Wilma J., R.N., Long, Barbara C., R.N. and Woods, Nancy,
      R.N. Shafers Medical Surgical Nursing, St. Louis: C. V. Mosby, 1980,
      p. 556-557
46.   Graedon, Joe. The People's Pharmacy. New York: St. Martin's Press,
      1976, p. 176-177
47.   American Review of Respiratory Disease 84:480, 1961
48.   Life and Health, June 1909, p. 375
49.   Pediatrics 69:117-118, January 1982
50.   Whaley, Lucille, R.N. and Wong, Donna L. R.N. Nursing Care of
      Infants and Children, St. Louis: C. V. Mosby, 1979 p. 494
51.   Weiss, Earle B. et. al. Bronchial Asthma: Mechanisms and Therapeu-
      tics. 2nd Edition, Boston, Little, Brown, 1985
52.   Guyton, Arthur, M.D. Basic Human Physiology. Philadelphia: W. B.
      Saunders, 1977, p. 82
53.   Brunner, Lillian, R.N., and Suddarth, Doris, R.N. The Lippincott
      Manual of Nursing Practice. Philadelphia: Lippincott, 1982, p. 622
54.   Griffith, H. Winter, et al., Information and Instructions for Pediatric
      Patients. Tucson, Az: Winter Publishing Company, 1980, p. 239
55.   Let's Live, February, 1978, p. 108
56.   The Lancet 2:775, October 7, 1967
57.   American Journal of Diseases of Children 35:13, 1928
      Drug Therapy, September, 1984, p. 123
58.   Brunner, LilliaN, R.N. and Doris Suddarth, R.N. The Lippincott Manual
      of Nursing Practice. Philadelphia: Lippincott, 1982
59.   Humbart, Santillo. Natural Healing with Herbs. Prescott Valley,
      Arizona: Holm Press, 1985, p. 274
60.   The Lancet 2:464, August 26, 1967
61.   Journal of the American Medical Association 130:249-256, 1946
62.   Graedon, Joe. The People's Pharmacy. New York: St. Martin's Press,
      1976
63.   Simon, Gilbert M.D. and Cohen, Marcia. Parent's Pediatric Compan-
      ion. New York: William Morrow, 1985
64.   Journal of Bone and Joint Surgery 45A:1152, 1963
65.   Pediatric Clinics of North America 33(6)1439-56, December 1986
66.   Journal of Bone and Joint Surgery 57B(1)69-71, February 1975
67.   Annals of Rheumatic Diseases 31:179-82, 1972
68.   Griffith, op. cit., p. 219
69.   Archives of Dermatology 113:952-953, July 1977
70.   American Journal of Diseases of Children 140(10)970, October 1986
71.   American Journal of Diseases of Children 120:32, 1970

72. Canadian Medical Association Journal 106:30, 1972
73. Clinical Trends in Family Practice, September-October 1978
74. Medical Tribune, April 9, 1980, p. 20
75. Gerrard, John W. Food Allergy. Springfield, Illinois: C. C. Thomas Pub Co., 1980, p. 177
76. Gerrard, op. cit.
77. American Family Physician 33:209, April 1986
78. American Journal of Diseases of Children 140:260-261, March 1986
79. Rocky Mountain Medical Journal 57:50-2, June 1960
80. Western Journal of Medicine 143(1)113, July 1985
81. Gerrard, op. cit.
82. Muenchener Medizinische Wochenschrift 84:585, April l9, 1937
83. Pediatric Clinics of North America 33(4)871-86, August 1986
84. Archives of Ophthalmology 68:446-449, 1969
85. Boyd-Monk, Heather and Steinmetz, Charles III. Nursing Care of the Eye. Norwalk, CT: Appleton Lange, 1987, p. 22
86. British Medical Journal 2:582-584, September 8, 1951
87. Gillis, S.S. and Kagan, B.M. Current Pediatric Therapy, 12th Edition, Philadelphia, W. B. Saunders, 1986, p. 486-487
88. Fraunfelder, Frederick and Roy, F. Hampton. Current Ocular Therapy. Philadelphia, W.B. Saunders, 1980, p. 433-434
89. Archives of Ophthalmology 36:464, October 1946
90. Archives of Ophthalmology 3:762-783, June 1930
91. American Journal of Ophthalmology 83:906-907, 1977
92. Homan, William. Caring for Your Child. New York: Harmony Books, 1979, p. 35
93. Schmitt, Barton, M.D. Pediatric Telephone Advice. Boston: Little, Brown, 1980, p. 121
94. Journal of the American Medical Association 154(5)390-394, 1954
95. Southern Medical Journal 53:830-860, July 1960
96. American Journal of Diseases of Children 121:219, March 1971
97. Journal of the American Medical Association 207(1)29, January 6, 1969
98. Hughes, James and Griffith, John F. Synopsis of Pediatrics. Sixth Edition, St. Louis: C. V. Mosby, 1984, p. 953
99. Simon, op. cit., p. 81-82
100. Medical Clinics of North America 30:121-133, January 1946
101. A.M.A. Journal of Diseases of Children 95(6)637-9, June 1958
102. Journal of the American Medical Association 260(9)1295, September 2, 1988
103. Kaye, Robert, Oski, Frank, and Barness, Lewis A. Core Textbook of Pediatrics, 2nd Edition, Philadelphia: Lippincott, 1982, p. 438
104. New England Journal of Medicine 268(26)1436, June 27, 1963
105. Whaley, Lucille F. and Wong, Donna L. Nursing care of infants and Children, St. Louis: Mosby, 1987 p. 1678
106. Journal of the American Medical Association 212(13)2231, June 29, 1970
107. Journal of the American Medical Association 212(13)2233, June 29, 1970

108. Pediatric News 19(7)6, July 1985
109. McKay, R.J., Behrman, R.E., and Vaughn, Victor C. Nelson Textbook of Pediatrics, 11th Edition, Philadelphia: W. B. Saunders, 1979, p. 98
110. Servonsky, Jane and Opas, Susan R. Nursing Management of Children. Boston: Jones and Bartlett, 1989, p. 497
111. Simon, op. cit., p. 213-216
112. A.M.A. Journal of Diseases of Children 91:27, 1956
113. New England Journal of Medicine 268(1)21-23, 1963
114. Medical Proceedings 10:439, October 3, 1964
115. Rudolph, op. cit., p. 1417
116. Hughes, James G. and Griffith, John F. Synopsis of Pediatrics. 5th Edition, St. Louis: C. V. Mosby, 1984, p. 397-399
117. Hutchison, James H. and Lockburn, Forrester. Practical Pediatric Problems. 6th Edition. London: Lloyd-Luke, 1986, p. 277-279
118. Griffith, H. Winter, M.D. Instructions for Patients. 4th Edition, Philadelphia: W. B. Saunders, 1989, p. 36
119. Smith, Marjorie, Goodman, Julie A. and Ramsey, Nancy. Child and Family: Concepts of Nursing Practice. New York: McGraw-Hill, 1987, p. 640
120. Griffith, H. Winter, M.D. Instructions for Patients. 4th Edition, Philadelphia: W. B. Saunders, 1989, p. 39
121. Chow, Marilyn, Handbook of Pediatric Primary Care. 2nd Edition, New York: John Wiley, 1984, p. 1035-6
122. Pillitteri, Adele. Child Health Nursing: Care of the Growing Family. Boston: Little, Brown, 1981, p. 1040-1041
123. Archives of Toxicology, Supplement 9, p. 69-73, 1986
124. The Lancet 2:1031-1034, November 2, 1974
125. Paris Med 46:394, Nov. 12, 1927
126. Allergy 42(2)85-91, February 1987
127. Stern, Jack I., M.D. and Carroll, David. The Home Medical Handbook. New York: William Morrow, 1987, p. 69-73
128. British Medical Journal 2:149-152, July 16, 1977
129. Buchman, Dian Dincin. Herbal Medicine. New York: Grammercy Publishing Company, 1979, p. 76, 77
130. Journal of Periodontics 12(2)107-127, Winter, 1988
131. Illingworth, R. S. Common symptoms of disease in children. Eighth Edition, Oxford: Blackwell Scientific Publications, 1984, p. 166
132. American Journal of Orthodontics 77(1)48-59, January 1988
133. Chow, op cit p. 677
134. Behrman, op. cit., p. 75
135. Burns, Including Thermal Injury 11(3)220-4, February 1985
136. Journal of the American Medical Association 173:1916-1919, 1960
137. Plastic and Reconstructive Surgery 81(3)386-389, March 1988
138. Behrman, Howard, Labow, Theodore A. M.D. and Rozen, Jack H. M.D. Common Skin Diseases. New York: Grune and Stratton, 1978, p. 9
139. Cutis 36(6)479-480, December 1985
140. British Journal of Dermatology 103:111, 1980
141. British Medical Journal 2:757-758, September 28, 1974

142. Griffith, op. cit., p. 43,
143. Avery, Mary Ellen and First, Lewis R. Pediatric Medicine. Baltimore: Williams and Wilkins, 1989
144. Griffith, op. cit., p. 312
145. Pediatric Clinics of North America 30:609, 1983
146. American Family Physician 36(1)135-136, July 1987
147. Avery, op. cit., p. 96-97
148. Archives of Disease in Childhood 56:292-294, 1981
149. Advances in Pediatrics 34:223-48, 1987
150. American Journal of the Medical Sciences 192:365-371, 1936
151. Canadian Medical Association Journal 88:854-855, April 20, 1965
152. Forfar, John O. and Arneil, Gavin C. Textbook of Pediatrics, 3rd Edition, New York: Churchill Livingstone, 1984
153. Hughes, op. cit., p. 740-741
154. Journal of the American Medical Association 207(2)312, January 13, 1969
155. Otolaryngology and Head and Neck Surgery 94(5)622-7, June 1986
156. Otolaryngologic Clinics of North America 15(3)649, August 1982
157. American Journal of Medicine 28:504-509, April 1960
158. Journal of American Veterinary Medical Association 193(3) 312-315, August 1, 1988
159. Rudolph, op. cit., p. 611-613
160. Family Centered Care of Children and Adolescents. p. 832
161. Servonsky, op. cit., p. 726-728
162. Avery, op cit p. 433-435
163. Acta Paediatrica Scandinavica 75:340-342, 1986
164. American Journal of Diseases of Children 28:421, October 1924
165. Canadian Medical Association Journal 127:963-965, November 16, 1982
166. Canadian Medical Association Journal 133:114-115, July 15, 1985
167. American Journal of Diseases of Children 79:936, 1950
168. Journal of Pediatric Gastroenterology and Nutrition 2(Suppl 1)S304-309, 1983
169. The Lancet 2:1265, December 18, 1926
170. McFarlane, Judith, Whitson, Betty Jo, and Hartley, Lucy M. Contemporary Pediatric Nursing: A Conceptual Approach, New York: John Wiley, 1980, p. 424-425
171. Nutrition Abstracts 4:399, 1934-1935
172. Schmitt, Barton D., M.D. Your Child's Health: A Pediatric Guide for Parents. New York: Bantam Books, p. 335-338
173. Shamansky, Sherry L. et al. Primary Health Care Handbook: Guidelines for Patient Education. Boston: Little, Brown, 1984, p. 316-317
174. Parents, November 1986, p. 3611
175. Griffith, op. cit., p. 194
176. Medical Tribune 27(17)10, June 18, 1986
177. Homan, William H., M.D. and Editors of Consumer Guide. Caring for Your Child. New York: Harmony Books, 1979, p. 45
178. Karelitz, Samuel M. D. When Your Child is Ill. New York: Random House, 1969, p. 113-115

179. Emergency Medicine Clinics of North America 3(4)785-808, November 1985
180. American Family Physician 36(2)149-52, August 1987
181. Buchman, op. cit., p. 102
182. Buchman, op. cit., p. 124
183. American Family Physician 37(2)61, 1988
184. Clinics in Perinatology 12(2)441-451, June 1985
185. Journal of Family Practice 19(1)107-116, 1984
186. Emergency Medicine, September 30, 1987, p. 47-48
187. American Baby, April 1987, p. 64-73
188. Pediatric Nursing 11:136, 1985
189. Servonsky, op. cit., p. 199
190. Pediatric Annals 16(10)817-820, October 1987
191. American Baby, September 1985, p. 38
192. American Family Physician 36(3)153, September 1987
193. Patient Care, March 30, 1985, p. 93-109
194. Denver Medical Times 21:94, 1901
195. Clinical Pediatrics 8(7)24A, July 1969
196. Kellogg, John Harvey, M.D. The Hygeine of Infancy. Battle Creek, Michigan: Good Health Publishing Company, 1916, p. 167-168
197. Patient Care, December 15, 1987, p. 152
198. British Medical Journal 289:660, September 1984
199. Journal of Family Practice 21(3)175, 1985
200. Wasserman, Edward M. D., and Gromisch, Donald S. Survey of Clinical Pediatrics. 7th Edition, New York: McGraw-Hill, 1981
201. Schmitt, op. cit., p. 435
202. Simon, op. cit., p. 201
203. Children, Winter, 1987, p. 51-52
204. Schmidt, Barton D., M.D. Pediatric Telephone Advice. Boston: Little, Brown, 1980
205. Chow, op. cit., p. 703
206. Pediatric News 19(7)6, July 1985
207. The Lancet 1:573, March 10, 1984
208. British Medical Journal 2:550, September 4, 1976
209. Medical Tribune 27(30)1, 16, October 29, 1986
210. Munchener Medizinische Wochenschrift, July 20, 1909, p. 139
211. Auris Nasus Larynx (Tokyo)9:81-90, 1982
212. Pediatric News 22(3)59, March 1988
213. Postgraduate Medicine 79(2)75-86, February 1, 1986
214. Hughes, op. cit., p. 374-379
215. Griffith, op. cit., p. 135
216. Schmitt, op. cit., p. 483
217. Simon, op. cit., p. 128-129
218. Chow, op. cit., p. 324-325
219. Journal of the American Medical Association October 28, 1974
220. Journal of the American Medical Association 260:1621, 1988
221. Servonsky, op. cit., p. 117
222. Clinical Pediatrics 36:872, November 1954

223. Moncrieff, Alan and Evans, Philip. Diseases of Children, Volume 1, London: Edward Arnold and Co., p. 538
224. New York Medical Journal, October 22, 1898
225. Stern, op. cit., p. 164-169
226. New York Journal of Medicine 57:265, January 15, 1957
227. Annals of Allergy 29:323-324, June 1971
228. Whaley, op. cit., p. 492-493
229. British Medical Journal 1(3147)601, April 23, 1971
230. Drug Therapy, March 1985, p. 93-98
231. Waechter, Eugenia H. Nursing Care of Children. Philadelphia: Lippincott, 1985, p. 885
232. British Medical Journal 298:1617-1618, June 17, 1989
233. Internal Medicine for the Specialist 9(7)92-100, July 1988
234. Gastroenterology 90(15 Pt 2)1445, May 1986
235. Hospital Tribune, May 8, 1985, p. 2
236. British Medical Journal 2:762-764, September 29, 1979
237. Gut 26:985-988, 1985
238. Crohn, Burrill, M.D. and Yarnis, Harry, M.D. Regional Ileitis. Second Revised Edition. New York: Grune and Stratton, 1958, p. 121-123
239. British Medical Journal 290:1786-1787, June 15, 1985
240. Internal Medicine News 17(3)3, 43, April 1-14, 1984
241. Scandinavian Journal of Gastroenterology 20(8)1014-8, October 20, 1985
242. Modern Medicine, June 1981, p. 42
243. Contemporary Pediatrics, October 1988, p. 51-70
244. Griffith, H. Winter, et al., Information and Instructions for Pediatric Patients. Tucson, AZ: Winter Publishing Company, 1980, p. 89-90
245. Karelitz, Samuel, M.D. When Your Child is Ill. New York: Random House, 1969, p. 294-299
246. American Baby, June, 1984, p. 40, 44
247. Evans, Marilyn and Hansen, Beverly. Guide to Pediatric Nursing: A Clinical Reference. New York: Appleton-Century-Crofts, 1980, p. 49-50
248. Forfar, John O. Textbook of Pediatrics, Vol. 1. New York: Churchill Livingstone, 1984 p. 536-538
249. Habenicht, Herald A, M.D. and Rhodes, Helen Metz. Doctor, What Can I Do? Washington, D.C.: Review and Herald, 1981
250. Kellogg, John Harvey. The Health Question Box or A Thousand and One Health Questions Answered. Battle Creek, Michigan: Modern Medicine Publishing Company, 1925, p. 891-892
251. Schmitt, Barton D., M.D. Pediatric Telephone Advice. Boston: Little, Brown, and Company, 1980, p. 133-136
252. Galton, Lawrence. 1001 Health Tips. New York: Simon and Schuster, 1984, p. 95
253. Pediatric Clinics of North American 8:123-6, February 1961
254. Scipien, Gladys M. et al., Comprehensive Pediatric Nursing. Third Edition. New York: McGraw-Hill, 1986, p. 868-870
255. Journal of Family Practice 2(2)85-89, April 1975

256. Schmitt, Barton, M.D. Your Child's Health: A Pediatric Guide for Parents. New York: Bantam Books, 1987, p. 474-476

257. Pediatric Annals 17(1)39-46, January 1988

258. Tackett, Joyce Marie and Hunsberger, Mabel, Family Centered Care of Children and Adolescents. Philadelphia: W. B. Saunders, 1981, p. 947

259. Archives of Disease in Childhood 41:199, 1966

260. Pediatric Dermatology 1(4)322-5, April 1984

261. Pediatrics 66:532-536, October 1980

262. Canadian Medical Association Journal 139:284-285, August 15, 1988

263. Silver, Henry K. et al., Handbook of Pediatrics, 11th Edition. Los Altos, CA:Lange Medical Publishers, 1975, p. 200-201

264. Clinical Pediatrics 26(3)154-155, March 1987

265. Indiana Medicine 77:610, 1984

266. Riggs, Maribeth. Natural Child Care. New York: Harmony Books, 1989, p. 135

267. Pediatrician 14(Suppl)21-6, 1987

268. Clinical Pediatrics 12(7)391-392, July 1973

269. Your Health, April 23, 1985, p. 2

270. Chow, Marilyn P. et al., Handbook of Pediatric Primary Care. New York: Wiley, 1984, p. 607

271. Journal of Pediatrics 57(6)586, December 1960

272. Pediatric News 21(3)3, 65, March 1987

273. Postgraduate Medicine 65(2)163-168, February 1979

274. Archives of Disease in Childhood 59:260-265, 1984

275. Symposium Observer, May 23, 1988, p. 1

276. Pediatric Annals 16(10)821-9, October 1987

277. Griffith, op. cit. p. 149

278. Emergency Medicine 20(3)138, 1988

279. Fox, Jane A. Primary Health Care of the Young. New York: McGraw-Hill, 1981, p. 602-605

280. Medical Times 114(7)95, July 1, 1986

281. Journal of Diarrhoeal Disease Research 4(1)20-25, March 1986

282. Riggs. op. cit. p. 121

283. Canadian Medical Association Journal 121:509, 564, September 8, 1979

284. New England Journal of Medicine 315:768, September 18, 1986

285. Journal of Pediatrics 30:742, 1950

286. Pediatric News 22(2)66, February 1988

287. Archives of Pediatrics 35(7)406, July 1918

288. Habenicht, op. cit., p. 67

289. American Family Physician 36(3)252, 1987

290. Journal of the American Medical Association 244(3)270, July 18, 1980

291. Pediatric Annals 14(1)15-18, January 1985

292. Grundfast, Kenneth M.D. and Carney, Cynthia J. Ear Infections in Your Child. Hollywood, Florida: Compact Books, 1987

293. Carroll, David L. and Stern, Jack I. M.D. The Home Medical Hand-

book. New York: William Morrow, 1987

294. American Journal of Otology 8(6)495, November 1987
295. Archives of Otolaryngology, Head and Neck Surgery 114:1007-1011, September 1988
296. Journal of Family Practice 22(1)39-43, January 1986
297. New England Journal of Medicine 308:297-301, February 10, 1983
298. Journal of Allergy and Clinical Immunology 83(1)239, January, 1989
299. Pediatrics 51:154-6, January, 1973
300. Journal of Laryngology and Otology 103:559-561, June 1989
301. Archives of Oto-rhino-laryngology 242(1)113-7, 1985
302. Annals of Otology, Rhinology and Laryngology 89(3 Suppl) 312-315, May-June 1980
303. Riggs. op. cit. p. 55
304. International Journal of Pediatric Otorhinolaryngology 17(2)119-125, May 1989
305. Medical Times, October, 1979, p. 28s
306. Acta Paediatrica Scandinavica 71:567-571, 1982
307. ORL; Journal for Oto-Rhino-Laryngology and Its Borderlands 49:254-258, 1987
308. American Journal of Nursing 81(8)1480-1483, August 1981
309. International Journal of Pediatric Otorhinolaryngology 12:39-47, 1986
310. American Family Physician 39(5)36, May, 1989
311. Schmitt, Barton D., M.D. Your Child's Health: A Pediatric Guide for Parents. New York: Bantam Books, 1987, p. 339-342
312. Buchman, Dian Dincin. Herbal Medicine. New York; Grameray Publishing Company, 1979, p. 148
313. Rudolph, op. cit. p. 834-836
314. Rudolph, Abraham. Pediatrics, 18th Edition. Norwalk, CT: Appleton and Lange, 1987, 443-446
315. Evans, Marilyn and Hansen, Beverly. Guide to Pediatric Nursing: A Clinical Reference. New York: Appleton-Century-Crofts, 1980, p. 56-57
316. Annals of Allergy 35(4)221-9, October 1975
317. Lancet 1:1340-2, June 20, 1981
318. Comptes Rendus des Seances de la Societe de Biologie et de ses Filiales 142:1033-1034, 1948
319. British Medical Journal 3:153-5, July 16, 1967
320. Pediatric News 22(2)56, February 1988
321. Maurer, Harold M., M.D. Pediatrics. New York: Churchill Livingstone, 1983, p. 188-189
322. Servonsky, Jane and Opas, Susan R. Nursing Management of Children. Boston: Jones and Bartlett, 1987, p. 501-502
323. Chow, op. cit.
324. Tackett, Joyce Marie, and Hunsberger, Mabel., Family Centered Care of Children and Adolescents. Philadelphia: W. B. Saunders, 1981, p. 1094-1095
325. Scipien, Gladys. Comprehensive Pediatric Nursing. Third Edition. New York: McGraw-Hill, 1986, p. 609
326. Waechter, op. cit., 1063

327. Pediatric News 22(5)24, May 1988
328. Developmental Medicine and Child Neurology 30:391-406, 1988
329. Rudolph, Abraham. Pediatrics, 18th Edition, p. 1658-1660
330. Patient Care, April 15, 1984, p. 11
331. Rudolph, op. cit., p. 1814
332. Renshaw, Thomas S. Pediatric Orthopaedics. Philadelphia: W. B. Saunders, 1986
333. Tachdjian, Mihoran O. The Child's Foot. Philadelphia: W. B. Saunders, 1985
334. Pediatric Nursing 5(4)21-22, July-August 1979
335. Avery, Mary Ellen and Lewis R. First. Pediatric Medicine. Baltimore: Williams and Wilkins, 1989, p. 1269
336. Schmitt, op. cit.
337. Canadian Medical Association Journal 139:706, October 15, 1988
338. Pediatric Annals 14(1)31-36, January 1985
339. Pediatric Annals 6(7)68-72, July 1977
340. Riggs. op. cit. p. 50
341. Annals of Allergy 37(1)41-46, July 1976
342. Griffith, op. cit., p. 158
343. DeAngelis, Catherine. Pediatric Primary Care, 3rd Edition, Boston: Little, Brown, 1984, p. 237
344. Servonsky, op. cit., p. 749
345. Clinical Pediatrics 33:69, February 1951
346. Tackett, op. cit., p. 621
347. Servonsky, op. cit., p. 710-713
348. Gastroenterology 95:534-9, 1988
349. Nelson, Christine A., M.D. and Pescar, Suan. Should I Call The Doctor? New York: Warner Books, 1986, p. 496-497
350. Clinical Pediatrics 20:7, 1981
351. Scipien, op. cit., p. 1073
352. Behrman, op. cit., p. 896-897
353. Homan, op. cit., p. 92
354. Behrman, op. cit., p. 885
355. Simon, op. cit., p. 250-251
356. Hughes, op. cit., p. 748-750
357. Homan, op. cit., p. 147
358. Griffith, op. cit., p. 202
359. Simon, op. cit., p. 322
360. British Medical Journal 282:1163, April 4, 1981
361. Archives of Disease in Childhood 66:232-234, 1981
362. Winter, op. cit., p. 161
363. Chow, op. cit., p. 574-575
364. American Family Physician 27(1)189-191, January 1983
365. DeAngelis, op. cit., p. 282-282
366. Simon, op. cit., p. 273-276
367. Speer, Frederick. Food Allergy, 2nd Edition, Springfield: C. C. Thomas, 1983, p. 34
368. Griffith, op. cit., p. 10
369. Infectious Diseases in Children 1(2)6, February 1988

370. Rhinology 24(4)265-9, December 1986
371. Graedon, Joe. The People's Pharmacy. New York: St. Martin's Press, 1976, p. 164
372. Medical Journal of Australia 2:378, October 6, 1979
373. Journal of the Minnesota Medical Association and Northwestern Lancet, May 1, 1906
374. Journal of Asthma 22(2)93-97, 1985
375. Science News, August 12, 1939, p. 107
376. Internal Medicine News 21(6)2, March 15-31, 1988
377. Acta Paediatrica Scandinavica 71:135-140, 1982
378. DeAngelis, op. cit., p. 282
379. Postgraduate Medicine 81(8)223-230, June 1987
380. Seminars in Neurology 8(1)51-60, Spring 1988
381. Austin, Glen, M.D. The Parent's Medical Manual. New York: Prentice-Hall, 1978, p. 125-130
382. Internal Medicine News 18(7)3, September 1-14, 1985
383. Schmitt, op. cit., p. 327-329
384. Patient Care, October 15, 1982, p. 48-80
385. Child Development 33:43-56, March 1962
386. Child Development 42:399-413, 1971
387. Diseases of the Nervous System 21:203-8, April 1960
388. Practitioner 222:676-679, May 1979
389. Pillitteri, op. cit., p. 1361
390. Medical Times 107(6)76, June 1979
391. Griffith, op. cit., p. 183-184
392. Pryse-Phillips, William, M.D. and Murray T. J. Essential Neurology. Garden City, New York: Medical Examiner Publishing Co., 1978, p. 227
393. Lewis, Sharon and Collier, Idolla. Medical Surgical Nursing: Assessment and Management of Clinical Problems. New York: McGraw-Hill, 1983, p. 1012-1020
394. Servonsky, op. cit., p. 742-745
395. Whaley, op. cit., p. 1436-1440
396. American Journal of Diseases of Children 139:453-455, 1985
397. Western Journal of Medicine 140(2)278-280, February 1984
398. Science News Letter, November 21, 1941, p. 334
399. Journal of Clinical Gastroenterology 7(6)539-552, 1985
400. Mayo Clinic Health Letter, September 1984, p. 3-4
401. The Health Letter 33(7)4, April 14, 1989
402. Parents, May 1989, p. 19
403. The Lancet 2:1344, December 23, 1968
404. New England Journal of Medicine 306(18)1115, 1982
405. Journal of the American Medical Association 84:1233-1234, 1925
406. Journal of the American Medical Association 57:396, July 29, 1911
407. British Medical Journal 2:709, September 10, 1977
408. Annals of Emergency Medicine 17(8)872, August 1988
409. Life and Health, February 1914, p. 89
410. Waechter, op. cit., p. 977-979

411. Archives of Disease in Childhood 57:875, 1982
412. Apgar, Virginia, M.D. and Beck, Joan. Is My Baby All Right? New York: Trident Press, 1972, p. 281-287
413. Journal of Bone and Joint Surgery 71B:4-5, January 1989
414. Avery, op. cit., p. 1273-1275
415. Schmitt, op. cit.
416. Riggs, op. cit., p. 168-169
417. The Lancet 2:900-903, October 28, 1972,
418. Clinics in Sports Medicine 1(3)515-527, November 1982
419. Patient Care, August 15, 1986, p. 203
420. Brain and Mind Bulletin 5(20)1, September 1, 1980
421. Servonsky, op. cit., p. 490
422. Science News 132:168, 1987
423. Journal of American Medical Association 260(15)2256, October 21, 1988
424. Archives of General Psychiatry 40:317, March 1983
425. Rook, Arthur. Textbook of Dermatology, Vol. 1, New York: Blackwell, 1979, p. 549-551
426. Canadian Medical Association Journal 139:706, October 15, 1988
427. Kinderarztl. Praxis 11:354, November 1940
428. Griffith, op. cit., p. 280
429. Drug Therapy, December 1983, p. 68-81
430. DeAngelis, op. cit., p. 370-371
431. Life and Health, February 1972, p. 17, 33
432. Pillitteri, op. cit., p. 837-838
433. Griffith, op. cit., p. 200
434. Crook, William G., M.D. Answering Parent's Questions. Springfield, II: C. C. Thomas, 1963, p. 191
435. Brown, Jeffrey L., M.D. The Complete Parent's Guide to Telephone Medicine. New York: Perigree Books, 1982, p. 111
436. Pediatric Clinics of North America 26(2)315-326, May 1979
437. Brace, Edward R. and Bacanowski, John, M.D. Childhood Symptoms. New York: Harper and Row, 1985, p. 169-170
438. Griffith, op. cit., p. 206
439. Griffith, op. cit., p. 198
440. Habenicht, op. cit.,
441. Waechter, op. cit., p. 897
442. Servonsky, op. cit., p. 709
443. Internal Medicine News 19(8)77, April 15-30, 1986
444. Medical Letter 11:60, July 11, 1969
445. Dermatology News, May 1988
446. Journal of the American Medical Association 26:144, Jan 18, 1896
447. Riggs, op. cit., p. 138-139
448. Rudolph, op. cit., p. 1812
449. Pillitteri, op. cit., p. 1034
450. Habenicht, op. cit.
451. Christian, Henry A., M.D. Principles and Practice of Medicine. 16th Edition, New York: Appleton-Century, 1947, p. 800
452. Practitioner 145:332, 1940

453. Schmitt, op. cit., p. 477-478
454. Forfar, op. cit., p. 1542-1543
455. Journal of Pediatrics 91(6)998-1000, 1977
456. Behrman, op. cit., p. 1929
457. Christian, op. cit., p. 545
458. Tijdschrift voor Geneeskunde 4(42)1478-1483, 1946
459. Rudolph, op. cit., p. 596-601
460. Schmitt, op. cit., p. 346
461. Griffith, op. cit., p. 199
462. Good Health 18(2)33-35, February 1883
463. Whaley, op. cit., p. 863-864
464. Shamansky, op. cit., p. 229
465. Griffith, op. cit., 514-515
466. Griffith, op. cit., p. 124
467. Journal of Reproductive Medicine 25(4 Suppl)198-201, October 1989
468. Archives of Surgery 46:611-613, May 1943
469. Journal of the Missouri Medical Association 28:382-384, 1931
470. Moor, Fred, M.D. Manual of Hydrotherapy and Massage. Mountain View, California: Pacific Press, 1964, p. 42, 45
471. Budoff, Penny. No More Menstrual Cramps and Other Good News. New York: G. P. Putnam Sons, 1980
472. American Family Physician 35(3)100, March 1987
473. Clinical Pediatrics 23(6)318-320, June 1984
474. Internal Medicine news 21(22)75, November 15-30, 1988
475. Journal of General Internal medicine 3:267-276, 1988
476. Evans, op. cit., p. 144
477. Schuartz, M. William. Principles and Practice of Clinical Pediatrics. Chicago: Year Book Medical Publisher, 1987, p. 795-797
478. American Journal of Diseases of Children 142:586-587, June 1988
479. Simon, op. cit., p. 181-189
480. Austin, op. cit., p. 178
481. Clinical Pediatrics 12(8)468-470, August 1973
482. Nurse Practitioner 11(4)41-51, April 1986
483. Pediatric Research 25(4 Pt. 2)99A, April 1989
484. Barness, Lewis A. M.D. Manual of Pediatric Physical Diagnosis. 5th Edition, Chicago: Year Book Medical Publishers, 1981, p. 216-217
485. Pediatric News 20(7)7, 1986
486. Avery, Gordon B., M.D. Neonatology: Pathophysiology and Management of the Newborn. 3rd Edition, Philadelphia: Lippincott, 1987
487. Nursing84, October 1984, p. 17
488. Canadian Medical Association Journal 104:526, March 20, 1971
489. The People's Doctor 4(7) Undated
490. Cooney, David O. Activated Charcoal: Antidotal and Other Medical Uses. New York: Marcel Keker, 1980
491. British Journal of Obstetrics and Gynecology 91:1014-1018, 1984
492. Pediatric Research 17(10)810-814, 1983
493. Journal of Pediatric Nursing 4(1)48-53, February 1989
494. Texas Medicine 70:70-72, December 1974

495. New York Medical Journal, May 8, 1915, p. 951-952
496. American Journal of Diseases of Children 138:1086, November 1984
497. British Medical Journal 297:592, September 3, 1988
498. Linday, Hal. More FYI. New York: M. Evans, 1983, p. 153-154
499. Simon, op. cit., p. 330
500. Kellogg, John Harvey. Health Question Box, p. 663
501. Good Health 20:27, 1885
502. Postgraduate Medicine 81(1)217-224, January 1987
503. A.M.A. Journal of Diseases of Children 99:819-821, 1960
504. Carroll, op. cit., p. 65-67
505. Denver Medical Times 21:32, 1901
506. Contemporary Pediatrics 5(5)50-57, May 1988
507. Tachdjian, op. cit., p. 1619-1625
508. Clinical Orthopaedics 77:134-143, June 1971
509. Journal of the American Medical Association 240(15)1607 October 6, 1978
510. American Journal of Clinical Nutrition 4:216, 1956
511. Pediatrics 75(5)807-812, May 1985
512. The Behavior Therapist 2(2)1, July 1978
513. Circulation 55-56(Suppl 3)111, October 1977
514. Journal of Pediatric Gastroenterology and Nutrition 1(4)485-8, 1982
515. Behrman, op. cit., p. 90
516. Hunter, Letha Y. and Funk, James Jr., Rehabilitation of the Injured Knee. St. Louis: Mosby, 1984, p. 409
517. Lovell, Wood W. and Winter, Robert B. Pediatric Orthopaedics. 2nd Edition, Philadelphia: Lippincott, p. 1116-1117
518. American Family Physician 33(5)181-185, May 1986
519. British Journal of Haematology 34:341, 1976
520. DeAngelis, op. cit., p. 246
521. Journal of the Royal College of General Practitioners 31:740-742, December 1981
522. Pediatrics 31:1056, 1963
523. Brace, op. cit., p. 75-76
524. Christian, op. cit., p. 73
525. Bahana, Sami L. and Heiner, Douglas C. Allergies to Milk. New York: Grune and Stratton, 1980, p. 74
526. American Journal of Ophthalmology 18:331-333, 1935
527. Maternal Child Nursing 10:111-113, March-April 1985
528. Humbart, Santillo, B. S., M.H. Natural Healing with Herbs. Prescott Valley, AZ: Hohm Press, 1985, p. 269
529. Rossiter, Frederick, M.D. The Practical Guide to Health. Nashville: Southern Publishing Association, 1913
530. Finska Lakaresallskapets Handlingar 65:354, May-June 1923
531. Medizinische Klinik 21:507, April 3, 1925
532. Griffith, op. cit., p. 258
533. Journal of Parasitology 30:26-33, February 1944
534. American Family Physician 38(3)159-164, September 1988
535. Habenicht, op. cit., (pleurisy)
536. Griffith, op. cit., p. 203-240

537. Journal of the American Medical Association 39:441, 1902
538. Buchman, op. cit., p. 173
539. Humbart, op. cit., p. 343
540. Buchman, op. cit., p. 172-173
541. Journal of the American Medical Association 81:598, 1923
542. Griffith, op. cit., p. 270
543. Kellogg, John Harvey, M.D. The Hygiene of Infancy. Battle Creek, MI: Good Health Publishing Company, 1916, p. 166-167
544. Homan, op. cit., p. 103
545. The Lancet 2:281, August 13, 1949
546. Rudolph, op. cit., p. 836
547. Schmitt, op. cit., p. 343-344
548. Journal of the American Medical Association 55:1602, October 29, 1910
549. Nutrition Abstracts 5:1108, 1935-1936
550. Cutis 34(5)492, 1984
551. Journal of the American Medical Association 117:317, 1941
552. North Carolina Medical Journal 47(5)253-255, May 1986
553. Sidi, Edwin, M.D. Psoriasis. Springfield, II: C. C. Thomas, 1968, p. 197
554. Archives of Dermatology 116:893-897, August 1980
555. Deutsche Medizinische Wochenschrift, December 21, 1906
556. Internal Medicine News, February 1-14, 1987, p. 58
557. New England Journal of Medicine 312:246, January 24, 1985
558. Hurwitz, Sidney, M.D. Clinical Pediatric Dermatology. Philadelphia: Saunders, 1981, p. 83-89
559. Forfar, op. cit., p. 436
560. Surgical Clinics of North America 58(3)505-512, June 1978
561. Griffith, op. cit., p. 263
562. Diseases of Colon and Rectum 20(1)40-42, January-February 1977
563. American Journal of Diseases of Children 142:338-339, March 1988
564. Behrman, op. cit., p. 945-946
565. Surgical Clinics of North America 52:1055-1065, 1972
566. Journal of the American Medical Association 32:80, 1899
567. Whaley, op. cit., p. 564-565
568. Schmitt, op. cit., p. 228-229
569. Fox, Jane A. Primary Health Care of the Young. New York: McGraw-Hill, 1981, p. 345
570. Primary Care 11(2)243-251, June 1984
571. Clinical Research 29(4)754A, 1981
572. Scandinavian Journal of Rheumatology 15:219-223, 1986
573. Arthritis and Rheumatism 30(Suppl 1)542, January 1987
574. Journal of the Royal Society of Medicine 78:410-413, May 1985
575. International Archives of Allergy and Applied Immunology 78:145-151, 1985
576. British Medical Journal 1:2027-2029, June 20, 1981
577. Arthritis and Rheumatism 28(4)Suppl S14, April 1985
578. Gut 28(10)A1398-A1399, October 1987

579. Medical World News, August 3, 1981, p. 24
580. Journal of the American Medical Association 246(4)317-318, July 24-31, 1981
581. Forfar, op. cit., p. 1752-1755
582. Globe, July 19, 1988
583. Humbart, op. cit., p. 345
584. Griffith, op. cit., p. 265
585. Rudolph, op. cit., p. 590
586. Homan, op. cit., p. 146
587. Kempe, C. Henry. Current Pediatric Diagnosis and Treatment, 9th Edition, Norwalk, CT: Appleton and Lange, 1987, p. 837
588. Journal of the American Medical Association 236:1136, September 6, 1976
589. Journal of Pediatrics 44:386-371, 1954
590. Medical Journal of Australia 1(2)60, January 23, 1982
591. Journal of the American Medical Association 236:2864, December 20, 1976
592. Rudolph, op. cit., p. 1041-1045
593. Evans, op. cit., p. 15-16
594. Smith, op. cit., p. 776-781
595. Chow, op cit., p. 764-771
596. Griffith, op. cit., p. 105
597. Karelitz, Samuel M.D. When Your Child is Ill. New York: Random House, 1969, p. 316-321
598. Buchman, op. 75, 174
599. Homola, op. cit., p. 48-49
600. Hospital Practice, January 30, 1986, p. 92-102
601. Pediatric Clinics of North America 35(5)1091-1101, October 1988
602. Laryngoscope 54:120-129, 1944
603. Journal of the American Medical Association 111:1744-1746, November 5, 1938
604. Phipps, op. cit., p. 331-332
605. Ear, Nose and Throat Journal 64:162-167, April 1985
606. Whaley, op. cit., p. 736
607. American Journal of Psychiatry 136(9)1214-1215, September 1979
608. Psychiatrica Neurologica (Basel) 152:306-312, 1966
609. Archives of General Psychiatry 37:1406-1410, 1980
610. Simon, op. cit., p. 315
611. American Family Physician 27(2)373, February 1983
612. New York State Journal of Medicine 82:1685-1687, November 1982
613. Whaley, op. cit., p. 1343-1344
614. Evans, op. cit., p. 166
615. Shamansky, op. cit., p. 151-152
616. Smith, op. cit., p. 636-637
617. Pillitteri, op. cit., p. 1028-1029
618. Schmitt, op. cit., p. 248-251
619. Speech Foundation of America. If Your Child Stutters. 3rd Edition, Memphis, TN: Speech Foundation of America, 1989
620. Boyd-Monk, Heather and Steinmentz, Charles G. III. Nursing Care of

the Eye. Norwalk, CT: Appleton and Lange, 1987, p. 164
621. Griffith, op. cit., p. 130
622. Marlow, op. cit., p. 851
623. Evans, op. cit., p. 219-220
624. Humbart, op. cit., p. 348
625. Whaley, op. cit., p. 775-776
626. Schmitt, op. cit., p. 398-399
627. Kempe, op. cit., p. 317-318
628. Canadian Medical Association Journal 137:1077, December 15, 1987
629. Shamansky, op. cit., p. 144-145
630. Patient Care, May 30, 1987, p. 28-36
631. Schmitt, op. cit., p. 156-157
632. Pillitteri, op. cit., p. 1151
633. Griffith, op. cit., p. 125
634. Journal of the Medical Association of Georgia 68:464-466, June 1979
635. DeAngelis, op. cit., p. 278-379
636. Tackett, op. cit., p. 508
637. Moncrieff, Alan and Evans, Phillip. Diseases of Children, Vol. 1, London: Edward Arnold and Co., p. 488-489
638. Annals of Allergy 54:342, 1985
639. Whaley, op. cit., p. 309
640. Hoekelman, op. cit., p. 1790
641. Pediatric Clinics of North American 29(1)95-103, February 1982
642. Pediatric Annals 12(11)821-824, November 1983
643. Current Problems in Pediatrics 8(6)29-41, April 1978
644. British Medical Journal 2:903-904, October 6, 1962
645. Psychiatric Annals 18(7)409-413, July 1988
646. Griffith, op. cit.
647. Archives of Pediatrics 55:703-709, November 1938
648. Interstate Medical Journal 22:145-155, 1915
649. International Clinics 3:179-190, September 1924
650. Journal of the American Medical Association 245(15)1583-1585, April 17, 1981
651. Sharrard, W.J.W. Pediatric Orthopaedics and Fractures, Vol. 1, Oxford: Blackwell, 1979, p. 578-579
652. Simon, op. cit., p. 198-199
653. Blockley, N.J. Children's Orthopaedics--Practical Problems. London: Butterworths, 1976, p. 2-3
654. McCrea, John D. Pediatric Orthopaedics of the Lower Extremity: An Instructional Handbook. Mount Kisco, NY: Futura Publishing Co., p. 1985, p. 149-152
655. Schmitt, op. cit., p. 161
656. Kempe, op. cit., p. 340
657. Bracce, op. cit., p. 290-291
658. Barness, Lewis A. M.D. Manual of Pediatric Physical Diagnosis. 5th Edition. Chicago: Year Book Medical Publishers, 1981, p. 90
659. The Lancet 1:846-847, April 15, 1972
660. Medical Hypotheses 19:291-293, 1986

661. Nelson, op. cit.
662. Archives of Pediatrics 4:439-466, January-February 1954
663. Habenicht, op. cit.
664. Evans, op. cit., p. 231
665. Hubart, op. cit., p. 262
666. Griffith, op. cit., p. 305
667. Journal of the American Medical Association 114:964, 1940
668. Journal of Epidemiology and Community Health 32:97-101, 1978
669. Lakartidningen 84:847-8, 1987
670. Scipien, op. cit., p. 1083-1084
671. Barnett, op. cit., p. 1644-1647
672. British Medical Journal (5257)929-933, October 7, 1961
673. Servonsky, op. cit., p. 736-742
674. Postgraduate Medical Journal 62:773-778, 1986
675. Journal of the American Medical Association 109:2017, December 11, 1937
676. Servonsky, op. cit., p. 706-709
677. Journal of American Medical Association 182(8)851-852, November 24, 1962
678. Scipien, op. cit., p. 1077
679. Medical Self-Care, March-April 1988, p. 22
680. Clinical Pediatrics 7(3)174, 1968
681. Journal of Urology 131(5)1013-1016, 1984
682. Griffith, op. cit., p. 208
683. Servonsky, op. cit.
684. Griffith, op. cit.
685. Journal of American Medical Association 189:241, July 20, 1964
686. Obstetrics and Gynecology 6:447-448, 1955
687. The Lancet, May 1984
688. Pediatrics 52:241-245, 1973
689. Schmitt, op. cit., p. 510-511
690. Brace, op. cit., p. 303
691. Journal of the American Medical Association 249(4)473, January 28, 1983
692. Avery, op. cit., p. 655-658
693. Scipien, op. cit., p. 1124
694. Smith, op. cit., p. 945-947
695. Hoekelman, op. cit., p. 765-767
696. Pediatric Annals 16(1)69-76, January 1987
697. Southern Medical Journal 36:442-449, June 1943
698. Science Digest, April 1988, p. 92
699. Servonsky, op. cit., p. 200
700. Nelson, op. cit., p. 489-494
701. Moncrieff, op. cit., p. 871
702. Simon, op. cite., p. 124-125
703. Morrow, op. cit., p. 417-418
704. Zuckerman, Barry S. and Suckerman, Pamela. Child Health: A Pediatrician's Guide for Parents. New York: Hearst Books, 1986, p. 99

705. New Orleans Medical and Surgical Journal 71:141-145, 1981
706. Pediatric Annals 16(1)69-76, January 1987
707. Comprehensive Therapy 13(8)34-40, August 1987
708. Plastic and Reconstructive Surgery 68(6)975-976, December 1981
709. Hospital Medicine, November 1980, p. 47
710. Graedon, op. cit., p. 100
711. Buchman, op. cit.
712. Buchman, op. cite
713. Cleveland Clinic Quarterly 29:156, 1962
714. Nelson, op. cite., p. 1560-1561
715. Archives of Dermatology 111:930, July 1975
716. Rudolph, op. cit., p. 518-521
717. Barnett, op. cit., p. 627-633
718. Whaley, op. cit., p. 1365
719. Forfar, op. cit., p. 1378-1379
720. LaPresse medicale 56(15)189, 1948

SYMPTOM INDEX

GENERAL INDEX

MORE BOOKS FROM
FAMILY HEALTH PUBLICATIONS

OF THESE YE MAY FREELY EAT JoAnn Rachor --- 2.95
THE COUNTRY LIFE VEGETARIAN COOKBOOK Diana Fleming -------------------- 9.95
TASTE & SEE: ALLERGY RELIEF COOKING Penny King ----------------------------- 11.95
COUNTRY KITCHEN COLLECTION Silver Hills Institute ----------------------------- 11.95
100% VEGETARIAN: EATING NATURALLY FROM
YOUR GROCERY STORE Julianne Pickle -- 6.95
NEW START LIFESTYLE COOKBOOK Weimar Institute ------------------------------- 19.99
BEST GOURMET RECIPES Five Loaves Deli and Bakery --------------------------- 15.95
THE BEST OF SILVER HILLS Eileen & Debbie Brewer ----------------------------- 11.95
COOKING BY THE BOOK Marcella Lynch -- 14.99
COOKING WITH NATURAL FOODS Muriel Beltz ------------------------------------- 14.95
COOKING WITH NATURAL FOODS II Muriel Beltz ---------------------------------- 14.95
EAT FOR STRENGTH (Oil Free Edition) Agatha Thrash, MD ----------------------- 8.95
ABSOLUTELY VEGETARIAN Lorine Tadej -- 8.95
TOFU COOKERY Louise Hagler -- 15.95
TOFU: QUICK AND EASY Louise Hagler --- 8.95
NUTRITION FOR VEGETARIANS Agatha & Calvin Thrash, MD ---------------------- 14.95
NATURAL HEALTH CARE FOR YOUR CHILD Phylis Austin, Thrash & Thrash ----- 9.95
HOME REMEDIES Agatha & Calvin Thrash, MD ----------------------------------- 14.95
NATURAL REMEDIES Austin, Thrash & Thrash, MD -------------------------------- 6.95
MORE NATURAL REMEDIES Austin, Thrash & Thrash, MD ------------------------- 6.95
FOOD ALLERGIES MADE SIMPLE Austin, Thrash & Thrash, MD -------------------- 4.95
PRESCRIPTION: CHARCOAL Agatha & Calvin Thrash, MD ------------------------- 6.95
FATIGUE: CAUSES, TREATMENT AND PREVENTION Austin, Thrash & Thrash --- 4.95
ANIMAL CONNECTION Agatha & Calvin Thrash, MD ------------------------------- 6.95
DIABETES & THE HYPOGLYCEMIC SYND Agatha & Calvin Thrash, MD ----------- 14.95
NATURAL TREATMENTS FOR HYPERTENSION Agatha & Calvin Thrash, MD --- 14.95
POISON WITH A CAPITAL C Agatha & Calvin Thrash, MD ------------------------- 3.00
PROOF POSITIVE Neil Nedley, MD -- 49.00
EATING FOR GOOD HEALTH Winston Craig, PhD ------------------------------------ 9.95
THE USE & SAFETY OF COMMON HERBS & HERBAL TEAS Winston Craig ---- 8.95
MOOOOVE OVER MILK Vicki Griffin, PhD -- 9.99
NEW START Vernon Foster, MD -- 13.95
DON'T DRINK YOUR MILK Frank Osld, MD -- 7.95
DIET FOR ALL REASONS (Video) Michael Klaper, MD -------------------------------- 21.95
YOU CAN'T IMPROVE ON GOD (Video) Lorraine Day, MD --------------------------- 19.95

Please attach name and address
and phone number.

Subtotal _____

MI residents add
6% sales tax_____

Remit check to:
Family Health Publications L.L.C.
8777 E. Musgrove Hwy.
Sunfield MI 48890

Shipping:
$2.75 1st book
.75 each addl._____

Total Amount Closed_____